Praise for
Post-Traumatic Thriving

"Written with both frankness and compassion, Dr. Bell's guide is simultaneously scientific and holistic, lending readers a path not only for getting through trauma, but also achieving their highest potential because of it."
—Vicki Pepper, Radio Host & Reporter, KFRG-FM

"The inspiring stories here, coupled with psychological science, will serve as beacons of hope for many who have experienced trauma. This book d ispels the common misconception that trauma always leads to weakness. In fact, it can lead to strength!"
—Dr. Wendy Walsh, Host of *The Dr. Wendy Walsh Show*, iHeart Radio; Assistant Professor of Psychology, California State University

"Never has there been a more impactful book at a more needed time than this one. *Post-Traumatic Thriving* offers the latest information on the science of trauma, how to overcome traumatic events, while offering real life stories of resilience from survivors. While we all experience trauma in one form or another, this book will teach you not only how to survive life, but how to thrive!"
—Marianne Pestana, Former Producer at PBS, Host of *Moments with Marianne*, iHeart Radio

"Bell's stories and philosophy of resilience are not only an inspiration for those recovering from trauma or who have hit rock bottom, but a practical guide to a more fulfilling life for all of us."
—Joshua Siskin, Marriage and Family Therapist

"It's an insightful, thought-provoking read that inspires and gives hope to anyone who reads it, that you can overcome what life deals you and thrive."
—Kelly McFarland, Editor of CelebMIX

"Dr. Bell weaves the theory and science of trauma and the detailed processes of recovery, healing, and ultimately thriving throughout the stories of eleven persons ... His grounding in science, his clearly illustrated diagrams of process, and the detailed experiences of the trauma victims, including his own trauma, will provide hope for many ..."
—Walter Schumm, PhD, Professor of Applied Family Science, Kansas State University

"An authoritative and extremely timely look at resilience and wellbeing. Rooted in the science and packed with great anecdotes and guidance, this is an invaluable book for anybody who wants to understand the issues and put them into practice in their own and other people's lives."
—Mark Eltringham, Publisher, Workplace Insight

"Randall Bell's *Post-Traumatic Thriving* effectively shows real people struggling against the lasting effects of past events to legitimize trauma. Easy-to-understand graphs and techniques offer hope to overcome even the worst crises. Clear, concise and comforting."
—Meyla Bianco Johnston, Editor, Alpaca Culture Magazine & Turn of Phrase Writing and Editing

"Dr Randall Bell's work with victims of trauma has earned him the nickname "The Master of Disaster", but the message in this book is

that there's always hope, and that it is possible not just to survive but thrive. His insights are of relevance to every one of us, since nearly everyone has been stressed or tormented at some point in life. This is a very important testimony to the resilience of some people, and a tool to help all of us deal with the traumas which we will all, sooner or later, face."
—Geraldine Comiskey, Freelance Journalist (Ireland)

A power filled book of stories that can heal or help to bring restoration to anyone that takes time to connect. It is so masterful to read how others are impacted by the world today.
—Cassandra McCann, Blogger, Cassandra M's Place

"No one can avoid traumatic events, anyone can thrive again, you need character. Dr. Randall Bell shows how you can learn. Connect with others but always stay who you are."
—Patrick van Schie, Director of Telders Foundation (Holland)

"Dr. Bell's book, *Post-Traumatic Thriving* uses real-people stories and offers effective methods and advice for learning how to move on, how to be better, and mostly how to thrive. Bell emphasizes the need for communication, the differences between guilt and shame, and forgiveness versus forgetting. *Post-Traumatic Thriving* is a must read for anyone who has had 'life happen.'"
—Chelle Cordero, Author, Courage of the Heart

"Never dry nor clinical, Bell traces the paths towards healing of twelve individuals, injecting research and science along the way. Besides providing fundamental tools on how to navigate trauma and heal, *Post-Traumatic Thriving* is a book of great hope and that is the book's greatest accomplishment and for his readers, their greatest gift."
—Cindy Ross, Author, Walking Toward Peace: Veterans Healing on America's Trails

"Dr. Bell masterfully explains how to thrive in the face of adversity. You will know how to empower yourself when trauma rears its ugly face. Through the use of real-life examples and scientifically backed advice, Dr. Bell provides clear cut direction on how you can navigate through anything. Dr. Bell provides clarity in a time of chaos and uncertainty!"
—John Poehler, Published Author, This War Within My Mind, Award-Winning Mental Health Advocate and Blogger

"Dr. Bell does a great job breaking down what happens to us when we are affected by a trauma. Then, he explains how to begin the healing process so that we can live a life without our trauma weighing heavily on us. I recommend his book, *Post-Traumatic Thriving: The Art, Science, & Stories of Resilience,* to anyone who has suffered and wants to thrive in their life post-trauma. It can be done, let Dr. Bell be your guide."
—Sarah Bowen, Retired Elementary School Teacher, Creator of "My Service Dog Tails" Blog

". . .a well-researched, relatable and surprisingly raw view of how we as people experience, process, deal and move forward from traumatic events."
—Fred Varley, Freelance Journalist (London)

"*Post-Traumatic Thriving: The Art, Science & Stories of Resilience* is a must read for those who cannot break past the barrier of suffering through your own traumatic experiences."
—Marie Parachutist, Blogger, Esthetician and Freelance Writer

"After witnessing trauma victims recover and show incredible resilience in the face of darkness, Randy Bell felt compelled to write this book to give others hope and information about how others can do the same. . . . [A] useful read for everyone, because no one escapes this earth without experiencing some sort of trauma or knowing someone else who has."
—Erica Berman, PhD, Psychotherapist, Healthy Life Lessons Blog

Post-Traumatic Thriving

The Art, Science & Stories of Resilience

Post-Traumatic Thriving

The Art, Science & Stories of Resilience

Randall Bell, PhD

CORE IQ

Publishers Group West
Distributor
Berkeley, California

PostTraumaticThriving.com

POST-TRAUMATIC THRIVING: The Art, Science & Stories of Resilience
Randall Bell, PhD

Copyright © 2023 by Core IQ Press
All rights reserved.

Visit our website and podcast at @PostTraumaticThriving

Post-Traumatic Thriving ™ is a trademark of Randall Bell, PhD

No part of this book may be reproduced in any manner without written permission of the publisher except for brief quotations embodied in critical articles or reviews.

Library of Congress Control Number: 2020946042

ISBN 979-8-218-02264-8 (Hardcover)
ISBN 978-0-9967931-9-3 (Softcover)

Printed in the United States of America
10 9 8 7 6 5 4 3 2 1

Edited by Kim Haman, Luna Corbden, and Brian Banashak
Book design by Firewire Publishing

The End

AND THEN IT HAPPENS. We wake up in this new place. It feels right. The old triggers now pass harmlessly through our minds. Our hearts are calm. We are grounded. Our vision is clear.

We are at peace with where we have been. We are at peace with what we have been through. We are at peace with the people around us. And we are at peace with where we are headed.

Our souls are ignited. Our old traumas are now the fuel to do something remarkable.

And now that we know how our story ends, let's look at the journey that led us here.

Table of Contents

Important Notice

THIS BOOK ADDRESSES TRAUMA. In the pages ahead, we will discuss both trauma and a path to healing. It is essential to understand that reading about trauma can itself be re-traumatizing. Several case studies and interviews are included with details of raw and disturbing events, along with a path to healing and ultimate growth. There is no attempt to downplay or soften the events described. Some incidents and language are graphic.

These discussions may be triggering to those who have experienced severe trauma. In other words, these discussions could prompt episodes of revisiting the emotions of your trauma.

When dealing with these topics, we urge you to be mindful of your mental well-being and remind you to practice self-care. We will follow a healing process, but we must take it step by step. Read each step in the order presented and avoid prematurely skipping ahead. We must "feel to heal" and process each stage. A doctor must clean out a wound before applying the stitches and bandages. Putting a bandage over an untreated wound only makes the problem worse. Premature actions can be problematic since each step has essential elements for authentic healing.

Nothing in this book should be considered to be medical, legal, or therapeutic advice. When dealing with trauma, *please remember to always consult a competent, trained, and licensed healthcare or mental health professional.*

And know that you are not alone. If you or someone you know is having suicidal thoughts at any time, confidential help is available at no cost:

For the US National Suicide Prevention Lifeline, call 1-800-273-8255 or go online and chat anytime, day or night. https://suicidepreventionlifeline.org/chat.

For domestic abuse, call the National Domestic Abuse Hotline at 1-800-799-7233.

Additionally, Crisis Text Line provides 24/7, free, and confidential support via text message to people in crisis. Text HOME to 741741 in the US and Canada, 85258 in the UK, or 50808 in Ireland.

For people who identify as LGBTQ+ and are feeling hopeless or suicidal, please contact The Trevor Lifeline at 1-866-488-7386.

For military personnel or veterans who are feeling hopeless or suicidal, please call the Veterans Crisis Line at 1-800-273-8255 and press 1, or for vets or their families, call the National Veterans Foundation Hotline at 1-888-777-4443.

Preface

A WAVE OF TRAUMA

HAVING STUDIED DISASTERS SINCE 1986, I thought that I had seen it all. Then COVID-19, or the Coronavirus, hit, and it impacted nearly everyone. While the virus was severe, I was more concerned about people's reactions to it. We managed to survive the swine flu, bird flu, SARS, and a host of other pandemic risks. Every year, the seasonal flu typically results in hundreds of thousand deaths globally. Yet this seemed different, and it was.

Arguably, every person on earth was traumatized by the Coronavirus. Hoarding and panic buying hit hard, along with a devastating blow to the stock market and the shutting down of schools, businesses, and government services. Everything from Disneyland to the Las Vegas Strip was closed, along with all sports and conventions. Hoarders, motivated by greed, fear, and deep insecurity, loaded up on paper towels, toilet paper, and hand sanitizer—not understanding that the production for all of these items had never stopped. All they accomplished was to fill up their closets while depriving their neighbors of the basics they needed. This behavior fueled even more anxieties.

When the virus hit, I was called by the media and did two television interviews in one day. The first one was with a New York network that was not allowing any guests in the studio. I did the interview on my cell phone in my kitchen. I did the second one from the studio in Hollywood. This interview stood out because this virus potentially impacted every person on Planet Earth. During the commercial breaks, the anchors were freaking out because, unlike the fires and crimes that they reported on every day, this one personally affected them and their families. That's when it hit me. This was different. Within a few days, the whole country shut down.

The pandemic alarmed everyone. While I knew the situation was serious, I instinctively knew that most of us were going to survive. Even in those initial days, I was optimistic that, despite all the fear-mongering, we would emerge from the shutdown. The vast majority of humans on Planet Earth are kind, caring people. I knew that some would be proud of themselves, while others could have done better.

Whether each of us became infected, nearly everyone was stressed and tormented. Perhaps from this experience or other unresolved traumas, we need resolution. While all of our experiences differ, the solutions follow an established, practical course for healing, which is the path we will follow.

TRAUMA TRIAGE

Triage is a term used for an imminent emergency, such as someone with a gunshot wound being rushed by ambulance to the hospital. This person may have a history of untreated heartburn, but the doctors don't worry about that. They dismiss the side issues and focus on the emergency. They stop the bleeding and treat immediate problems. Likewise, we can't address past issues if the trauma is going on right now. We need to stop the trauma.

So we must pause and ask if we are currently being traumatized. We may legitimately look to the past for our problems and the future for solutions, but we should not overlook the present. We cannot heal from trauma when we are in it. Along with the past, it is time to take stock of our present situation.

One friend told me, "I wish self-help books and my therapists had done 'triage.' All those years I was with my abuser, I was in therapy and reading books. No one, not a single person, asked me, "Do you think you might be undergoing trauma right now? Do you think your recovery from previous traumas might be hampered by the fact that you are presently not safe?"

There seems to be an assumption that everyone has escaped their trauma and are dealing with things squarely in the past. But many people are presently being traumatized and need tools or the suggestion to make getting to a safe place a top priority. Abuse and trauma can start to feel "normal" after a while, so we need a reality check.

Before you read this book, please pause and ask yourself this question, "Am I safe *now*?" If not, please get to a safe place. If you are not in a safe place in your life, reach out to online resources, self-help materials, free support groups, and free tools like journaling and meditation. But whatever you do, get to a safe place. Then you can move forward with your healing.

SECTION I

Dive Stage | We Get Knocked Down

When trauma strikes, the darkness comes in multiple stages. Many people will experience some or all of them; however, there is no specific order, and any stage can be revisited at any time. It is normal to skip around or to be immersed in several stages at the same time.

In 1969, the Swiss-American psychiatrist Dr. Elisabeth Kübler-Ross of the University of Chicago published her groundbreaking research that outlined the stages of grief. We will address all of them, along with others:

- **Shock:** The sting of trauma is a feeling of stunned disbelief that paralyzes us to the core. The blood rushes from our brains and puts us in the fight-flight-freeze mode. It is nature's way of protecting us and getting us to safety.
- **Denial:** Trauma can be so overwhelming that we suppress, dodge, hide, and avoid the inevitable. This protects us from being overloaded with too much grief at one time.
- **Anger:** Tragedy may fill us with rage, hate, resentment, or blame. These negative emotions are normal, but we must not use them to hurt ourselves or others.

- **Bargain:** Still wanting to avoid the pain, we may attempt to negotiate, dodge, or seek ways around facing the trauma.
- **Depression:** Once we see that the trauma is real, it can bring on feelings of stress, utter hopelessness, or despair. This is normal, but we must not remain stuck here.

The essence of these stages is that they bring a spectrum of suffering. The hallmark error is to continually dodge the pain. There is a time and place for avoidance. However, to heal and grow, we cannot dodge the pain forever. Yet it is normal to dodge it in pieces. We work hard, then we rest. Or sometimes even rest first, then work hard. And to keep our moods balanced, we come close to the edge of being triggered, but stay in a place where we can come back, or be brought back, without falling all the way in. It is a wash, rinse, and repeat process.

We work to understand that our grief is normal and can even be healthy. We reject society's norm to mask our pain and put on a happy face. Instead, we take a more thoughtful approach. Suffering is our opportunity to stare our moral compass in the eye and deal with the problem in a dignified way.

CHAPTER I

Shock

When people are hit with trauma, they are often overcome with an overwhelming feeling of disbelief and paralysis to the core.

THE DIVE STAGE

LIFE IS GOOD. SURF'S UP! Everything is cruising along smoothly. We scored high on the last school quiz. We received some recognition at work or even a raise. We have lovely friends. We have been on time for our appointments, the family is getting along, and our puppy has not peed on the carpet in more than a week.

Then it happens. As Elkhart Tolle observes, every movie can be described in three words, "Something goes wrong." And just like the movies, it hits us at the most inconvenient time and catches us off guard. It upsets everything. It roars through our life like a tornado. When it passes, it leaves us stunned and wondering what just happened.

What is it? It is trauma, in all of its forms. It slaps us right in the face, and hard. The "dive stage" is the moment of sirens and emergency status. There is an outcry of disbelief. Feelings, actions, and emotions are at their most intense. Anxiety is at overload levels.

This may be a one-time event, such as an assault, or prolonged, recurring events, such as ongoing neglect or abuse. Either way, it profoundly hurts.

The immediate reaction to trauma is to go into shock. Shock proceeds the first of the five stages of grief. Shock is nature's way of protecting us from overwhelming pain or fear in a terrible situation. When our bodies go into shock, there are emotional and physical responses. Our eyes and ears immediately send signals to the brain, which triggers the secretion of epinephrine, more commonly known as adrenaline, a powerful stress hormone stored in our adrenal glands located right above our kidneys. The heart quickly pounds to circulate massive amounts of blood throughout our bodies. Our breathing escalates, and we often hyperventilate. Or, some people hold their breath and stop breathing when they are scared like a little bunny hoping that the tiger cannot see them. We become hyper-focused, which means that our overall memories may become limited later, and we do not experience the full reality of the situation.

As babies, we had what is called a "reptilian" or instinctual brain. We just eat, sleep, and poop. As we grow, so does our brain. Our limbic, or "mammal brain" comes next, and, finally, our cortex or "rational human brain" develops. Yet this inner "reptilian" core always remains and continues to regulate our most basic instincts. During trauma, it kicks into gear. People usually first call for help, and then go into a fight-flight-freeze stage, where any of these options become very real. Trauma directly and measurably impacts the brain. Trauma affects our ability to think clearly.

In shock, our minds become somewhat numb, foggy, and disconnected from reality. It is almost as if we are watching a movie or having an out-of-body experience. The blood supply is being diverted to the muscles to fight or run, and the objective centers on mere survival. We may feel nauseous or anxious, and our muscles and chest can feel tight. We can feel rage, intense anger, or the urge to scream. Some find superhuman strength.

In this state of traumatic shock, we are often overcome with an overwhelming feeling of disbelief and paralysis to the core. This surge of adrenaline is nature's way to numb the pain and help us survive and get to a safe place. Many of us have experienced an electrical blackout where the power grid is overloaded, the circuit breaker trips or the fuses burn out. Televisions, computers, refrigerators, and electric clocks all shut down. When trauma overloads our brain and emotional system, a similar phenomenon occurs. Normal operations shut down. Often people feel as if they are "looking at themselves from the outside." The human brain physiologically performs far differently under these conditions. Shock is not in one's imagination. Shock is real.

UNRESOLVED TRAUMA

Unresolved trauma is the most significant problem facing humankind. Our present stress is from our unsettled trauma. When trauma hits, the most critical decision we make is to choose whether to be a victim, aggressor, survivor, or thriver.

By college age, up to 85% of us have been impacted by at least one trauma. In all its forms, trauma shatters our reality. Perhaps with COVID-19, even more feel they have been traumatized. It smashes our life's assumptions and turns our world upside down. Our past traumas are impacting our current state of mind and the relationships of those we love. Ultimately, the quality of our lives, family, career, and community depend on our ability to process trauma successfully.

Today we see crime, alcoholism, drugs, anger, anxiety, abuse, and violence everywhere. Recovery centers are packed with patients. Extremist political and religious groups regularly trap more members. Jails and prisons are jammed on an industrial scale.

As dangerous as these are, they are all secondary problems. The common issue underlying each of these conditions is unresolved trauma. Addictions, fanatical extremes, workaholism, and mass incarceration are just the symptoms.

Anger, guilt, cynicism, self-righteousness, greed, and anxiety are all secondary reactions. Anger gives you a feeling of power and produces adrenaline, which is physiologically addictive. Violence, aggression, shame, and rage are ancillary emotions. Scores of people self-medicate in an attempt to numb the pain and shield themselves from harsh realities. Yet, despite these efforts to dull the pain, many of us continue to wallow in our misery.

We may or may not be responsible for our trauma, but we are responsible for our healing. When we focus on and address unresolved trauma, we gradually replace "self-medication" with "self-care." It is a messy process, and sometimes it feels like the directions say to rinse and repeat. At times we take one step forward and two steps back, but we keep going. If we unlock the secret of healing from unprocessed trauma, we can heal our world, nation, families, and ourselves.

It is a tall order. Still, the fields of psychology, physiology, and social sciences have become so advanced that we now have the verifiable and measurable research that brings authentic solutions. We understand brain chemistry. We can heal and have peace. We *can* repair the world, and at a minimum, we can change our world. We can achieve post-traumatic thriving.

TRAUMA AND THE BRAIN

Our body's brain functions, nervous system, and chemistry are remarkably complex; however, when it comes to trauma, it is helpful to understand some fundamentals. Our central brain's physiology includes hormones, endorphins, and neurotransmitters, or "HENs."

The interactions of these hormones, endorphins, and neurotransmitters regulate emotions widely, ranging from rage to bliss. There are about 50 hormones which are primarily stored in eight major glands and secreted into our bloodstream. There are also over 20 endorphins, which are chemicals mainly stored in the pituitary gland and secreted into our bloodstream. Finally, there are over 40 neurotransmitters, which are chemicals stored along with our nervous system and released by nerve impulses.

Trauma involves four significant categories of HENs, and by using

THE HUMAN BRAIN AND TRAUMA

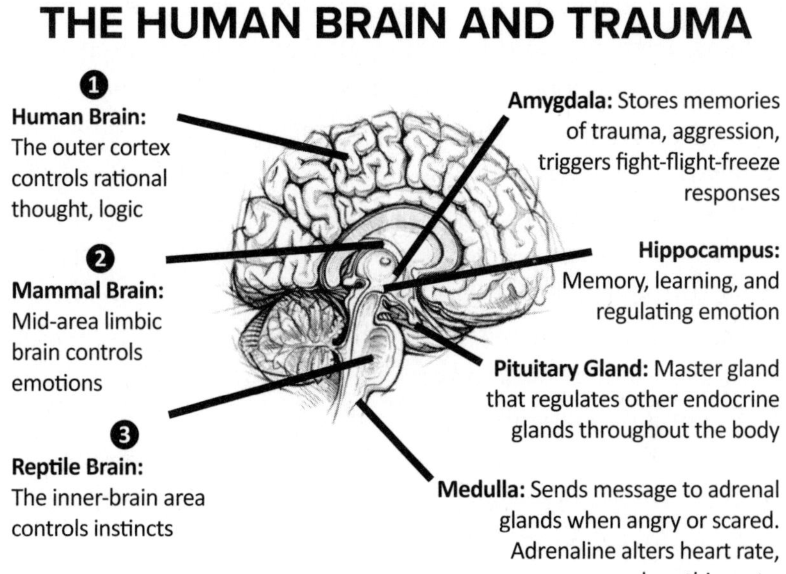
1
Human Brain:
The outer cortex controls rational thought, logic
2
Mammal Brain:
Mid-area limbic brain controls emotions
3
Reptile Brain:
The inner-brain area controls instincts
Amygdala: Stores memories of trauma, aggression, triggers fight-flight-freeze responses
Hippocampus:
Memory, learning, and regulating emotion
Pituitary Gland: Master gland that regulates other endocrine glands throughout the body
Medulla: Sends message to adrenal glands when angry or scared. Adrenaline alters heart rate, breathing, etc.

HEN: Hormones - Endorphins - Neurotransmitters

- **Hormones** include about 50 chemicals primarily stored in eight major glands and are secreted into our bloodstream.
- **Endorphins** include about 20 chemicals primarily stored in the brain's pituitary gland and are secreted into our bloodstream. They are used primarily for pain relief and are considered both hormones and neurotransmitters.
- **Neurotransmitters** include about 40 chemicals stored along our nervous system and are released by nerve impulses.

SODA: Serotonin - Oxytocin - Dopamine - Adrenaline

- **Serotonin** is related to well-being. It is a neurotransmitter that is released by various activities, such as eating certain foods, exercise, meditation, sleep, and music.
- **Oxytocin** is a hormone associated with feelings of love and social bonding. This hormone is released by the pituitary gland when people snuggle and connect socially.
- **Dopamine** is a pleasure-related neurotransmitter and hormone produced in the brain's hypothalamus. It is released during actual and anticipated pleasurable experiences such as eating, sex, finishing tasks, and certain drugs.
- **Adrenaline** (fear and anger) and **Cortisol** (stress) are released during sports or exercise or by fear or anger. The brain's medulla triggers the adrenal gland, located above the kidneys, and releases these hormones into the bloodstream causing an increase in heart rate, muscle strength, breathing, sugar metabolism, etc. This is the classic flight-fight-freeze response.

the acronym SODA, they are easy to remember. SODA stands for serotonin, oxytocin, dopamine, and adrenaline. Serotonin is related to well-being. It is a neurotransmitter released by various activities, such as eating certain foods, exercise, meditation, massage, sleep, laughter, and music. Oxytocin is a hormone associated with a feeling of love and social bonding. This "cuddle" hormone is released by the pituitary gland when people snuggle or connect socially. Dopamine is a pleasure-related hormone regulated by the hypothalamus, located at the base of the brain, near the pituitary gland. It is released during pleasurable situations such as food, sex, and certain drug use. Feelings of happiness result from a mix of serotonin, oxytocin, dopamine, and endorphins. A key to healing is to understand that specific activities are proven to result in these chemical releases. This is not wishful thinking. This is science.

Adrenaline and cortisol are released when we play sports or exercise. Strong emotions such as fear or anger cause the brain's medulla to send a message to the adrenal gland, which is located above the kidneys, and releases adrenaline into the bloodstream. Adrenaline is a hormone that causes an increase in heart rate, muscle strength, blood pressure, and sugar metabolism. This is what produces the classic fight-flight-freeze reaction.

In ordinary life, our brains encode information, send it down an established pathway, process it, and store the experience as a narrative, or story, at some level in our memories. Our brains are always alert with a variety of routine chemical, electrical, and neurological impulses during a typical day. These impulses tell us to do something, pay more attention here, and forget there. Under normal circumstances, the only messages are those that need attention. We are mindful, fully aware, and mentally present. When our brains are in this mode, we are merely processing specific facts, figures, details, and realities. Our outer brain cortex is busy processing our senses, logic, and facts. Generally, in our "mammal brain", we process our emotions. We work and have fun. Life goes on.

When trauma hits, the brain activities change. The focus shifts to our inner "reptilian" brain that is responsible for our most basic instincts. Facts, standard memory, and general knowledge are pushed away, and a flood of high emotion and sensations take over. Powerful chemicals and hormones are pumped directly into our bloodstreams, both by our brain and some of the eight main glands located throughout our bodies.

To survive, our brain turns down rational, explicit decision making and switches to implicit emotions. In other words, we switch from an ordinary, logical world to a world of raw instinct. Sensing danger, our brain tells us to run, freeze, or fight like hell.

In this state of shock, our memories can be distorted. This is fundamental to understanding the healing process. We first react to trauma with shock because it is impossible to wrap our heads around the situation. It is simply overwhelming. If we see an accident, we are so stunned that we freeze on the spot with our mouths hanging open and our eyes wide. If we are in the accident, we are paralyzed even further. Our normal thought processes are put on hold, and we cannot fathom what is going on. Some people recover quickly and take action. Others stay frozen.

Because we "simply cannot believe it," we may shut down. We may dodge discussions of the topic and repress the thought so profoundly that we cannot recall it later. Since our brain did not perform normally during the trauma, the information was not customarily processed and stored. Our memory of the experience is fragmented, repressed, forgotten, or just scrambled up. Consequently, rather than store the information and move on, our brains may continue to send mixed signals that we are still in danger. In an attempt to protect us moving forward, our senses continuously scan our surroundings looking for any slight similarity to the traumatic situation. We become hypervigilant to prevent the trauma from happening again, even though we may no longer be in any actual danger.

Specific triggers can bring out the trauma all over again. Particular words, images, smells, or experiences can set off the amygdala within our brain, which secretes hormones and triggers adrenaline as if the trauma were occurring again. Our heart rate races, we sweat, our breathing speeds or freezes up, and our muscles tense to get ready to fight or run.

Exposure to an event may not be traumatic to one person but can cause trauma to another. What hits to the core of one person may be shrugged off by someone else. Some are inherently more or less prone to the lasting effects of trauma. We all handle tragedy differently. Your trauma is valid. Everybody's hurt is legitimate.

MASTER OF DISASTER

I write this book from three perspectives. First, I write this as a regular person who has experienced trauma. Second, I am writing as an academic researcher, and third as someone who has had a unique career dealing with traumatic situations up close. I understand the academic science of trauma. I also feel it.

I was born with a congenital heart defect, and at the age of 11, I had open-heart surgery, and I feared for my life. Since that first trauma, I have had others. Statistically, I know that more are coming.

Perhaps you have had more trauma than I, or maybe less, but it's not a competition. We are all in this together. We all have traumas, they all hurt, and they all require an effort to heal.

In 1986, I founded what later became Landmark Research Group, LLC, to help communities navigate the aftermath of natural and human-made disasters. For more than three decades, I have studied thousands of disasters in 50 states and on seven continents. I have been hired by the federal governments of the United States, Canada, and Australia to help resolve some of the biggest problems that have faced humanity. In the aftermath of a disaster, I compute the economic damages, and to do this, I get to know the people involved. I have personally seen raw trauma up close, all over the world.

My work has given me unique access to people and places that are impacted. I have visited and researched sites like the nuclear meltdown in Chernobyl, coral bleaching in Australia, global warming in Antarctica, chemical leaks in Bhopal India, and the site where a Dow Chemical accident killed at least 20,000 people and injured

500,000 more. When it comes to disasters and newsworthy topics like the World Trade Center, Flight 93, Sandy Hook, BP Oil, Hurricane Katrina and Hurricane Harvey, OJ Simpson, JonBenét Ramsey, Heaven's Gate mass suicide cult, and the COVID-19 pandemic—I have worked on them all and hundreds of others. Over the years, the media has called me by the nickname, *Master of Disaster.*

With this experience, I have learned that behind every statistic is a person. As much as I enjoy pouring over numbers and raw data to research economic damages, I have taken the time to sit at many kitchen tables, curbs, and coconut tree logs with the people behind the statistics to learn their stories. I have become long-time friends with many of them and have followed their journeys of recovery and resilience. For years, I have volunteered in homeless shelters, jails, prisons, battered women's shelters, and recovery centers. Much of what we will discuss is a result of these conversations and relationships, intermixed with academic research.

If there is anyone who has "been there" to tell you how harsh the world is, I can. Having seen many get back up and thrive, my experiences have given me some insights and passion for helping others do the same.

Having sat in prisons and jails, I have learned that there are indeed some evil people whom everyone, including themselves, have given up on. Surprisingly, most of the people I meet in jail, or prison desperately want to heal from their trauma and take responsibility for their harm. Most hardcore inmates and addicts are just like the rest of us who do not want to face the truth about our childhood traumas, lousy fates, false beliefs, or bad choices. When we learn that a person's behavior has more to do with their internal struggle that it does with us, we learn grace. When we cut some slack and give ourselves and others some grace, we heal and grow.

"IT CAN'T HAPPEN TO ME"

In talking with thousands of folks all around the world, I have observed that, in general, there are two types of disasters and two great lies.

The first type of disaster is externally inflicted. We did nothing wrong. The situation just happened. Our community suffers a massive earthquake. We are diagnosed with a severe illness. We are the victim of a crime. We are abused.

The second kind of disaster is that which is self-inflicted. In this case, we made a terrible choice and harmed others—or ourselves. Our arrogance damages our careers. We caused an accident that results in injuries. We made a mistake that negatively impacted our lives. We bullied someone to make ourselves feel better. We lost our temper and lashed out. Our greed hurt someone. Our judgmental viewpoint harmed a friendship. Our aggressiveness hurt a relationship.

In either case, the first great lie we tell ourselves is, “It cannot happen to me.” That is, until it does.

The second great lie is, “There is no hope.” Let me say that there is hope. On top of that, the more efficient our recovery and healing, the more time we can spend thriving. We don’t want to rush our recovery and relapse, but the right concepts can help us move forward.

In life, it is reasonable to need time alone, to have unsettled thoughts, get angry, mourn a loss, and go through ups and downs. However, it is not healthy to get stuck in a cycle of dysfunction. Those who suffer from abuse, inflicted by others or self-inflicted, tend to display a cluster of unhealthy behaviors. Our self-esteem is damaged, so we over-apologize, break down over small issues, seek validation, are hypersensitive, suppress our feelings, or become over-vigilant and defensive. These reactions are entirely natural as our brain is reacting to the trauma and trying to protect us. Some of these reactions can be beneficial at the right time or in small doses. The key is being mindful and observing what is helpful, harmful, or neutral.

As we process the trauma and implement new self-care practices, our objective is to be triggered less frequently and respond in a reasonable way. To enjoy the benefits of thriving, we must appreciate that understanding the trauma response is a precursor to healing. In other words, we must understand what is going on physically and emotionally when a trauma event is experienced. Then, to ultimately grow, we must take steps to regulate our emotions and take deliberate steps to reduce our anxiety. We must learn how to control intrusive thoughts, or allow the intrusive thought to flow through us, so we can translate what that thought is trying to tell us. We create a new narrative within the constructs of healing and steady growth. Our ultimate objective is to develop new life principles that are solid and build a foundation for enjoying life while meeting the challenges that lie ahead.

Let's not wallow in how *it is*. I want to tell you how it *can be*. In this rough world, I see a vision where people who have suffered through trauma are understood and understand themselves. I see a world where everyone is better equipped to work through their injuries successfully. I see a world where homeless people can get back on their feet, incarcerated people can be rehabilitated, victims can process their grief, addicts can start to treat the real issues that they are trying to numb, and those who lost a loved one can heal.

When I was a kid, my friends and I would go in the backyard with a magnifying glass and light leaves on fire. There is enough energy in just a few inches of sunlight that, when focused, can ignite a flame. Think about what you are going to focus on today. The power of focus is remarkable. The things we focus on catch on fire, and the things we do not concentrate on blow away.

So, what should we focus on first? I focus on how life can be. We can navigate the path to healing. The principles are simple, but they are not easy. This path is not a theory or a new concept. There are clear, established steps to post-traumatic thriving. This means that in the aftermath of our traumas, we not only get back up but use the experience to grow in entirely new ways. Many have already successfully traveled it, and you are next.

When I visit a disaster site, at first I do not attempt to provide answers or fix anything. That would be destructive at this stage. Instead, I observe and conduct a full assessment of the situation. The process can take many weeks or months, but my team and I uncover every aspect of the disaster we can find. After the "assessment" stage comes the "repair" and "ongoing" stages. But if we attempt to repair before we assess, we skip the essential step and turn that focused sunlight to light the fire in the wrong areas.

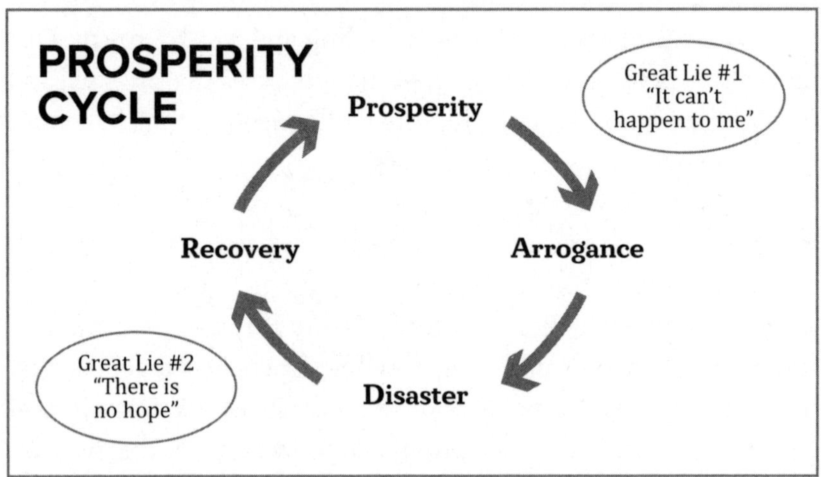

We will spend considerable time assessing and exploring the various stages of the trauma itself. But first, to build anything, we need to create a foundational structure. I know that it is tempting to jump ahead to the solutions in the chapters ahead, but we have to lay a solid foundation so that we can enjoy authentic growth. We must face and process each stage and own the stage we are in. As we do, we will grow in awareness.

HANDLING SHOCK

Shock can hit us through being in an accident, witnessing a crime, consuming news stories, being stopped by the police, undergoing dental or medical procedures, fighting litigation, breaking up a relationship, learning of an unexpected death, or even reading about the trauma of others. Shock is a medical condition. Do not underestimate it. If you or anyone you know goes into severe shock, call 911 immediately.

Depending on the cause, symptoms, or signs of severe shock may include:

- Anxiety
- Confusion
- Difficulty breathing
- Fainting
- Heartbeat irregularities or palpitations
- Outbursts and screaming
- Pale, cold, clammy skin
- Rapid heartbeat
- Shallow, rapid breathing
- Thirst or a dry mouth
- Unconsciousness

At a minimum, ask for help and sit down if possible. Reach out and accept support.

When a shock hits, the most visible sign can be altered breathing. Take slow, deep, regular breaths to avoid hyperventilating and to keep a level amount of oxygen flowing to your brain. Focusing on your breath can also ground you. We can likewise be in a lightheaded or foggy mental state. Do your best to keep as calm as possible and think before taking any action.

Though we have been impacted by trauma, our bodies are not intended to have cortisol and adrenaline continually flowing in our veins. In this state, our system becomes overloaded, often resulting in chronic fatigue.

Shock is intense, so we must give ourselves time to allow our rational mind to return. It may be challenging to listen accurately and follow instructions while in shock, so we need to take it slow. If we are told to do something, perhaps we can slowly repeat back the instructions. Merely understanding what shock is and that it is reasonable can help to make the event somewhat less frightening.

LETTING LOVE IN, AT LAST

Slowly, John's world started to come back into focus. After the initial shock, it took several long minutes. During that time, the boy became aware of his older sister's arms around him. He listened to the far-off sobs of his other sisters; at first, they sounded muted, as if his ears were stuffed with cotton. Their sobs grew louder—or rather, the roaring train sound in his ears had finally started to diminish, and he could hear the girls' weeping more clearly.

It could not be possible.

But it was true; his mother was dead. A heart attack had taken her. She was just 51 years old. At 16 years old, John was parentless; only one year earlier, in 1981, his father had died of a diabetic coma.

John was born in late 1965 to a working-class Catholic family in Buffalo, New York. The youngest of five children—and the only son—John was doted on by his sisters—Phyllis, Fran, Gladys, and Kate. His parents, Edith and Joe, loved him dearly. However, his father's alcoholism sometimes upended the household, and the children lived in trepidation of the mercurial temper that overcame Joe when he was drinking. The siblings never knew which version of their father to expect—the strict but kind dad who entertained them by playing the flute, or the frightening specter whose rages sent them running to their rooms.

John's mother was a teacher. Like her husband, she was strict and stoic. To Edith, getting an education was the most important goal a person could have, and she saw to it that John put his energy into getting good grades. She also saw John's pure musical talent. When he was 13, Edith gifted him his first electric guitar and amplifier and money for lessons.

Instead, John used the money to buy beer. He learned a few chords from some older boys in the neighborhood. Combined with his natural gift for music, John learned to play pretty well—without a single lesson.

When John's father died, his guitar became his solace. He played for hours on end, continually experimenting with new chords, creating sounds that had previously only existed in his head. Following his mother's sudden death just 18 months later, John fell into a deep depression.

John's sisters and his cousin, John Guljas, tried to step into the parental roles, but the teenager was reeling. Even before his parents' untimely deaths, John had experimented liberally with alcohol. He and his friends were a rowdy, fun-loving group who spent most of their free time together—and much of it drinking. But a falling out of some sort happened—probably caused by one of those arguments over something unimportant to one person but of vital importance to another—and his group of friends dissolved.

At the time John lost both parents, he had no peer group support and was still drinking. Flush with social security survivor cash, John decided to move into his own apartment while he was still a high school student. He resisted his sisters' attempts to parent him, though to their credit, they never gave up.

Loss. Loneliness. Depression. Alcohol. It was a combination that could crush even the most resilient spirit. But John had something else—his music. During these dark days, it was his only comfort.

John coped with his pain the only way he knew—drinking and playing the guitar. He didn't receive counseling—in the dim days of the early 1980s, that was simply not cool. He learned from his dad to suppress his feelings. His mom taught him that the only way to get through grief was to keep moving forward, no matter the pain, just as she had done after his father died.

He did make new friends, which alleviated some of his loneliness. He laughed, did teenager stuff, and drank a lot. But at night, by himself in his apartment, he listened to music, played his guitar, and wondered where it was all going.

While John was still in high school, he and some other guys decided to pool their talents. They started a band they called the Beaumonts. The band didn't stay together long though—it dissolved, falling victim perhaps to the members' lack of focus and general teenage boy distractions.

In 1985, shortly after the Beaumonts broke up, John met a guy named Robby whose love of music equaled his own—and who had the same talent as well. Robby was outgoing and friendly, a contrast to John's shy and somewhat reserved persona. The guys decided to take a shot at forming a band of their own.

Driving from gig to gig in an old van, the new band performed at a breakneck pace, hitting bars and clubs up and down the Eastern seaboard. John and Robby—along with drummer George Tutuska—took every gig that came their way. They worked hard and partied hard. The band caught the attention of a small label called Celluloid, which released their first album in 1987. They were a punk band when they started, with Robby on lead vocals.

It took nearly a decade before the band, the Goo Goo Dolls, really gained traction with the broader public, despite releasing four albums in that time. In the meantime, they played around Buffalo's underground music circuit and across the country, opening for punk bands such as Bad Religion, Motorhead, Doughboys, and The Dickies. They also got a lot of play on college radio stations, creating a devoted fanbase.

In 1993, John Rzeznik and Robby replaced George Tutuska with Mike Malinin. The trio worked well together, creatively, and on a personal level. In 1995, when the Goo Goo Dolls released their album, *A Boy Named Goo,* John was the lead on vocals and their sound morphed from punk to alternative rock. The song, "Name," embodied their unique sound. It was an instant hit and cemented the band as one that was poised for greatness.

Greatness came with the release of the song, "Iris," which John had written for the *City of Angels* movie soundtrack. Their eighth album, *Let Love In,* released in 2006, sold more than 83,000 copies its first week. The Goo Goo Dolls hit a record twelve top ten hits in the Adult Top 40 with their third consecutive single from the album, "Let Love In." By the mid-90s, the Goo Goo Dolls had

BRAIN WAVES

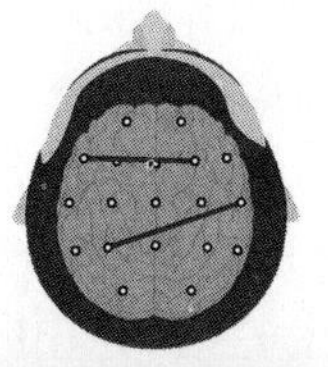

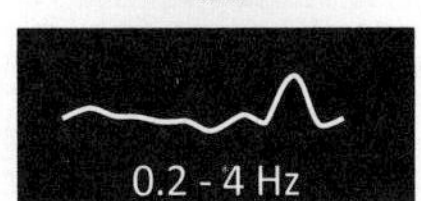

DELTA

These slow, loud brainwaves are generated in dreamless sleep and deepest meditation. They are a source of empathy and stimulate healing and regeneration.

THETA

Theta waves occur most often in sleep (drifting off or waking up) but are present in deep meditation. They are the gateway to learning, memory, and intuition. They focus on internal signals versus the external world and can hold fears, troubled history, and nightmares.

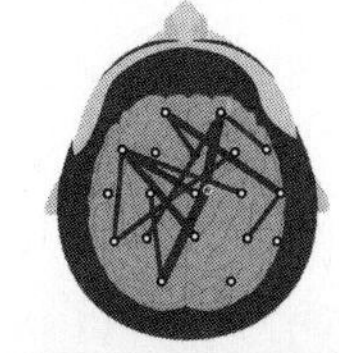

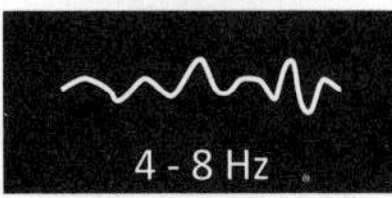

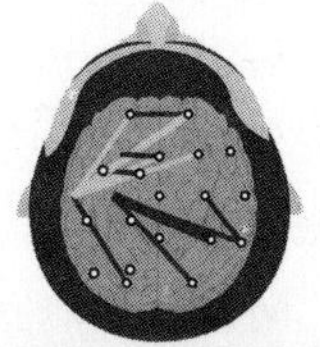

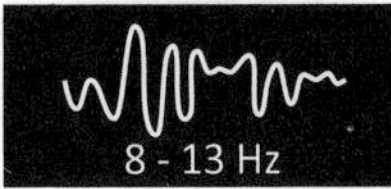

ALPHA

Alpha waves are dominant during quietly flowing thoughts and some meditative states. They are a resting state for the brain and help us be in the present. They aid mental coordination, calmness, alertness, learning, and mind/body integration.

BETA

Beta waves dominate the normal waking state of consciousness. They are present when we are alert, attentive, engaged in focused mental activity, judgment, problem solving, or decision making. Beta waves are directed towards cognitive tasks and the outside world.

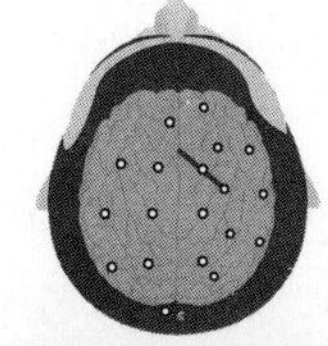

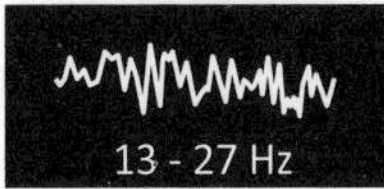

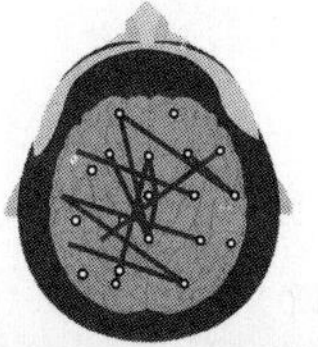

27 - 100 Hz

GAMMA

These are the fastest moving brainwaves. They pass information in the brain, and we must be quiet to tap into them. They relate to simultaneous processing of information from different brain areas.

become one of the biggest bands in the world. Of course, they had no way of knowing this would happen back in 1985. Back then, they were just two guys who found something in each other that they never expected—understanding.

The unprocessed trauma of John's parents' deaths a year apart when he was only 16 gnawed at him. Like his father, he drank to excess. When he was young, and the band was taking the music scene by storm, his alcoholism was dismissed by friends as "hardcore partying." But he drank to stifle the pain.

The drinking did not stop, and every day John was drunker than the day before. It got so bad that at one point, Robby, who got sober in 2004, ended his friendship with John, even though they continued to write songs and tour together. Yet this devastating blow—losing his relationships with the one person who understood his deep commitment to music more than anyone else ever had—was not enough to stifle John's drinking. He dabbled in drugs, too. It wasn't just his connection with Robby that suffered; John's first wife, Laurie, whom he had married in 1993, left him. His second wife, Melina, whom he had married in 2013, was considering leaving him. It was just too much.

Somehow, though, his performances never deteriorated while everything else in his life did.

At last, on November 16, 2014, John decided it was time to *stop*. The night before, John had realized that the alcohol would someday contribute to his early death, just as it had his father's, but the idea of dying didn't scare John at all. So, he took a drink, and another, and another, until he blacked out.

John had tried rehab before, going to high-end places with luxuries such as massage tables, yoga classes, and steam baths. However, none of those approaches helped him cope with the reason he was an alcoholic—his unprocessed trauma.

This time, things were different. He signed up for an old-school rehab center that focused on therapy, the Twelve Steps, and spirituality. The therapists spent a great deal of time working with him to

SITTING IN THE FIRE

Society and perfectionist cultures tend to downplay the difficult experiences in life. Internal pressure builds up when we "suck it up," "sweep it under the rug," or dodge the real conversations. Not only does this prevent healing, the pressure builds up like a volcano.

"Sit in the fire" means that we are honest and have the difficult conversations about what is real. We candidly discuss the details of the trauma, without sugar-coating or glossing over anything.

Opening up to these vulnerable conversations allows us to relieve the pressure. The process is called "Sitting in the fire" because the raw words often burn with emotion. During these moments, we can be tempted to mask the hurt with humor, sarcasm, or some other distraction, but we must just sit in the fire.

The ultimate goal is to have a conversation with a trusted person or group where we can express what really happened. It is remarkably healing to sit in the fire, and there are basically three options:

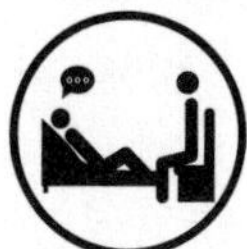

1. **THERAPIST:** The ideal way to have a dialogue and process trauma is with a trained therapist. A competent therapist will allow us to express the full extent of the trauma without judgment and will keep the conversations confidential.

2. **TRUSTED FAMILY MEMBER OR FRIEND:** We can confide in a trusted person; however, there are two important criteria. First, the person must simply listen within interrupting or being judgmental. Second, they must be trustworthy and keep our conversations strictly confidential. If these conditions are not met, this could lead to being re-traumatized.

3. **JOURNAL:** Until we find a therapist or a trusted person, we can journal our experiences. We write about life before our trauma, the trauma itself and what has happened since. Maintain the journal and continue to write about the experiences as additional thoughts come to mind. Writing things down organizes our thoughts and emotions. Make written lists of what you need.

deal with past issues, including the loss of his parents. As the end of his three-month stay approached, John readied himself for the outside world. He created a plan to repair the relationships he had destroyed. He also allowed himself to believe in an idea that he had only dared dream about, which was to start a family.

The Goo Goo Dolls rose higher and higher throughout the 1990s and 2000s and have enjoyed steady popularity ever since. They have racked up dozens of awards, including five Grammys, three Radio Music Awards, and a Billboard Music Video award.

Yet the story does not end there. After years, John is still proudly sober. He and Robby have picked up their friendship where they left off and are even closer than ever. Melina, seeing that this time John was genuinely committed to staying sober, decided not to leave. They both reinvested themselves in their marriage. In December 2016, two years after John's last drink, they welcomed a beautiful baby girl into their home.

Once I had the pleasure of meeting John Rzeznik in his dressing room. I was backstage at a rock concert with a friend, and John invited us in. Far from having a rock star ego, he was kind, calm, and humble. We sat and talked about his years spent with his band driving an old van at a time when not many people noticed their music. He was open about the fact that he had lots of guitars strung to different chords because he never took lessons. John had lost both his parents but had used that trauma as the fuel for his journey for post-traumatic thriving. Like other thrivers I have met, he was far from loud and proud of his success. Instead, he was reflective, gentle, and had a grateful heart. His past pains turned up the volume of his current joy.

"Everything happens for a reason," John once shared. "If you stand right where you are now, and you look down and back to everything, to all the events that led up to you sitting in this room right now, you will see where the order is. And where you are right now is pretty amazing. Where we all are, where I am right now, is amazing."

When ordinary coal is placed under extreme pressure, a diamond is created. All of us are the same. We know about John's success, but his background is like many others. He faced a lot of trauma, from his father and mother dying when he was a boy to going through alcoholism and a difficult first marriage. Trauma is widespread, and John has had his share of what I call the "Difficult Ds": death, disease, disability, drugs, divorce, despair, depression, deceit, disaster, destruction, desertion, and dysfunction.

John turned his world around by using the principles we will explore here. *He kept going.* He finally listened to his inner voice and sought real help. Success is not final. Failure is not fatal. It is the courage to continue that counts. Albert Einstein said, "You never fail until you stop trying." We never go wrong when we turn off the noise and listen to our inner voice.

THE "DYNAMIC DUO" OF HEALING

In the pages ahead, we will visit each stage of grief and then explore new ways of thinking and self-care practices that will allow us to heal and ultimately thrive. However, many of us are hurting right now, so we will introduce two powerful concepts: the "dynamic duo" of resolving unprocessed trauma. They are simple, yet they are scientifically proven to be effective.

First is the concept of "grounding," which simply involves controlled breathing exercises. Grounding is similar to Lamaze, mindfulness, yoga, meditation, and related practices, but simply focuses the mind on breathing and being mentally present right now. Accordingly, we will refer to any type of meditation, mindfulness, or breathing exercises simply as "grounding."

Some people associate meditation with religious practice or some mystic thing, but that is not what is meant here. There are at least twenty-one published studies from Harvard Medical School alone about the positive, measurable effects of grounding. These are simple breathing exercises that are profoundly successful and proven to be effective by brain scans and medical studies. Controlled breathing is shown to moderate the brain's electrical impulses and generate

GROUNDING

Grounding is an exercise that can help improve your memory, lower blood pressure, control anxiety, and reduce stress. Choose the steps below you are comfortable with and spend 60 seconds or 60 minutes grounding. The time does not matter.

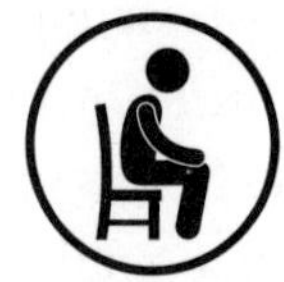

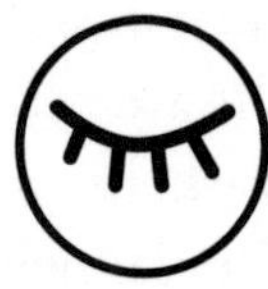

1. Sit comfortably in a chair with both feet planted on the ground.
2. Hands can rest gently on your lap.
3. Close your eyes and bring your attention to your breathing. Take 3-5 slow, deep breaths in and out.

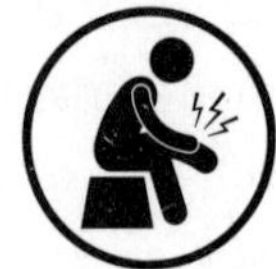

4. Conduct a complete body scan. Focus attention on what you're physically feeling beginning at your toes and moving upwards towards your head.
5. Where in your body are you feeling pain, discomfort, or stiffness? Explore why you are feeling this.
6. Bring your attention to each of your 5 senses, one at a time.

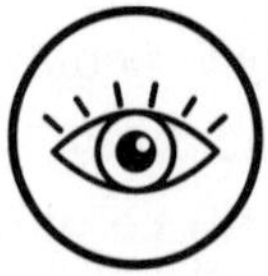

7. Focus on what you touch, hear, taste, or smell.
8. Finish by taking 5-7 deep, slow breaths in and out.
9. Open your eyes. You are now grounded!

emotional healing and clarity. Simply start following the steps for grounding once or twice a day.

Second, healing is never a solo exercise. Trauma occurs when we keep our secrets to ourselves. To heal, we must express ourselves, and we call this practice, "Sitting in the Fire." This means that we express our trauma, pains, and fears with a trusted person. Here there are three options: (1) find a good, licensed therapist, (2) talk to a good friend who is non-judgmental and keeps your information confidential, or (3) write or journal your experiences, thoughts, and feelings. Expression through art, music, or other creative outlets is also valid.

While it may be useful to rely on friends at times, we need to be aware that it might emotionally weigh on them. We should be considerate of their limits and mental health. There should be open communication with them to be sure that they are all right with these discussions. At a minimum, they should be allowed to take time off from heavy topics, and the ability to say "no" to specific conversations.

Seeing a therapist is healthy. There is no legitimate stigma in seeing a therapist. When we need medical help, there is no shame in seeing a doctor. Being in therapy does not mean that something is wrong with us, but that we are doing the right thing in seeking authentic, personal growth. We want clarity in complex circumstances. We want to learn new tools, heal from past traumas, and move forward with a fresh perspective. Seeing a therapist means that we dare to face reality and take intelligent, decisive action.

Starting now, it is essential that we do not bottle up our feelings or "brush them under the rug." Follow the steps to "Sit in the Fire" at least once a week.

My plan is focused on one thing, and that is your authentic healing. Countless times I have seen the most horrific traumas healed over time with just these two practices. We will discuss much more, but make this "dynamic duo" a regular exercise beginning right now.

Our Stories of Shock

In conducting this research, I sat down with several people, or their spouses, who had successfully navigated through a trauma. Each person started by hitting rock bottom. As we progress in this journey, we will see that rock bottom is a great place to start building.

DEBBIE

If there was ever a "perfect life," Debbie appeared to have it. A pretty brunette with an infectious smile and engaging personality, Debbie was the kind of person that others couldn't help but adore. She grew up in a loving home and was surrounded by close friends.

In high school, she was a cheerleader, part of the "popular crowd." She was kind and genuinely interested in other people, whether they were the captain of a winning team or the quiet student focused on studying. Her friendliness drew others to her—including the man who would eventually become her husband. They knew each other in high school, reconnected after college, and married.

During the next two decades, life was generally pretty enjoyable. She was married to a loving man who was deeply invested in their family, active in her church and admired by her friends, and her children were excelling. Her spacious home was the "hang out" destination of all the neighborhood kids. She appreciated her good fortune and looked forward to the future.

Now that the kids were grown, or nearly so, she was finally pursuing her dream of being a therapist. She completed her graduate degree and had started an internship. It was going well. *Everything* seemed to be going well.

One morning before she headed out to her internship, Debbie and her husband, Gary, made plans to go on a walk later in the afternoon. When Debbie arrived, she saw her husband's truck in the driveway. She went inside, calling for him so they could go on their planned outing.

Debbie wandered through the house, growing increasingly worried when she couldn't find him. She went into the master bedroom, rounding the corner into the bathroom. There she saw her husband's feet in the shower—but he wasn't standing on them. He was lying down. At first, Debbie couldn't comprehend what she was seeing. After several long moments, Debbie suddenly realized what he had done. She shrieked in horror.

Her husband of nearly 30 years, her lover and her hero, the person she had built a life with, lay dead on the shower's cold tile floor. He had shot himself.

Debbie immediately went into shock. She screamed, "Oh, f___ no! She screamed again, panic building. Her heart pounded, and she couldn't catch her breath. Her brain simply could not absorb the magnitude of what was in front of her. It was too much.

The funeral passed in a blur. So many people, so many tears. She moved through it as best she could. The next day, Debbie began the task of going through her husband's records, seeking information about their insurance policies, bank accounts, and the like. As she poured through some papers in the garage, she discovered a horrifying secret her husband had been keeping from her—and it was as soul-crushing as his unexpected death.

She discovered that for the last several years, her husband had led a secret double life. He was a gambling addict; even more devastating, he was a sex addict and spent thousands of dollars on prostitutes. And there was more: their savings—nearly a million dollars—was completely wiped out. Gone. There was nothing left.

JOHN

John loved his life on his scenic island, living with his wife and children. Their home was located on a beautiful blue lagoon in a tropical paradise. It was a simple life. He and buddies went fishing, while their wives cooked taro roots found all over the island. The children ran around and collected coconut crabs.

There was a small school in the village, along with a beautiful wooden church that everyone attended. There were no jails and no need for police. The worst thing that ever happened on the island was when someone drank too much, and they would just get tied to a coconut tree until they sobered up. There was no crime, no IRS, no debt, and no mortgage to pay. Food was everywhere. The villagers would joke that the dozens of smaller, outer islands were their "refrigerators," full of delicious chickens, pigs, fruits, and vegetables, just for the cost of picking them up. There was always a lot of laughter and kids playing. Everyone knew everyone. John thought of it as heaven.

One day, John got up to make coffee for his wife and himself. As he enjoyed the sunrise and the smell of fresh coffee brewing, he was startled by what he called "a second sunrise." There was a giant glowing ball of fire on the horizon. He had no idea what was going on. He was baffled.

This tropical village had never seen snow, but soon large flakes started sprinkling down. Later that afternoon, his daughter and her friends were dancing and spinning in grey ash.

A few days later, his daughter was taken to a military hospital in Bethesda, Maryland, suffering from extreme nausea, internal bleeding, a high fever, and severe weakness. A few days later, she died. Then John learned from some visiting military men that atomic bomb tests had been conducted across the lagoon. John, along with his wife, family, and neighbors, were stunned that they had been used as human guinea pigs in the United States nuclear test programs. He was in shock.

SUSAN

Susan had always believed that focus, determination, honesty, and faith were the foundation of a successful life. She built her life on these values.

After college, Susan earned her MBA. From there, she spent time working in international sales where she excelled. But she was drawn to acting—the idea of telling stories to a wide audience, of *being someone else* to tell a story, was irresistible. So she approached a career as an actor with the same tenacity and determination that had defined her life so far.

She had some successes, primarily in commercials, where her pretty, friendly face proved the perfect vehicle to sell various products. But the work was not as consistent as she would have liked, nor as fulfilling. She didn't want to leave the entertainment industry, though. She began to consider other roles she could play to get stories out there.

Susan was intrigued by the business side of the profession. Soon, she found herself working on the "other side of the camera." With her business acumen and communication abilities, Susan began rising rapidly through the ranks. She reached the producer level, a role she equated to being the Chief Operating Officer of a large corporation. She was good at it, even being voted one of the top 250 women in the film business by *The Business of Film magazine.*

Despite her professional success, Susan was an extremely down-to-earth person. She was proud of what she had accomplished, but Susan didn't hold it over other people's heads or act as if she were better than anyone else. When people were intimidated by her high-profile job, she went out of her way to make them feel comfortable. She loved to laugh and spend time with the people she loved.

Her husband, Peter, was a successful actor. While he wasn't necessarily a household name, he had appeared in dozens of movies. If you ran into him on the street, you would know you had seen him somewhere before. He also ran a movie prop business out of their home, which did quite well. He focused primarily on supplying authentic props for western-themed movies. Peter had outbuildings full of saddles, boots, rifles, and everything else to supply a movie.

All in all, life was good. They had fulfilling careers, a lovely hillside home built in the 1930s, plenty of friends, and travel. Susan was content. In the back of her mind, she had many aspirations for the future but wasn't moving forward because they seemed a little risky. She was happy with her level of success and didn't want to rock the proverbial boat too much. Better to keep things as they were.

One evening, Susan came home late from work. It was dark outside and the roads up to her home were dimly lit. As she approached her house, she sensed something was wrong but couldn't quite put her finger on it. Just a sense that something was "off." She pulled into the driveway. The house looked fine from the outside though, so she went in.

As soon as she opened the front door, a strange, earthy smell hit her. She fumbled for the lights. They snapped on. Susan just stood for a moment. What was all over the floor? And wait—were those things *leaves?* And was that a small tree branch? *What the —?*

Suddenly she realized what it was. *Mud.* Mud everywhere. It covered the floor. It flowed through the table legs and oozed up into couch fabric. It had absorbed into the lower part of the walls, so that it almost looked like a line of dark moss.

She was astonished. She walked further into the house. Each step led her to a sight more astonishing and distressing than the last. Every single room of her house was full of mud from a major landslide.

Her home, her beautiful, unique, lovely home, where she and Peter had made so many wonderful memories, was completely destroyed.

SHAD

Shad entered active duty in the US Army in 1968 as a captain after receiving his master's degree in psychiatric social work from Florida State

University. At 23, he was about a half decade older than the other troops. He served as a social work-psychology officer for I and II Corps in the Republic of Vietnam. It was a good role for his—naturally empathetic and kind, yet firm and pragmatic character. Shad was devoted to helping his fellow soldiers process the trauma of all they had seen.

Shad served as a medical services officer attached to a MASH (Mobile Army Surgical Hospital) unit. The battlefield had been relatively quiet for the past few days. There was nothing to make the unit leaders think that an attack was imminent. As the officer on duty, Shad settled in for the night, checking in on patients and making sure that the medics were ready for anything that might happen. It looked like it was going to be an uneventful evening.

A few hours later, complete chaos suddenly erupted. The enemy had attacked. US troops fought bravely, but the enemy had surprise on their side. Before Army troops could gain the upper hand, more than 35 young men were grievously wounded. They were brought in, one after the other—an endless rush of broken, burned, and shot-up bodies. Shad had never seen such carnage.

Initially, Shad froze in complete and utter shock. He stood immobile as the MASH unit filled with the wounded. Their cries and screams of pain drowned out his thoughts. Suddenly, he felt a hard slap across his face—a surgeon raised his hand, ready to slap him again if Shad didn't come out of his daze. Shad just stared at him. The surgeon slapped him once more. The second slap snapped him out of his shock, and he got to work.

The scene was something from a nightmare—one soldier, missing his body from the hips down, grabbed Shad and begged, "Where are my legs? Where are my legs?" Another lay calmly on his bed, talking to Shad about various things, blissfully unaware that he had been shot in the head and most of his brains had spilled out. At last he asked Shad, perhaps seeing the expression on Shad's face, "Am I going to die?"

The answer, tragically, was yes. That young man—no older than 19—died shortly after that, along with 15 others. Throughout that long night, Shad and his team of medics performed triage, allocating treatment to those they thought would survive. It was a harrowing experience that would ultimately shape Shad's life.

He had helped many soldiers work through trauma as a counselor; now he had to learn to deal with his own.

GERI

Pregnant with her first child, Geri's mom was filled with delight and anticipation. She sat on her front porch, imagining what it would be like to hold her soon-to-arrive baby girl in her arms.

Suddenly, from out of nowhere, a car jumped the curb. It flew over the lawn and knocked down a maple tree, causing Geri's mom to run off the front porch in a state of sheer panic. That's when she tripped and fell. She and her growing baby barely survived the accident. Her recovery was long and arduous.

Soon after, her sweet baby girl was born. But because of the accident, little Geri was born with cerebral palsy. During her childhood, she experienced orthopedic walkers, physical therapy, special schools, and the trauma of being bullied by other children.

TANYA

By the time Tanya was twenty years old, she had suffered more traumatic losses than the average person three times her age.

While she was in high school in the 1980s, six of her classmates, all friends or acquaintances, suddenly and tragically lost their lives – two in cliff-diving accidents, one from leukemia, two in car accidents and one in a skiing accident. She went to six funerals in four years.

Tanya, a profoundly empathetic girl who felt things on a "cellular level," was utterly devastated. She had no idea how to process what she was feeling. All she knew was that her friends from the neighborhood, schools, and Catechism classes were suddenly and irrevocably gone.

During that time, the primary responders to help students grieve were academic counselors and teachers who did the best they could to help, but that wasn't their expertise. There seemed to be no process in place to deal with the losses.

Tragically, another loss was right around the corner—two years after high school, in 1989, her best friend was killed in a hit-and-run in Laguna Beach. The perpetrator was never found.

Each tragedy was a devastating trauma that built on the one before. But it was the 1980s—long before the lingering effects of unprocessed trauma were fully understood. Tanya's parents were from the World War II generation and did not really know how to process feelings. So, according to what they knew, they encouraged Tanya to carry on and reassured her that this too will pass. She went to the funerals, cried, said her goodbyes, consoled her friends, and that was it. The next day they went back to class and moved on.

After her best friend was killed, 20-year-old Tanya sank into a deep depression coupled with an eating disorder. The more her feelings tried to bubble to the surface, the more she stuffed them down. She used food to distract herself, putting on more than 70 pounds.

After a three-year struggle, Tanya moved to San Diego for a fresh start and enrolled at the University of California. She was, as she puts it now, "tired of feeling sick and tired" and decided to lose weight. Soon enough, she was down to a svelte 150 pounds on her 5' 10" frame.

But the move to San Diego did nothing to alleviate her depression. It grew worse. To shake herself out of her misery, she signed up for a full load of classes. Without the familiar structure of home, it took her a while to adjust, and on her first day of class, she grew overwhelmed and suffered a panic attack, losing consciousness outside her classroom door.

She dedicated herself to study and work. But she still felt like she needed to do more, so she took a second job. She also frantically tried to keep up an active social life—anything to keep her from allowing those feelings to escape from the place where she had carefully hidden them away.

It was getting to be too much. *It would be so much easier,* she thought, *if I didn't exist. No!* She wasn't suicidal. Yet one day, listening to a presentation in her "Psychology of Suicide" class about a talented, athletic, beautiful, young woman who had unexpectedly died by suicide, Tanya felt powerfully connected to that girl. While the rest of the class questioned why someone with everything going for them would end their own life, Tanya understood. She felt the girl's pain. She saw it mirrored in her own.

Her parents begged her to come home, but she wouldn't. She was tough—she was of German stock, after all, and Germans don't let anything as trivial as emotions derail their plans.

On Christmas Eve 1993, Tanya sat in her apartment alone, wrapped in blankets. Though her family had begged her to come home for the annual holiday celebration, Tanya had no motivation to move from the couch. Her heart weighed like a stone in her chest, and her body felt like it was tethered to the ground. She couldn't move. She was filled with hopelessness.

It was then, at her darkest moment, that her older sister Nicole called. Tanya saw her sister's number flash on the handset. Of all the people in the world, Nicole was probably the only one for whom Tanya would have picked up the phone.

"I can't do this," Tanya sobbed. "I don't understand what happened to my life. I don't understand God or why so many terrible things have happened!"

Nicole, ten years her senior, seemed to be everything that Tanya was not: confident, happy, and living a great life after navigating through a tumultuous, painful divorce. Soon enough, Tanya would find out that none of this was true, but at this moment, that's what Nicole represented to her.

Nicole listened to Tanya as she cried. Then she said simply, "Delete the need to understand everything. We don't need to understand *everything*. Some things just 'are.'"

It was as if a lightbulb went off in her head. Her sister's words made sense. She roused herself from the couch, changed clothes, and made the hour and a half drive home to her parents' house, where the family was gathered for their Christmas Eve celebration.

Tanya's sister was Nicole Brown Simpson. By June 1994, Nicole was dead. Her brutal murder, allegedly at the hands of her ex-husband, football star turned actor, OJ Simpson, garnered international headlines, and turned the entire Brown family inside out. Every member of their tightknit family suffered unimaginable trauma.

The murder of the beautiful 35-year-old mother, daughter, and sister was horrifying enough, but what followed launched the family into a greater nightmare.

The trial of OJ Simpson for Nicole's murder was dubbed the "Trial of the Century." The eight-month trial exposed the family—and that of Ron Goldman, a friend of Nicole's who had stopped by Nicole's house on his way home from work to return a pair of glasses—to a hideous scenario that left images in their minds long after the trial concluded. The media circus that surrounded the trial turned several of the trial's key players into reality stars. Judge Lance Ito, Prosecutor Marcia Clark and Defense Attorney Johnnie Cochran captured the attention of television viewers across the world.

The whole situation was sordid, tragic, and appalling. When the jury returned a verdict of "Not Guilty" in an egregious display of jury nullification, the entire Brown family lost faith in the American justice system.

Each member worked through the trauma of Nicole's murder in different ways: forgiveness, activism, addiction. For Tanya, her sister's death added one more layer to the complex trauma she was already dealing with. Tanya felt alone and fell victim to a controlling relationship that necessitated a restraining order. Many people throughout the years have asked Tanya, "How did you get through it?" She would reply, "Obviously, I did not because I attempted suicide ten years later."

Tanya found some comfort in becoming involved in the fight against domestic violence. When her father, Louis Brown, retired from the organization he founded, The Nicole Brown Simpson Foundation, he passed the torch to her older sister Denise, and Tanya was at her side, attending fundraisers, helping plan strategy, and soliciting donations.

But more blows were to come. In 2000, Tanya's dearest friend Troy, who had struggled on and off for years with addiction issues but had finally gotten sober, died in a fall during his bachelor party weekend. It was too much for Tanya. Tanya, who had been through so much and felt like she was coping so well, felt complete shock and despair.

JC

Smart, hard-working, intuitive, and gifted with natural humor that drew people to him, 17-year-old JC seemed like a great young adult with a limitless future. He had taken the SATs in preparation for college and was now fielding several scholarship offers from colleges around the country. He was poised for success.

However, his natural charm and easy smile disguised an unstable and challenging life. He lived in Oakland, California, a poverty-stricken area that was a hub of gang activity. JC's earliest memories were of people wandering in and out, at all hours, of the apartment he shared with his mother and sister. At nine years old, JC witnessed his aunt die of a drug overdose in his mother's arms. He stood mere feet away in shock, trying to make sense of it all. Shortly after that traumatic incident, his mother's drug addiction spun out of control, leading to JC and his siblings entering into the foster care system. After many years in the system, his father was able to prove himself able to care for JC and his younger sister and regained custody. Despite everything, JC was determined not to succumb to the life for which his childhood and neighborhood seemed to prime him.

He did all the right things—he played sports, he had a girlfriend he was deeply in love with, and he was planning a future. One Saturday morning, while sitting in his kitchen window seat, he looked around at his family members and stated with pride, "Wow, I'm the only one here that has not been locked up."

That would soon change.

Later that week, JC's girlfriend and a buddy approached him about robbing a woman his girlfriend knew well—her stepmother. The woman was controlling and abusive. JC's girlfriend hated her with a passion. He had interacted enough with the stepmother to know she had serious issues with his girlfriend and the two of them being together. Given how horrible the woman was and how terribly she had treated his girlfriend—even to the point of trying to pressure JC and his girlfriend to have sex in front of her—JC agreed to take part in the robbery.

Why did he agree to go along? Everything was going so right for him; it was just a matter of months, and he would have been able to leave Oakland and his past behind for good.

JC's girlfriend rationalized that her stepmother deserved to be robbed. JC's girlfriend pitched the plan as a great way to get even, to make her pay for all the bad things she had done. Out of a sense of wanting to prove to his girlfriend how much he loved her, JC went along with the plan.

But there was another, deeper reason JC agreed to take part, something JC was hardly aware of on a conscious level. JC had been sexually abused by his aunt as a young boy. While he had managed to suppress the memory, he never dealt with the trauma for the most part. He never told anyone. How could he? The environment he grew up in was hyper-masculine. To admit that something like *that* had happened to him—no, he just couldn't. The interaction with his girlfriend's stepmother had triggered the emotions of deep shame and anger that JC wasn't ready to address.

A few weeks before the robbery, the woman had tried again to coerce JC and his girlfriend to perform sexual acts for her perverse pleasure. The long-suppressed memory of the abuse rose, zombie-like, from the deep place within himself where it was buried. So, when JC's girlfriend proposed robbing her stepmother, JC felt she deserved it. Having been victimized himself, he was able to victimize her.

A few days later, JC, his girlfriend, and their friend entered the stepmother's house. They were startled to find that she was at home. Instead of running away, they decided to go ahead with the plan. The three teenagers tied the stepmother up with rope and placed a bedsheet over her head. JC and his friend made quick work of the robbery and dashed out with whatever valuables they could grab. JC didn't think twice about leaving his girlfriend behind with her stepmother—it was part of the plan. But what occurred next was not something they'd agreed upon. JC's girlfriend, filled with rage over years of abuse, and without JC's knowledge or approval, snapped and suffocated her stepmother with a pillow.

The robbery took place exactly one week after he had boasted to his family about being the only one who hadn't been locked up.

Several hours later, the police showed up at JC's door.

Under California law, because JC participated in the original crime, the robbery, he was considered just as guilty as his girlfriend of committing the murder. It all happened so quickly—he was charged—not as an *accessory* to murder, but the *murder* itself. JC was baffled and confused—he couldn't wrap his head around it. He was okay with taking his punishment for robbery—he admitted he did it and was prepared to pay the price. But murder? No, it wasn't possible.

JC was tried as an adult, even though he was just 17. That was bad enough—but then, he learned that the chief witness against him was his girlfriend. He couldn't believe that she would betray him that way. Yet here she was on the witness stand telling the jury that the murder was his idea. He was devastated. How could she do that to him?

At the trial's conclusion, JC sat, terrified, waiting for the jury to deliberate the outcome. They emerged far too soon in JC's opinion. Had they even discussed all the evidence? How could they, when it took so little time for them to return to the courtroom? JC waited, anxious, for the jury foreman to speak. "Guilty." Even as the words left the man's mouth, JC couldn't fathom what had just happened. It had to be a nightmare. How had it all come to this?

Shortly after being found guilty, the iron gate slammed shut behind JC, as he faced a life sentence in prison.

LEO

Leo was a friendly, quiet kid who grew up on a vegetable farm.

It was a tough childhood. His parents were stern and unaffectionate, demanding that Leo and his sister perform non-stop chores. His father was fond of saying, "Leo, you are only as good as the work you accomplish." There was no time for birthdays and celebrations at Christmas were meager. Nonetheless, Leo was calm about it and just went about his chores and schoolwork. Occasionally, at night, if all his chores were done, his dad would let him tinker with radios and batteries on the workbench. But this rarely happened.

One evening he cleaned the family's flatbed truck after delivering the tomatoes and lettuce to the market. As he hosed it off, he slipped and fell right into a picket fence where a spike went right into his eye.

Now Leo had a glass eye. But that was not the end of it. One day Leo was fixing an amplifier and had his head stuck inside a speaker box. Without warning, someone switched on the power. A 200-decibel shrill rang, and Leo's eardrums were shattered. He described it as if he could feel his eardrums quickly melt away. The only way he could hear anything was with powerful hearing aids.

Now Leo had to go through life half-blind and mostly deaf. But that was no excuse as far as his father was concerned, and there were always more chores to do.

JOE

Joe grew up in New York. If a movie were to be made of his life as a young boy, it would be filmed in sepia tones and filled with scenes of 1960s and 1970s New York City middle-class neighborhoods. There were kids running up and down the street, dads sitting on the steps smoking and talking shop, and moms calling from the window, "Come on in, dinner is ready!" All the families on the street knew and protected each other.

But, like a movie subplot, Joe's life as a boy in New York City had a dark undercurrent. His father, whom he loved with the fierce loyalty and unfailing admiration of someone who doesn't know the object of his affection, had been in prison since Joe was just five years old. His memory of him was spotty, although his mother filled in the rest, and she made him sound like a hero. She loved her husband very much; she visited him regularly in prison and wrote him near-daily letters. Joe had vague recollections of his father hitting and shouting at his mother, but took her at her word. When his father came home from prison when Joe was 11, he was overjoyed.

But the father he had hoped for—the one who would play ball with him and be his buddy—was not the one who came home. Though gregarious and friendly, Joe's father, whom everyone simply called "Jimmy from Queens," had a dark side. He drank and frequently abused Joe's mother. Joe's love for his dad was mixed with a feeling of unease and nervousness. He never knew who was coming in the door—the dad he loved or the dad he feared.

And then there was his father's choice of professions. The neighborhood Joe lived in was a center of organized crime. There was the Irish Mafia, the Italian Mafia, and the Jewish Mafia. The boldest and brashest tended to rise to the top and make the most money. And those who weren't in the Mafia cooperated with the Mafia. It was, in some ways, like the movies.

Joe's father occasionally spoke of getting out of organized crime. Organized crime was, after all, the thing that had cost him all those years in prison. Yet the siren song was too hard to ignore.

Joe's dad and some buddies concocted a plan sure to make them some money and establish Joe's dad as the boldest and brashest of them all. Together, the group decided to kidnap men in the neighborhood who belonged to the Mafia. His dad figured that this would never be reported to the police.

Indeed, his dad and the others did start the kidnappings, and at first, everything went well. Their very first kidnapping, of the Lucchese crime family capo, Frank Manzo, brought in $150,000—a king's ransom in the early 1970s. There was a new car in Joe's family's driveway, expensive gifts, and even a family vacation that Joe never forgot. But soon enough, the money started to run out. Joe's dad and his friends decided to plan another kidnapping. Following the abduction of Frank Manzo, Joe's dad and the crew conducted two more successful kidnappings of members of organized crime.

There are different versions of what happened next.

In one version, the one widely published in the newspapers, Joe's dad made arrangements to kidnap a Gambino crime family loan shark known as "Junior." But Junior fought his attempted kidnappers. Two young boys witnessed the kidnapping, recorded the license plate, and turned it over to a relative with connections to organized crime.

It got worse. At a stoplight, Junior jumped from the car and ran for his life. Shots rang out and Joe's dad was dead within seconds.

In another version, Joe's dad wasn't responsible for Junior's kidnapping at all. It was another crew of kidnappers. But Joe's dad got fingered because one of his previous victims had seen Joe when his blindfold slipped and identified him to the Gambino family. In this version, the Gambino Family decided to make an example of Joe's dad, whether or not he was Junior's real kidnapper.

Carlo Gambino, the crime boss of the Gambino Family, ordered Joe's father killed. The person who carried out the act was a young up-and-comer named John Gotti.

To 11-year-old Joe, none of that mattered. All he knew was that his dad was dead. All the daydreams he had of a loving dad, a buddy, someone to play ball with, were destroyed by a single bullet.

In the end, John Gotti received only two years in prison for the murder of Joe's dad, James "Jimmy from Queens" McBratney.

ERICA

Erica grew up in the beautiful city of Budapest. She was engaged to a wonderful man.

She was looking forward to her wedding day. One day, she walked home from work and was startled that the house was empty. Typically, her mom would be cooking dinner, and her siblings would be playing games or doing their homework. Yet today, her mom, dad, sister, and brother, along with her entire extended family, had vanished.

She quickly learned the Nazis had taken them all. The Nazis would typically knock at the front door or kick it in and tell everyone that they had five minutes to be outside, or they would be shot. They then loaded them onto a truck and took them to the brickyard, where they had a makeshift prison.

The Nazis were not yet well organized, and Erica was caught and escaped more than 20 times. She was in constant shock and horror. Her fiancé was missing.

Erica was surrounded by Nazis. The trauma was chronic. Jews, like herself, almost expected to lose their family, friends, and loved ones. She said, "You were not looking to see who was missing, but you were so happy when you found somebody alive. You almost expected them to be gone."

As the war raged, she finally found a spot where the Nazis would not find her. She hid in the basement of a hospital. To survive, Erica ate potato skins out of the garbage. When the war finally ended, she learned that her family was gone forever.

TOM

Tom was born gifted both intellectually and physically. He was tall and exceptionally athletic. On top of that, he was intelligent, and he whizzed through his school lessons like he had heard it all before.

Tom worked diligently to ensure that he made the most of his talents. As a boy, his above-average intelligence was noted by his teachers. He was invited to apply to one of the most prestigious private schools in the country, especially designed for intellectually gifted children.

As Tom grew from boyhood to his teenage years, he became even more focused and determined. Perhaps these traits were no better exemplified than on the athletic field.

His interests gravitated toward track and field. With his tall build and strong, broad shoulders, he decided to give "shot put" a try. Shot put involves "putting" (pushing rather than throwing) a heavy spherical ball, called a "shot," as far as possible. The shot weighs 16 pounds.

It is a challenging sport. Tom was strong, but being good at shot-put requires more than just strength. There is also technique and consistency. It takes hours of grueling practice to get it right. Tom put in the hours, day after day, week after week. When his dad came to pick him up from practice, Tom would beg to be allowed to "put" just a few more times. Tom's coach had never seen a high schooler work so hard to perfect his technique. Tom put his heart and soul into every practice. If he came home with aching muscles, he knew he had made progress. At night, it was rare when he didn't down a couple of aspirin.

The effort paid off. Tom started winning competitions everywhere he went. As a senior in high school, he won the national championship.

To Tom, winning was great. It validated all the hard work he had put in. But shot put was about more than just winning. He truly loved the sport. It was a part of his soul.

Coaches started talking to Tom about trying out for the 1980 Summer Olympics Track and Field team. The idea held immediate appeal for Tom. Making the team would be the pinnacle achievement.

Tom started training even more passionately, and the Olympic Team was in sight. His family and friends were ecstatic. Tom would be representing his country in the 1980 Summer Olympics. He would be on the field, competing against the best the rest of the world had to offer. He would do his country proud. He would bring home the gold. He couldn't wait. All his effort, all the years of training, all the nights of aching shoulders, and the practices spent perfecting his technique was finally about to pay off.

And then, the Soviet Union invaded Afghanistan. In protest, several countries—including Canada, West Germany, Japan, Turkey, Kenya, and the United States—boycotted the 1980 Summer Olympics, which were to be held in Moscow that year.

Tom didn't care about international politics. It didn't matter if

Russia had failed to withdraw its troops by an agreed-upon deadline. The only thing that mattered to Tom was the Olympics. His dreams were dashed.

TRAUMA TRIANGLE

The world of *trauma drama* can suck us into a cast of characters including perpetual victims, offenders, and rescuers. We may be in a legitimate state of trauma for a while, but we do not want to get stuck there:

- **Victims** are the prey who remain helpless and give up. Their state seems hopeless and they refuse to take action to change. Victims get off the trauma triangle when they say "Enough!" and get the help they need to solve their problems, and practice self-care.
- **Offenders** are predators who bully and persecute others. They get out of the trauma triangle when they stop being domineering and harsh and hold themselves accountable.
- **Rescuers** are enablers who sweep in to declare, "You need my help!" They get out of the trauma triangle when they become a supporter and offer encouragement while never doing anything that someone can do for themselves.

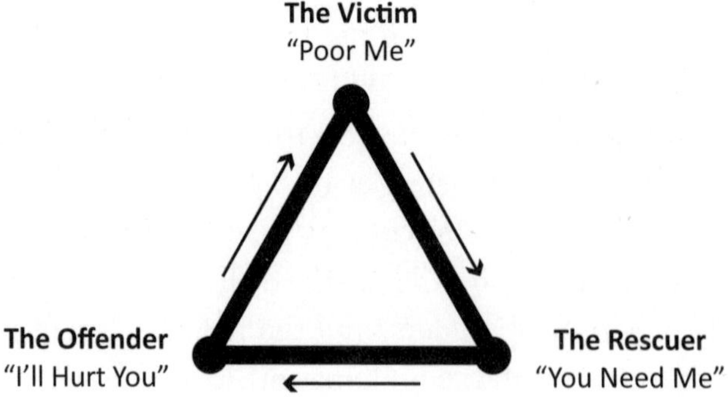

Adapted from the *Trauma Triangle* by Dr. Stephen Karpman.

MY STORY

When I was seven years old, I had a conversation with my mother that I remember vividly. I was in the kitchen, peeling an orange. My mom sat on our trendy orange-colored leather couch reading the *Los Angeles Times*. She said, "Honey, you should read this article about a man who had the same heart surgery you are going to have, and look, today he is bowling!"

I was in shock. Even though regular visits to the cardiologist were just a part of my childhood, I had never heard mention of surgery. I thought, "What is so wrong with me that it's newsworthy that this guy is bowling with the same condition I have? What is wrong with me?" I felt numb and went into complete shock and disbelief.

* * *

Shock is the start of trauma, but it is not the end.

The principles we will discuss ahead are grounded in decades of verifiable, scientific research that emerged from research conducted at UCLA in the 1970s by Richard Bandler and Dr. John Grinder. They developed Neuro-Linguistic Programming (NPL) or the "art and science of personal excellence."

This began a revolutionary area of study. In essence, "neuro" means understanding our brain functions and neurological pathways. "Linguistic" is our ability to communicate. "Programming" is focused on behavior. The combination of these three elements contributes to our personal and professional growth. This early research expanded from UCLA to Brown, Princeton, Harvard, Stanford, Yale, Vanderbilt, and numerous other universities.

Today, the science is solid. I have personally spent time with heroin addicts who now have beautiful lives. I've worked with homeless people who now have great jobs and have reconnected with their families. I know prison inmates who were released, went to college and graduated with honors. I have sat at the kitchen table with ridiculously rich and famous people whose arrogance destroyed them, and only later did they reconnect with humanity. I have met many women who suffered from domestic violence, only to call the police, get away, heal, and move on.

No matter how hard the shock hits, you can recover. No matter how long you have been beaten down, you can get up. No matter how long you have traveled in the wrong direction, you can turn around. No matter what, you can thrive if you choose to. Yes, we are in the shock stage, but as Winston Churchill said, "When you are going through hell, keep going."

CHAPTER 2

Denial

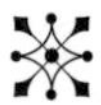

Denial is about dodging, hiding, and avoiding the inevitable. It can prevent us from getting the help we need. Taken too far, denial becomes more than a normal response and causes us to live a lie. We will never heal from a trauma that we fail to acknowledge.

A RIVER IN EGYPT

DENIAL IS NOT A RIVER IN EGYPT. It is an expected part of trauma where we say to ourselves and others around us, "I can't believe this happened!"

How we recover —and even if we recover— is dependent upon the path we take. Until that healing occurs, there will be triggers that bring negative emotions back, such as specific words, tastes, sounds, or a visit to the site of the original trauma itself. Seemingly innocent actions can trigger panic and negative emotional flashbacks that seem to come out of nowhere.

Trauma and stress hurt. When the shock and numbness begin to wear off, we often do everything possible to dodge, suppress, avoid, and hide from reality. It's a natural thing. If we avoid conflict to keep the peace, we start a war inside ourselves. Yet gradually facing reality, and even embracing it, is the key to healing.

While computers, satellites, and smartphones are remarkable technologies, the human brain is far more powerful. Our brain generates electricity in the amount of 15 to 25 watts—enough to power a lightbulb! Human brain waves are primarily divided into gamma, beta, alpha, theta, and delta waves. Gamma brain waves are the most intense and include moments of awareness. At the other end of the spectrum are delta waves, which are the most relaxed ones that occur when we are in a dreamless sleep state or deep meditation. When we are awake and alert, the human brain operates in the beta state in ordinary life. When we are relaxed, such as watching television, we are in the alpha state.

The body operates in two modes, which are the sympathetic and parasympathetic nervous systems. The parasympathetic nervous system is a decelerator. This is our "rest and digest" mode. The sympathetic nervous system is an accelerator. It activates our fight-flight-freeze responses. When an injury occurs, it turns on all our sympathetic brain functions, including our automatic physiological tasks such as flexing our muscles, adjusting our heart rate, and breathing.

Once activated, we can get stuck in the fight-flight-freeze mode. Hyper brain activity and denial are a continuation of the brain's protective reaction. Denial is a normal psychological reaction when we are experiencing grief, and when a devastating, life-changing event happens to us. In this stage, we cannot absorb the full reality of the situation or do not believe it. The numbness of shock stays with us as we refuse to accept what is in front of us.

In this stage, we often say things like, "I don't believe it," "No, No, No!" "They can't be dead," "My candidate would never do that," "There is no way that my church leaders would lie!" "I can't imagine that, after 14 years, my company fired me!" "He couldn't leave me!" "I can't believe we lost all that money!"

In this state of denial, we can have a selective memory or pretend that nothing happened. We are overwhelmed and unable to cope with the magnitude of the problem. We protect ourselves by acting as if nothing is wrong. When we are in denial, it is evident to others around us.

Denial provides brief relief from the full impact of the trauma. It gives us the chance to absorb and adapt to the situation over time rather than all at once. It protects us from having to deal with the full onslaught of destructive emotions.

Often, denial is presented as a "blame thing." Society uses the concept of denial as evidence of some moral failing. For example, when an alcoholic is in denial of their alcoholism, society uses denial as a point of judgment. This does not help. Denial can be a natural response to issues that are too painful to face right now, and thus may be beyond our control. Denial can be an instinctive, subconscious, automatic response that the brain uses to hide a memory without our choice or effort. It is not necessarily a choice and, therefore, not always a moral issue. We must curb our self-judgment so that we don't wrongly accuse or feel accused.

In our recovery, we may learn to be grateful for some of our mind's responses that we once stood in judgment of. Indeed, some coping mechanisms are problematic in specific ways, but they do the job of protecting us. If we want that behavior to go away, we acknowledge it and tell the behavior it is no longer needed, as we have found other ways to protect ourselves.

While denial has its benefits, it also has its limits. Remaining in a state of denial is damaging because it keeps us from acknowledging or dealing with reality and moving forward. It can also cause us to underestimate or minimize the magnitude of the issue. Denial prevents us from getting the real help we need, and, taken too far, denial can cause us to live a lie. We cannot process or heal from a wound that we do not acknowledge.

There are multiple forms of denial, from the young mother who witnesses a hit-and-run accident and cannot remember the details, to the college student who drinks excessively before an exam. It includes the shopaholic that goes further into debt to the older person who fails to get his affairs in order. It encompasses the dad who can't believe his daughter is a drug addict to the single mom who will not accept that she is addicted to opioids.

Denial comes in many other forms. *Rationalization* is where we give a brief acknowledgment of the situation but quickly explain it away. It's easy to *blame* another for the situation or make *excuses*. Pope John Paul II said, "An excuse is worse and more terrible than a lie, for an excuse is a lie guarded." Still, another is to *minimize* the condition and treat it less seriously than we should. Finally, denial can cause us to *dodge* and fail to face the trauma at all. These are all forms of denial and can lead us away from mindful awareness and cause some problems to get worse. To cure trauma, we must talk about its real roots. We must anchor our minds in the present while visiting the painful past.

IT'S JUST A CUT

Suppose when you are cutting some carrots, you slip and deeply cut your finger wide open. It hurts! There is shock, intense pain, and blood splatters all over the kitchen. Our natural response is to panic, quickly wash it off, and cover up the cut with a bandage as fast as possible.

The wound is evident, but if we deny the full reality and quickly minimize it, we'll find that our improperly dressed wound is ultimately going to be retraumatized. We are just kicking the can down the road, and, eventually, it will be far worse than the original cut. It is just a matter of time before our wound gets red, infected, and disgusting. Left untreated, the infection grows from just our finger to our hand, spreads up to our arm, and then starts attacking our entire body. We could quickly end up in the hospital, and, indeed, many have died from small, improperly treated wounds. Covering it up and suppressing it only brought temporary relief, and, ultimately, we will pay for our denial in a significant way.

The intelligent approach is to face reality. Though the cut hurts, we must open up the wound and douse it immediately with stinging antiseptic. We may need to get stitches, where our skin is pierced repeatedly

POST-TRAUMATIC THRIVING

The Post-Traumatic Thriving framework is founded on a range of sciences, including computational biology, neuroscience, game theory, neuro-linguistic programming, positive psychology, and psychophysiology.

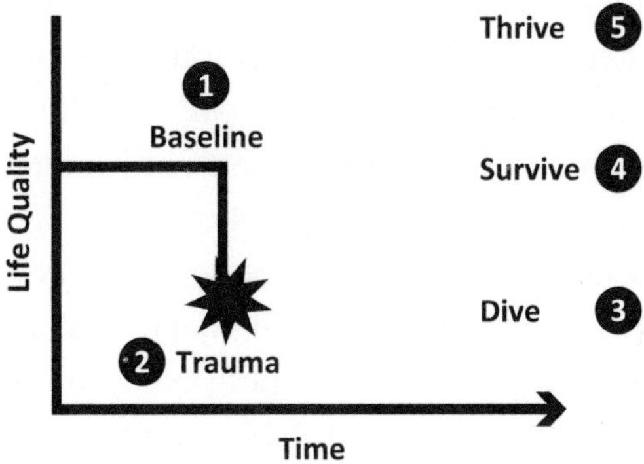

1. BASELINE. The baseline represents our average day-to-day lifestyle. We primarily use the outer (human-logical) brain and the mid (mammal-emotional) brain. Our inner (reptilian-instinct) brain operates in the background. Our parasympathetic nervous system (rest & digest or feed & breed) dominates over the sympathetic (fight-flight-freeze) nervous system.

2. TRAUMA. This may be a single (acute) event (e.g., accident or crime) or a recurring (chronic) event (e.g., abuse or lingering illness). During a trauma, our outer and mid brains yield to our inner (reptilian) brain's amygdala. Our parasympathetic nervous system is taken over by the fight-flight-freeze response. This is an evolutionary adaptive response to get us to safety. We are on high-alert and we may go into shock.

3. DIVE. We get stuck in the fight-flight-freeze mode although the trauma is over. Our inner (reptilian) brain dominates. Hormones, endorphins, and neurotransmitters (e.g., cortisol, adrenaline) continue to flood the bloodstream. Our breathing elevates and hearts race. Triggers continue to reactivate this response, even though the trauma is past and we are in no danger. We are prone to chronic anxiety, depression, addiction, or burnout.

4. SURVIVE. At this stage we heal. We stabilize as we complete the trauma cycle and let the brain know that we are safe. Our brains reset from the high-stress sympathetic to the baseline's parasympathetic nervous system. We do this through affirmations, exercise, grounding (deep-breathing) exercises, sitting in the fire (talking with a therapist or trusted person), and other activities.

5. THRIVE. Now awakened to our inner strength, we use the trauma's energy as fuel to do something new, vibrant, and fulfilling. We set goals for growth and development. The memory of our trauma passes harmlessly through our minds. We develop gratitude for the lessons we have learned.

© Copyright. Randall Bell, PhD. All rights reserved.

as the doctor sews it up. Properly cleaning and dressing an open, infected wound can easily hurt more than the original cut, yet we must do it. That is the only way to heal.

Emotional wounds involve a similar process. If we slap a makeshift Band-Aid on them, we are going to look fine for a while. But inside, something is going on. Those internal wounds are going to fester and spread. In the meantime, we mask the pain by self-medicating with drugs, alcohol, materialism, workaholism, self-righteous delusions, compulsive anger, or a host of other options.

We now have tripled up on our problems. First, the original wound is still there; second, there is damage from all the self-medication; and lastly, some forms of coping can lead to behaviors that worsen the problems or introduce new traumas. We now have a real mess.

We can mask our pain and stay in the trauma, or we can deal with it. It is time to face the music once and for all. It is time to face our choices and our misery.

FACING THE TRAUMA

Some employ "trickle truth" to situations rather than facing a complete truth all at once. This is a good thing. While the reality is harsh, gradually facing the entire trauma is the only way to truly heal. We must be heard, and a good therapist knows this and can regulate a healthy pace. The goal is to be able to confront traumatic events without being retraumatized.

As we navigate the denial stage, it is helpful to look at the specific types of traumas. Simply stated, trauma is the set of ongoing effects of an adverse event. These effects include depression, psychiatric disorders, post-traumatic stress disorder, a sense of betrayal, a lack of trust, or resentment. We may experience trauma in our roles as a victim, witness, first responder, soldier, or caregiver.

There are BIG traumas, called "acute" and little traumas called "chronic." Chronic traumas can be harder to recognize because one episode may go unnoticed. However, when these small traumas accumulate, the effect can be just as problematic as the big, or acute, ones. Trauma may be impersonal, interpersonal, or attachment-based.

Impersonal trauma includes events generally outside of our control, such as an accident or a natural disaster, like an earthquake or tornado.

Interpersonal trauma is the result of a negative interaction between people, such as abuse, rape, murder, or robbery.

Attachment trauma comes from attachment theory and emerges from one's dependence upon caregivers, mainly in infancy, childhood, and old age. This trauma could include caregiver neglect or mistreatment, physical or sexual abuse, abandonment, cruelty, or the lack of supervision and basic care. Childhood attachment trauma can be especially problematic, as it can alter a young person's psychological and social growth and development. Some of us perform well despite childhood attachment trauma, yet an injury in adulthood may make those issues reappear.

Commonly a trauma in adulthood brings back memories of childhood traumas. Thus, it is essential to deal effectively with each trauma as it comes, rather than let unresolved issues quietly pile up so that we feel vulnerable, alone, sad, and afraid. Leonardo da Vinci said, "It is easier to resist at the beginning than at the end."

DISSOCIATION

In ordinary, day-to-day life, we typically are aware of what is going on both inside our minds as well as in our surroundings. At times, we may become so absorbed in reading a book, playing a video game, watching a movie, playing an instrument, or painting a picture that we can become unaware of actions going on right next to us or even that someone is speaking to us. In everyday life, this kind of dissociation can occur during regular play or a creative experience. Yet, in cases of trauma, the experience is more intense and can create long-term issues.

Dissociation is a type of denial that involves a partial or complete loss of awareness of the horrible event we are experiencing. When faced with overwhelming trauma, some people dissociate—they mentally detach from the situation. Some call it an out-of-body experience and compare it to watching a movie. To the outsider, this may appear to be a "freeze" reaction, but others consider it a mental flight when a physical flight is not possible. Dissociation is yet another one of the tools that nature has given us to cope and protect us in the face of overwhelming stress.

Of the various kinds of dissociation, dissociative detachment is the most common. This is a feeling of being disconnected from ourselves, the outer world, or of reality itself. Many describe this feeling as a trance or dream. We are unaware, largely removed or detached from ourselves and the event, as if watching from the outside. We may completely block reality. With dissociative detachment, many lose track of time or have limited to no memory of the event.

Various dissociative detachment levels include having a sense that the world is not real, viewing events from above or through a tunnel, or serving as actors in a play. In the most extreme cases, we detach entirely and lose, at least temporarily, all memory. In other words, some traumas are so severe that we develop a form of profound amnesia.

Our memories of the trauma can be blocked from consciousness; however, certain places, smells, words, or people can bring these unpleasant memories back, sometimes in the form of flashbacks. In these cases, professional treatment can be valuable as the therapist can help us cope with these reemerging memories and the accompanying stressful emotions.

SUFFERING

Suffering hurts, but it is an inherent part of finding our inner voice and healing. While the last few decades have ushered in considerable academic and popular interest in psychology and post-traumatic growth, the roots of suffering can be found in ancient texts. Indeed, virtually all classical philosophy, religion, art, and literature focus on, and even celebrate, suffering. While modern society often emphasizes positive thinking and suppressing our pain, the real answers take us in the opposite direction.

Buddha declared that "life is suffering" and Greek mythology discusses suffering as a means of human transformation. Aristotle focused on the role of tragedy in literature. Islam states that suffering is required to reach a higher state. Christianity, by far the world's largest religion, is rooted in Christ's suffering as a gift to redeem the world.

All recognize that profound, positive, and permanent transformations are possible in the aftermath of trauma and suffering. All cultures universally admire those who overcome. Indeed, our very character is revealed in the way that we respond to challenges.

Suffering involves coming to a new reality where we do not have all the answers. The tree was bent and now grows differently. Some well-intended people chime in and say, "You have to get over it," and, "It will get easier." And we reply, "Really? Because it still hurts." We don't get over it; we get through it. In an instant, trauma changes our self-perception and our core world view. When trauma hits, we know that life will never be the same again.

People tell us to get over it, but it is not that easy. It still hurts, and the pain is there for a reason. The pain tells us that something is wrong. Validation is the remedy to denial and self-repression. Validation is a form of acceptance. Yes, this bad thing did happen, and it was as awful as it seems. It caused damage, and there is something that needs to heal.

Processing trauma is not a simple journey; it is complicated.

I am all for surviving and thriving, but there is an effort in the survivor community to abolish the word "victim." This is not always a good idea. There's a time to be a victim and a time to be a survivor. The danger in eliminating the term "victim" is that it also eliminates the perpetrator. It disregards the fact that a wrong has been committed. If we pretend we are all survivors, then there are no victims. It's as if some random thing caused our trauma rather than a person who should be held accountable. We have a society full of "survivors," but few who point out and say, "Those people are causing the damage."

In this regard, this attitude is too close to victim-blaming. That is, if we have been hurt but are still dwelling on it, there is something wrong with us. It is a form of "Why can't you just get over it?" The message is, "You need to move on to thriving in a hurry!" There is no room for hurting, being angry, grieving losses, holding the perpetrator responsible, seeking justice, and so forth. It is wrong to believe that it is the victim's fault for not immediately jumping to a position of strength. Sometimes, referring to ourselves as a "victim" is right, particularly when we want to make it clear that a person caused us harm, and we deserve that the damage be fully acknowledged.

The "no victims" mindset enables abusers. There are harmed people and responsible parties. We may use the term "survivor" at some point, but there is an appropriate time and place.

Seeing ourselves as a victim helps us let our feelings out. It allows us to sort out our feelings, separate ourselves from our abuser, and process that it was not our fault. An abuser's actions are morally on them. This allows us to accept the reality of our situation rather than put on a fake smile and pretend to be a strong "survivor" when we simply are not there.

We need to face our suffering, wrestle with it, and come to terms with it. Pain, trauma, and disaster are rooted in history and the human psyche. Trauma should not be suppressed. While heart-wrenching, we must experience the full impact of our suffering before we can move forward. Martin Luther King, Jr. said, "If you can't fly, then run. If you can't run, then walk. If you can't walk, then crawl. But whatever you do, you have to keep moving forward."

Trauma is not a mellow thing; it always generates a high level of energy. Some see themselves as hopeless victims and try to keep that energy inside, where it eats at them like cancer. Others become aggressive and use that energy to abuse others. Neither are good options because they keep us in an internal or external fight. However, what does work is to take that energy and convert it into high-octane fuel to power our productive agenda. It is terrible advice to "let it go" as that energy must go somewhere. As we heal, we will learn ways to take our hurts, fears, and pains and do something worthwhile with them.

Society demonizes the negative when we should see trauma for what it can be, a remarkable resource to fuel our dreams. It is not true that people stop pursuing dreams because they grow too old; they grow old because they stop pursuing dreams. Trauma causes some to shut down, but to thrive, we must move forward. We grow, or we die. Nelson Mandela said, "A winner is a dreamer who never gives up."

We must face our traumas and keep dreaming. I have visited with people in country clubs, prisons, posh restaurants, jails, golf courses, homeless shelters, beach resorts, and rehab centers. So far, I have not found a single person who is unable to use their suffering to their advantage. This is a universal truth.

Values give us direction, and our moral compass determines that direction. Suffering is our opportunity to examine ourselves and see what we are made of. The surprise comes when we wholeheartedly reject society's norm to mask our pain and put on a happy face. Instead, we need to embrace our suffering, see it as a valuable asset, and use it to propel ourselves toward something astounding. We do not throw our hurts and pains in the trash. We keep them to leverage them and learn from them.

Dr. Fiorindo Simone has said, "Telling a survivor of trauma to 'let go' is equivalent to expecting a person to fall off a building and walk away. It's not just a memory, it's a wound." As we respect our injuries and heal, our feelings are speaking. Our emotions are telling us something important, and we need to listen. *Anxiety* is telling us that we are stuck in the past, or worried about the future, and we need to stop and pay attention to right now. *Guilt* is saying that we made a mistake, but we are human. We should make amends the best we can, and move on. *Shame* is telling us that we are too concerned about what others think about us, rather than owning our story. *Grief* is telling us that we are compassionate, and still connected to humanity. *Anger* is showing us what we are passionate about, and what we should focus on changing. *Bitterness* is showing us the areas where we have yet to heal, while *disappointment* is telling us we broke out of our comfort zone to try something big. It didn't work out, but we should be proud of ourselves for trying!

Suffering is a sign of struggle, and struggle is life. We battle one another to get our needs met, as all creatures do. As humans, no matter how hard we try, we cause suffering, and we suffer. Suffering is a sign of life.

As therapist Daniell Koepke stated, "Your trauma is valid. Even if other people have experienced 'worse.' Even if someone else who went through the same experience doesn't feel debilitated by it. Even if it

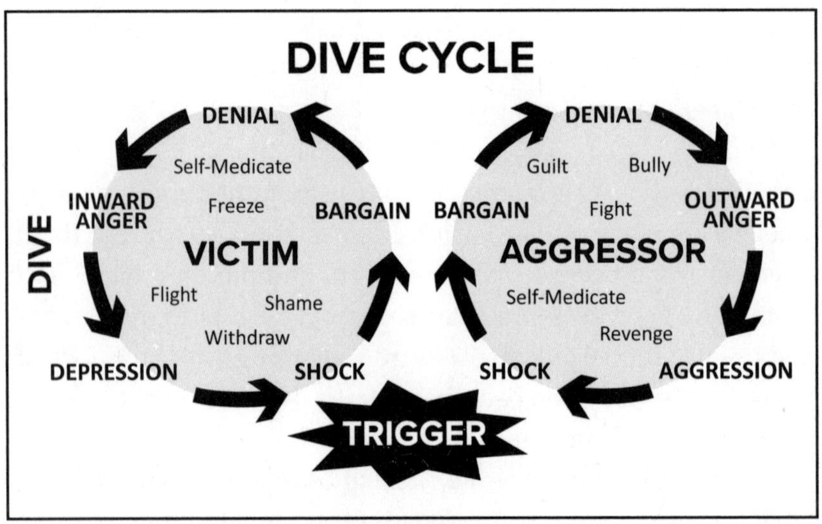

'could have been avoided.' Even if it happened a long time ago. Even if no one knows. Your trauma is real and valid, and you deserve a space to talk about it. It isn't desperate or pathetic or attention-seeking. It's self-care. It's inconceivably brave. And regardless of the magnitude of your struggle, you're allowed to take care of yourself by processing and unloading some of the pain you carry. Your pain matters. Your experience matters. And your healing matters. Nothing and no one can take that away."

Our Stories of Denial

DEBBIE

Debbie simply could not accept that her husband killed himself in the shower. It was incomprehensible. She had known him since high school. He was the father of their four children, and he had a successful career working for a large company. He served in the volunteer ministry for their church. He could not have done *that.* Not to himself, not to their children, not to her. Just. No.

Thinking back, though, Debbie knew there had always been a side of him that was a bit unstable. He had an issue with drinking, but, while Debbie was aware of it, she didn't know its extent.

Debbie admitted to herself that part of her attraction to him all those years ago was that she thought she could help him become a better man. She believed in her heart that her love would change him. With her at his side, he could tame that wildness in his soul—and, along with it, curtail his drinking.

For many of the years of their marriage, he did. She loved being married to him. He was a great guy—gentle, pretty easy going, and a wonderful father. He seemed to have successfully buried the past.

That is, until the last four or five years of their life together. Debbie instinctively knew something was wrong but could not put her finger on what it might be. Their marriage was solid. Their children were succeeding. His job—as far as she knew—was going well. On the surface, he was the epitome of the successful, middle-aged man. Yet in her deepest heart, she was unsettled. Perhaps it was in the way he sometimes stared off into space when they were together, his mind a million miles away. She had caught him mumbling to himself occasionally, but, then again, everyone did that from time to time. She hoped that he wasn't having a midlife crisis.

But in all her imaginings, she never could have fathomed how far he had fallen—to suicide.

And then, his secret life. The more she learned about it, the more she *had* to know. Gambling. Prostitutes. Lies. The evidence was right in front of her, but none of it made sense. The more she learned, the more her heart ached. She was in agony. But she couldn't stop herself—she had to know more.

This was a plotline from a television drama. This could not be her life.

JOHN

John was not happy about the US military detonating an atomic bomb near his home. He was angry that they did not tell them anything, nor did they come and take his family to safety. It was outrageous. He had enjoyed a perfect life in a tropical paradise where his only concern was what kind of fish they would be eating that night as a family.

As John and his fellow islanders stood dazed watching an atomic bomb detonate across the lagoon, they could not fathom the scale of what they had witnessed. After all, the United States was their friend; they were the good guys. The military personnel were nice men and women who dropped off cases of Spam, grape juice, and other wonderful things. They had made assurances that everything was fine, and the islands would return to normal in just a few short months. The grey fallout that showered the islands was just a harmless novelty like snowflakes that the children could play in. After all, there was no way that the Americans would harm these peaceful and cooperative local people.

SUSAN

A landslide had annihilated Susan's beautiful house. She walked from room to room in disbelief. Remarkably, the power was still on. Each time she flipped on a light, the damage was worse than she could have imagined. As she took in her ruined surroundings, she wondered if there had been an earthquake or something that had triggered a mudslide. But she would have heard about that on the news, right?

Susan and Peter had some horses who were, fortunately, fine. But Peter ran his company from their property and the outbuildings where he stored his supplies were destroyed. They lost their home and Peter's business in one fell swoop.

She thought of her husband who was out of town on business and would not arrive home for a few hours. She called some friends from her church who came within minutes and took her to a neighbor's home for the night.

Arriving at her neighbor's house, she saw that they had not had any damage. Whatever had happened seemed to affect only her home.

It all felt surreal. She was in shock. How had this happened—and who or what was responsible?

Her friends from church stayed with her that first night and prayed with her. Always a believer, Susan took great comfort in knowing that whatever had happened was the result of a plan that God created for her. She knew there would be challenges ahead, but, with His help, she would be okay.

After her husband got home a few hours later, he looked around at the walls of mud that now filled his home. Also in shock, Peter sat down on the couch in the one clean spot. He turned on the television to watch a show. Susan was baffled by his strange behavior but soon realized he was as devastated as she was. He was trying to find a normal moment the only way he could.

They could not live in the house the way it was. Friends immediately offered them a place to stay. The very next day, Susan began the difficult task of investigating what had happened. First, she called her homeowner's insurance to send an appraiser. That process alone took far longer than it should have. In fact, it took weeks. The company moved at a snail's pace.

For the next few weeks, she and Peter lived in a friend's guest room. Susan still went to her demanding job each day, and Peter worked to re-establish his business and assure his clients that their productions would go on as scheduled despite the landslide. In her free time, Susan spent hours on the phone trying to find someone who could help them navigate what had happened to their home and how to recover.

Despite her friends' support and generosity, Susan's emotions were fraying. When the appraiser finally did inspect the house, he said it was the worst situation he had seen where the house was still standing. The landslide, the inspector explained, came from the hill above them. There were no houses on the hill, just a narrow access road. And yes, there had been rains recently, but not in the volume required to loosen the dirt and rocks to the point where they went sliding down the hill. Something specific had triggered it.

Susan investigated further. She was relentless. She was shocked to discover that the City of Los Angeles owned the land on which the landslide originated. City workers had been doing grading work on property above her home. Their heavy machinery had triggered the landslide. Unbelievably, the City had not even contacted Susan and Peter to let them know what had happened. They just allowed them to find it on their own. They could not believe it.

SHAD

Shad left the Army when he completed his tour of duty. Initially, he was at loose ends. He went back to Alabama for a while but had trouble connecting with friends and family. He was restless and anxious. Shad's mind kept returning to that horrific night in Vietnam.

The more he thought about the Vietnam War, the more he became convinced that it was utterly pointless. Initially, he had believed in the United States' stated mission of preventing the spread of communism. But he came to realize that the war had nothing to do with winning hearts and minds. It was all about economic interests, national fears, and geopolitical strategies. The South Vietnamese didn't want the Americans there—and even if they did, so what? It had not been worth all the death and destruction.

The year he came back, Christmas of 1970, was the most overwhelming year of his life. "You went home alone," Shad recalls. "You don't know where you are. You don't know what to do. No one helps you transition back into civilian life. You were just expected to pick up where you left off, and that was that." The Army had trained him how to kill, but had not retrained him for a healthy life at home. It was too much.

Shad was looking for an escape. As he puts it, he wanted to "go to Mars" or as far away as possible. Los Angeles seemed a good enough alternative.

TANYA

Tanya's go-to emotion every time she experienced trauma was denial. When her friends in high school died, she did not know how to accept it. She continued telling herself it wasn't true. People were just lying. It was not until she attended their funerals that she fully absorbed what had happened.

When Tanya learned that her sister, Nicole, was brutally murdered, her first thought was that she was asleep and having a nightmare. Her denial was so deep that she scoffed at the idea Nicole was dead. Nicole was not dead—how could she be? She had finally rid herself of her horrible husband, she was starting to enjoy her life as a single woman, and she was making plans for a future. God would not take away someone with so much to live for and so much still to give.

JC

When JC was arrested for a murder committed by his girlfriend, he was in disbelief. He was nowhere near the crime scene when his girlfriend killed her stepmother. He was willing to accept punishment for the robbery. But he had not murdered anyone.

"Besides," he told himself, "this was the only crime I have ever committed." It was not like he had spent his youth selling drugs, assaulting people, or robbing people. He was not in a gang. He was a good student, and he had plans for a great life. On his bedroom dresser at home, there was a stack of admission letters from several universities.

There was no way, JC thought, that the jury would convict him of murder.

JC did not know that the night he and his girlfriend were arrested, even while he sat in the holding cell waiting to talk to the police, his girlfriend was doing some talking of her own—and most of it was about JC. In a desperate bid to save herself, JC's girlfriend had turned state's evidence against JC.

LEO

Leo had lost an eye to a picket fence and his hearing to an amplifier accident. He loved sports like any boy, but that was not in the cards. He could not deny his disabilities for long, but he could hide them. An eye patch was not for him, so he got fitted with a glass eye. He could not hide his problems from himself, but at least he could hide them from others. Who could blame him for wanting to?

JOE

Joe was traumatized by the sudden death of his father. Just a boy, he turned to his mother and grandmother in his grief. But the two women, perhaps in a misguided attempt to protect him from the truth, tried to distract him from his grief by giving him toys or his favorite foods. Joe learned to suppress his feelings rather than work through them.

Everyone around Joe was in denial. They never told him exactly what had happened to his father. They just said that he was gone and never coming back. Joe would not learn the truth for nearly another decade when he was 20 years old.

As he grew up, Joe's tendency to cover up his true emotions with a façade of bravado only increased. He grew up tall and strong. He was a gifted student and an even more gifted athlete. But his bitterness over the death of his father grew with each passing year.

It was made worse by the rumors about his father that swirled around his high school. Joe heard again and again that his father was a criminal. He had been gunned down in a bar, and his father's death benefited John Gotti in the world of organized crime.

Joe confronted his mother with these rumors, but she would not confirm or deny if they were true. Joe could not believe his father was the kind of person that others claimed him to be. There was no way. Yet on another level, Joe knew in his heart that his father had been involved in something very serious.

ERICA

As a young woman in Budapest, Erica noticed that many turned a blind eye to the horrible things the Nazis were doing. Yet horrible things kept happening, and people were quickly disappearing. She made her denial stage a very short one and faced the ugly reality right away. This kept her alive, one day at a time.

TOM

President Carter's move to boycott the 1980 Olympics was controversial. Many people, including members of President Carter's own political party, felt the move was merely symbolic and wouldn't do anything to stem Russia's military aggression. The United Kingdom, France, and Greece supported America's decision to boycott the Olympics but left the choice of whether to participate up to individual competitors.

Tom, his coaches, and his fellow Olympic teammates watched the developments with trepidation. For a time, it seemed that President Carter would relent. However, it became apparent that, folly or not, the President was committed to his decision.

Tom was in denial. After all, how could one person have such influence over Tom's dreams? Why could Tom not go on his own? There had to be a way that he could be part of the Olympics.

When his friends and family tried to comfort him by reminding him that he could likely make the 1984 team, Tom lashed out. Could they not see that he would never be able to make the 1984 team? He was 20 years old—four years was a lifetime away. He might lose his skills or strength. He might be injured. There could be other young, stronger men to whom he would lose. No, his only chance to be in the Olympics was now. In his mind, no one understood what he was going through. His life was ruined.

MY STORY

When I was 10, and my mom told me that I needed to have open-heart surgery, I went into a state of shock and denial. I just froze by the big picture window that overlooked the street and driveway, waiting for my dad to get home from work. I did not believe my mom. I did not know why she was lying to me, but I was sure she was.

The moment my dad got home, I bolted for the front door and down the steps. My dad did not even have time to get out of his car before I ran up to him. He turned off the engine and rolled down the window. I yelled, "Dad! Mom told me that I need to have open-heart surgery. That's not true, is it?" My dad just looked at me and said, "Yep, it is true. You need to have surgery next summer." My afternoon of denial was shattered.

CHAPTER 3

Anger

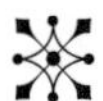

Trauma often fills otherwise calm people with a sense of uncontrollable rage, hurt, resentment, and blame. It is all right to be outraged at traumatic experiences, as long as we do not hurt ourselves or others.

MESSING WITH OUR HEADS

TRAUMA, AND THE ANGER IT CAUSES, is complex. While we know trauma will affect everyone at one time or another, everyone reacts differently.Some have a higher threshold to trauma than others, and an event that does not disturb one person will be disabling to another. Some have symptoms such as panic attacks, nightmares, flashbacks, alterations to behaviors, or chronic anxiety. Some bounce back to their baseline immediately, whereas others get stuck. Some completely fall apart, whereas others hide their pain beneath a functional exterior, yet they are suffering all the same. The rate at which one recovers from trauma is not a moral question. It is not a choice. It is based on genetics, temperament, circumstance, and chance.

One thing is for sure: no one reacts to trauma the same. Nonetheless, when trauma does hit, there are general patterns, and knowing the trends helps us navigate the path.

The emotion of anger is demonized by some in our society, in part because a person who is misdirecting their anger can cause a lot of damage. But anger is also a natural reaction to pain. It is a feeling that comes out of frustration for a problem that cannot be solved, pain without a known end, or tragedy without apparent hope. Anger fills us with a sense of movement, a motivation to act and try solutions we otherwise would not consider.

When those solutions are harmful, we might lash out and make the problem worse. But when we are mindful of anger, sit with it, and try to understand what it is telling us, anger can help us plot a more reasoned path forward.

In the moment, pain, anger, or fear might overwhelm our senses. We call for help, which may or may not come. Then comes the fight-flight-freeze response.

When the anger eventually subsides, the world may return to normal, but our emotions and neurochemistry do not. There are a variety of immediate responses to trauma:

- The "hit-and-run" injury hits hard, but then the person runs away from it and pretends it never happened.
- The acute "knockout punch" trauma involves a severe blow, from which the person is "out cold" for days, weeks, or longer.
- The "roller coaster" reaction is when the person has periods of incredible highs and then deep lows, and the ride goes on and on.
- The chronic "trickle" trauma is a low-grade, constant drain. The person simply never performs near their capacity again.

The single common denominator of these reactions is that we do not believe the trauma happened, and we certainly don't want to face it. Yet, when we do, the rage may come flooding back as if we are still facing the event.

Anger can be scary, especially when it makes us feel out of control. As with the other uncomfortable feelings of trauma, we may attempt to deal with the problem by repressing it and stuffing it down until we can no longer feel it. But anger repressed can be transformed into other damaging emotions or triggered by nontraumatic situations, causing us to lash out seemingly at random.

The bad news is that a chronic state of anger impairs both our physical and mental health. In other words, it is unhealthy to have adrenaline pumping through our veins when there is no actual danger. This is like slamming on the gas pedal of a car when it is parked in neutral.

The good news is that this process has been well-researched, and there are more effective ways to process the impulses. We can safely activate these traumatic memories, allowing them to harmlessly pass through our minds without setting off this fight-flight-freeze response. It is not the goal to suppress or forget a traumatic incident—the objective is to view the thoughts of the trauma dispassionately, the way we would view a nontraumatic memory, and remember without reliving the full horror over and over again. Even better, we can repurpose our trauma as fuel for ourselves in a positive direction.

ALL THE RAGE

We may not change when we see the light, but we may change when we feel the heat. In the fallout following a traumatic experience, outrage and anger are typical responses as the shock and denial wear off. The intense rage often fills otherwise calm people with a sense of uncontrollable hurt, resentment, and blame. This is a natural response to fear or frustration in some situations.

Anger can be directed towards those who have harmed our loved ones or us. We may be upset at the person or situation that caused the trauma, or more widely, at God, the universe, first responders, hospital staff, or anyone who happens to be around or trying to help. Overall, this anger stems from the need to protect ourselves from intense pain. Accumulated and unresolved traumas may also trigger anger.

A trigger is the stress response—any strong emotion or mental state—that is set off by conditions that recall prior trauma. A trigger could be a song, a picture, a smell, a place, a voice, a name, or other everyday events. For example, a car that backfires might cause a soldier to hit the ground. Their brain's amygdala prompts a physical reaction—to take cover from gunfire—before they can process the noise and realize it's just a car.

An unresolved trigger never goes away. Even in adulthood, childhood memories can trigger physical responses. Driving by our first home or old grade school can make our heart race, breathing increase, or blood pressure go up. This is not just "all in our heads." There is a real physiological reaction. Cortisol and adrenaline are being pumped into our bloodstreams, and our heart rates goes up, our breathing changes and all of these things can have an impact on our health. These stress responses are the body's natural defenses from peril—yet triggers can set off these same reactions when there is no actual danger. It is good practice to be aware of our physical responses and those triggers that cause them.

The triggers that bring anger or fear differ from person to person. Not everyone is triggered by the same things, nor does everyone have the same responses to trauma. For example, one soldier may have grown up on a farm where firearms were commonplace. Hearing a gun generally just meant that somebody was target practicing in the backyard. During his deployment, he did not experience any direct combat. Yet another soldier, who grew up in the city and saw few guns, trembled the first time he shot one as an adult. Also, he may have been in an active combat zone when he saw his buddies die. When the car backfires, the first soldier has no response, but the second hits the ground. The sound of the car backfiring brings back all the fear and anger of being shot at.

Our triggers can include driving by a school where we were bullied, hearing a parent bring up a painful family event, smelling the scent of aftershave, watching a situation on TV, hearing the sound of a dog barking, or running into an old love interest from an abusive relationship.

We all react to these situations differently, and all triggers are valid for those who experience them.

Unprocessed trauma can lead to an anger addiction or an intense craving for fear, where we crave the neurotransmitters it produces. Watching the news can generate anger or watching a horror movie can create the fear we crave. Once in this trap, we create thoughts and behaviors that deliberately bring more anger, and an ugly cycle continues.

IF YOU ARE PISSED, BE PISSED

In the aftermath of a trauma, some jump in with the advice, "Just get over it and calm down!" Never in the history of "calm down" has telling someone to "calm down" actually made them calm down! It does not work, as we need to process our anger and get it out of our system.

Anger is a natural, healthy part of processing trauma. Suppressing anger prevents healing. It keeps us in the battle. On the other hand, allowing ourselves to *feel* angry, to become aware of the sensation and what it is telling us, means that we can express our anger in healthy ways that do not hurt ourselves or cause additional trauma to others.

Anger takes a variety of forms, such as passive-aggression. Passive-aggressive behaviors are when someone has been hurt or traumatized but has become quiet and sullen about it. They outwardly act as if nothing is wrong, but clearly, something is. Instead of getting visibly angry, some people express their hostility in passive-aggressive ways that only result in hurt and confusion towards their target.

We need to sit with our anger and express it safely for as long as we need to. We need to experience all of our legitimate feelings. Do not allow others to tell you how to feel. Over time, you will feel less angry; and if not, consider working through the process with a therapist.

When we lose something that once brought us comfort and peace, there will be sadness, depression, and anger. When we experience loss, we grieve. When we lose a spouse, people will rally around and understand. Yet when we walk away from a relationship where we were deeply betrayed, many people struggle to understand. In a situation like this, the grieving process is incredibly lonely. We are heartbroken and sick with loss.

Both narcissists and empaths tend to have had early developmental trauma. The difference is that narcissists are fundamentally weak at their deepest inner core and succumb to heavy defenses that manifest as selfishness and control issues. At the same time, empaths rise above their torturous past with softened defenses and continue to be there for humanity. Yet, they may remain easy targets for abusers. Either way, we are not meant to stay wounded; we are meant to push through our anger. When we feel the rage and appropriately express it, we finally release our pain and move forward. This way, narcissists who grow up, take responsibility and apologize can connect with humanity, and empaths who stop tolerating others' bad behaviors can develop assertive self-respect.

Anger is a secondary reaction, so it is critical to look at the unresolved trauma underneath it. This takes raw honesty. There is no assumption that we will automatically heal. We must be willing to explore the dark corners of our grief. We must stay there until we find that critical comment or thought that hits us and allows us to move forward.

There are several healthy ways to deal with anger that neither harm ourselves or others. One is to write a scathing letter, but never mail it. This was an approach taken by Abraham Lincoln. We can go to the batting cages and crack the bat. We can go in our car and scream and yell. Exercising, pumping iron, or just taking a walk outside is outstanding for letting off steam and reducing stress. We can listen to our favorite music. We can go into a room by ourselves and dance to loud music. We can draw, paint, or create some form of art. We can take several deep breaths until we feel our blood pressure drop. Ultimately, we can rely upon the "dynamic duo" of talking to a trusted person and doing our grounding exercises.

MEMORIES OF TRAUMA

Dealing with the memory of traumatic events is an essential element of our healing, but there are some pitfalls. For example, we may obsess and become haunted by uncomfortable flashbacks. Furthermore, we may have distorted memories or be confused about what happened; or, we may have detached so entirely that we have no recollection of the trauma.

Trauma includes both implicit and explicit memories. *Implicit* memories are our conditioned emotional responses, while *explicit* memories are our conscious recollections of specific events. Trauma also includes *conditioned* responses, which means we construct a memory of our autobiographical self-narrative by including our memories, what others have told us, as well as what we infer happened. Even in the best of circumstances, our minds can be a mix of perfect recall and false memories. When trauma is introduced, memory issues are amplified. When we are in shock, angry, fleeing, or fighting, our sense of time and memories enter a new dimension. Predators often take advantage of this fact and will trick victims into making them question their memories, a type of manipulation called "gaslighting."

Our memories are compiled in much the same way as a video recording. Yet they can be distorted by time, triggered by certain words or smells, forgotten, or even repressed. Generally, our memories capture the gist of what happened, but the details may be fuzzy.

Flashbacks are intense recollections, where we relive painful, traumatic events. Flashbacks are often depicted in media as visual, but they can be composed of any or all senses, or even simply be an emotion flooding back. They can take place when we are awake or in our sleep as nightmares. The essence of healing is to engage in formal trauma treatment and focus upon mindfulness and grounding in current reality. It is essential to draw a sharp distinction between the past and the present. We acknowledge the past, yet we focus on the here and now.

When it comes to memory, the objective is to remember the

trauma but not to relive it. In other words, the goal is not to forget or repress a memory, but rather acknowledge it honestly and not allow ourselves to be retraumatized by it. To do this, it is often helpful to construct a written and meaningful narrative that helps us document what happened, put context around it, and attempt to make some sense of our honest history. In the process, we want to recall both the negative along with the positive. It is a blend of our recollections and what others can tell us to understand, but some of our history may never be fully known.

POST-TRAUMATIC STRESS DISORDER

In extreme cases, trauma can be so severe that it anchors itself inside of us. In essence, it hijacks our minds. The harm is so profound that we develop a disorder called post-traumatic stress disorder, or PTSD. Today, PTSD symptoms affect tens of millions of people around the world. While this condition was first noted in soldiers, it is a myth that PTSD affects only those who served in combat. PTSD can affect anyone.

PTSD has been documented for centuries going back as far as 2100 BC. In ancient times it was referred to as "nostalgia." During the Civil War, it was known as "soldier's heart." During World War I, it was called "shell shock." During World War II, it went by the name "battle fatigue."

If we have not seen violence ourselves, we may think of war as if we are watching a movie, drinking soda, and munching on popcorn in our air-conditioned seats. In reality, war is brutal. When I was in Israel doing research on terrorism, I accidentally wandered into an active war zone. Sirens went off, machine guns started blazing, and a bomb exploded. I was crouched behind a wall terrified, and from my response to this single incident, I cannot imagine what soldiers go through every day.

In the 1970s, as our soldiers began returning from Vietnam, a host of problems emerged. Combat veterans displayed severe physical, mental, emotional, and social effects. The symptoms included intense nightmares and flashbacks. Veterans were triggered by any number of seemingly harmless events, like the 4th of July fireworks or police sirens. "Vietnam Syndrome" has taken on a variety of meanings over the years, but it was first used to describe these new symptoms.

After centuries of seeing this condition, PTSD was first officially recognized as a mental health concern in 1980, only five years after the Vietnam War ended. According to US Department of Veterans Affairs estimates, PTSD afflicts almost 31 percent of Vietnam veterans, 10 percent of the Gulf War veterans, and 10 to 18 percent of Iraq and Afghanistan war veterans. People living with PTSD may have difficulty coping, holding down a job, or maintaining stable relationships. If left untreated, PTSD might lead to substance abuse or a host of other problems.

As a society, we train and program our soldiers to fight and kill. Yet when they come home, our society does little to deprogram this training. There are many horrible things about war, but the worst part should not be when a soldier comes home. These unseen wounds can be retraumatizing for years or decades. We often say to veterans, "Thank you for your service," but perhaps we should take the time to sit down, really listen to their stories and try to understand what they have been through. Like anyone who has experienced trauma, these wonderful people deserve to be heard. Today millions suffer from PTSD and related issues, and we as a society have significantly benefited from the research that came out of studying the "Vietnam Syndrome."

While the roots of understanding PTSD came from combat service, today we know that it can affect anyone. PTSD can result from domestic abuse, child abuse, bullying and cyberbullying, stalking, neglect, poverty, fire or natural disaster, secondary trauma from being a first responder or therapist, workplace abuse, and it can even impact the folks who filter reported posts on social media and see ugly material daily. Any of these can cause us to burn out quickly.

Complex PTSD or, C-PTSD, is caused by numerous smaller impacts or a series of larger ones. This can occur when repeated acts of sexual, emotional, or other abuse occur over an extended period.

Anger may not always be our first response. There may be anger, but we can also experience fear, anxiety, pain and despair, confusion, shock, and bargaining. At the same time, "love bombing," which is the use of flattery and praise, can keep us in a toxic relationship. These highs become part of the trauma.

For some, C-PTSD can be easier to minimize and dismiss. Superficially, years of smaller manipulations do not seem as severe. Yet chronic lack of safety, degrading messages, seemingly small acts of harassment, sexual trauma, disability, homelessness, family issues, or difficulty connecting can take a serious toll.

HALLMARKS OF PTSD

Scientists now know that PTSD can happen to anyone. It is a lasting consequence of traumatic ordeals (such as a sexual or physical assault, the unexpected death of a loved one, an accident, war, or natural disaster) that cause intense fear, helplessness and horror.

Recent research reveals chemical and physical changes that occur in the brains of people living with PTSD. In 2010, scientists from the University of Minnesota and Minneapolis VA Medical Center discovered that long-term, sustained stress causes the hippocampus, the part of the brain that connects and organizes memory, to shrink. PTSD also affects the prefrontal cortex which regulates fear and other emotions.

The hallmarks of PTSD are triggers that lead to flashbacks or nightmares that cause us to re-experience the full and shocking events of the original trauma. Other symptoms include:

- Panic attacks
- Eating disorders
- Cognitive delays and lowered verbal memory capacity
- Intense feelings of distress
- Nausea

- Sweating
- Pounding heart
- Invasive memories
- Flashbacks
- Nightmares
- Loss of passion
- Feeling detached or not feeling that we fit in; self-isolation
- Substance abuse issues resulting from attempts to self-medicate
- Long-term, stress-related health issues

PTSD is severe and requires professional intervention. Flashbacks and nightmares can bring extreme and profound stressful reactions where we are left vulnerable to reliving the full experience. In this condition, we feel the full force of the fear, helplessness, loneliness, and hurt of the first event. We relive it entirely in our minds, and these episodes are debilitating.

PTSD and traumatic memories are real. When I was retained to work on Hurricane Katrina, I saw people go from friendly and sociable to suddenly trembling and convulsing with just a single word. It is not anything to be embarrassed about, but it does need to be treated. It is entirely reasonable to want to avoid stirring up past and painful memories. Yet we are stuck in this condition, and we may feel helpless as to how to escape.

To complicate matters, we are dealing with two issues: the profound trauma of the past as well as ongoing traumas today that are the result of leaving the past trauma untreated. This hurts us as well as the people around us. When untreated, many traumatized people bring issues into their current relationships. A professional therapist can help with the priorities of today and the existing relationships, while also working to resolve the past traumas. It takes courage to address past and present traumas.

THE VICTIM CYCLE

Bullying is persistent and ongoing, happening sometimes up to three or four times a day. It is likely to continue into adulthood, unless the trauma that leads to the bullying is addressed. As noted in a study conducted by Utterly Global, children who were bullies in grades six to

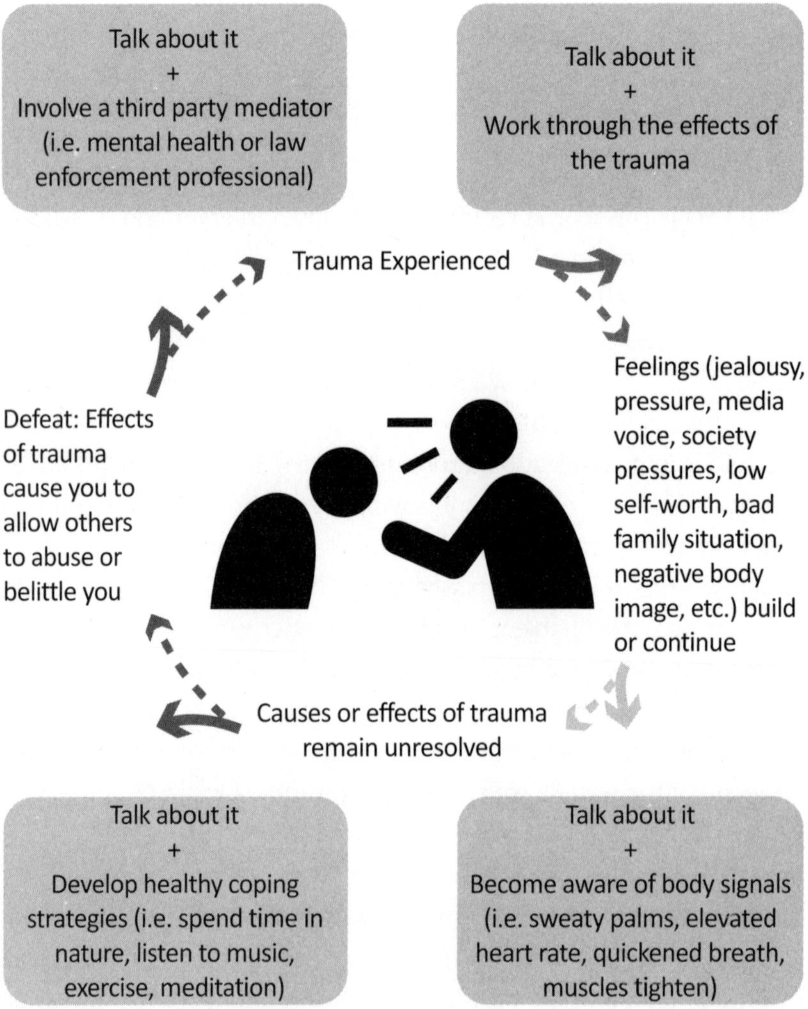

Talk about it
+
Involve a third party mediator (i.e. mental health or law enforcement professional)

Talk about it
+
Work through the effects of the trauma

Trauma Experienced

Feelings (jealousy, pressure, media voice, society pressures, low self-worth, bad family situation, negative body image, etc.) build or continue

Causes or effects of trauma remain unresolved

Defeat: Effects of trauma cause you to allow others to abuse or belittle you

Talk about it
+
Develop healthy coping strategies (i.e. spend time in nature, listen to music, exercise, meditation)

Talk about it
+
Become aware of body signals (i.e. sweaty palms, elevated heart rate, quickened breath, muscles tighten)

THE BULLY CYCLE

nine are 60% more likely to have a criminal conviction by the age of 24, and according to the National Institute for Occupational Safety and Health, workplace bullying causes $3 billion in lost productivity and a $19 billion loss in employment every year.

Talk about it
+
Involve a third party mediator (i.e. mental health or law enforcement professional)

Talk about it
+
Work through the effects of the trauma

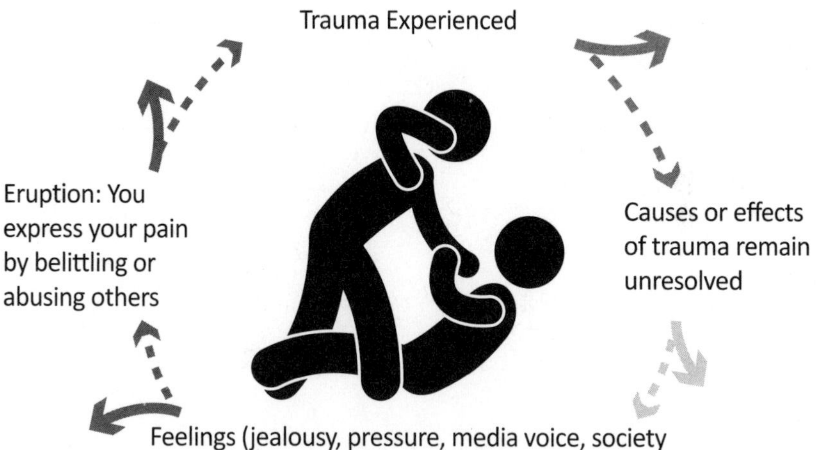

Trauma Experienced
Causes or effects of trauma remain unresolved
Feelings (jealousy, pressure, media voice, society pressures, low self-worth, bad family situation, negative body image, etc.) build or continue
Eruption: You express your pain by belittling or abusing others

Talk about it
+
Develop healthy coping strategies (i.e. spend time in nature, listen to music, exercise, meditation)

Talk about it
+
Become aware of body signals (i.e. sweaty palms, elevated heart rate, quickened breath, muscles tighten)

When we experience acute trauma, it is unreasonable to expect ourselves to account for every detail. Indeed, it is not even necessary to do so. Once the trauma is fully processed or deprogrammed, we may also choose to forget it, but only if we want to.

Our Stories of Anger

DEBBIE

In time, grief gave way to anger, and then, to rage. Debbie was pissed.

Before Debbie's husband died of suicide, she had absolutely no idea of his double life of gambling and prostitutes. He had carefully and intentionally crafted an entire life based on lies and obfuscation. He used Debbie's trust in him and in their marriage against her. She was furious at what he had done. The deception. The trickery. The way he had upended their whole life and turned it into a mockery of what it once was.

She had every right to be angry. At times she found herself shaking with emotion. But she was careful not to let that anger flow into other relationships. She did not take it out on their children or anyone else who did not deserve it. She did not blame herself, either. Her husband had made his choices for reasons of his own that had nothing to do with her.

She focused her anger squarely on her dead husband, where it belonged.

SUSAN

Even with the help of their friends, it took weeks for Susan and her husband to move everything out of their house that had been destroyed by a landslide. They did not clear the mud right away—the cost would have been astronomical. Their insurance company would not pay for a cleanup. Susan was on the phone, almost daily, asking in vain for some assistance. Tension mounted with each passing day as did her anger.

Susan and Peter's entire way of life was upended. And it was not just their lives—the lives of their animals were impacted too. Susan had to find alternative lodging for their horses while their stables were rebuilt.

A few weeks after the landslide, Susan received a letter from the City of Los Angeles. At first, she was relieved—had all her calls and messages paid off? Could it be that the City had decided to help them after all? Would City officials now do the right thing by taking responsibility for the damage they caused with their carelessness? She opened the letter with some trepidation, hoping for the best.

To her astonishment, the city sent her and Peter a letter informing them that they violated code for not clearing the landslide. Unbelievable. The letter threatened fines and potential legal action if they did not resolve the issue within a specific number of weeks.

Susan immediately reached out to the City. Officials there offered no solutions and took no ownership of the problem they created. They insisted that as the homeowners, it was her and Peter's responsibility to clean up the property.

To Susan, it was unbelievable. She was beyond angry at this point.

Susan reached out to her local congressman, sure he would help her. Instead, he shrugged it off. Feeling desperate, she contacted both FEMA and the Red Cross. Neither organization could provide any support at all.

Susan and Peter felt alone, devastated, and helpless in the aftermath of the event. Susan was upset enough with the situation before she discovered its cause. After she learned that the City of Los Angeles was at fault and everyone was dodging responsibility, she was livid.

SHAD

During the Vietnam War, Shad, a captain, was placed in charge of a MASH unit. A sudden battle ensued, and more than 70 young soldiers were brought in who were all terribly injured. Shad and his team of medics performed triage, trying to save those who had a chance of survival. Thirty-five young men died of their injuries.

That night of horror traumatized Shad. After the insanity of triage, he and his team had to strip the bodies and put them in body bags. To make sure each victim was identified correctly, they placed his dog tag in his mouth, using the metal grooves in the dog tag to secure it between each man's teeth. He never forgot that.

At the end of his tour of duty, he returned home to Alabama, where he felt disconnected and apathetic. These feelings were overshadowed, though, by his terrible, relentless anger. The war had been a terrible mistake—so many young lives taken, so many soldiers wounded, an entire country decimated, unrest at home, and protests. All of it ate at Shad. He was filled with anger at the politicians in Washington for their stupidity and shortsightedness. How could they not know that Vietnam was a lost cause? How could they continue to send more young men to their deaths, wasting so much potential?

Shad's head was still in the war. His self-isolation affected his relationships. He did not know how to communicate with family and friends at home, who were hurt by his distancing. They all wanted to give him love and support, but his anger was like a solid wall they couldn't break down.

GERI

Geri's primary emotion was love; therefore, anger was not her initial response, and she was driven mostly by compassion. While she knew she was different from the children in her neighborhood, Geri experienced so much love from her family that she had a solid foundation for growing and evolving. This served her immensely throughout her life.

Geri had an especially close relationship with her younger sister, Gloria. Gloria was beautiful and kind with dark hair and lively eyes. She was never embarrassed about Geri's disability. She was fiercely proud of all of Geri's accomplishments and passionately protective. She always made Geri feel deeply loved. They both loved one another deeply, and their bond never wavered into adulthood.

When Geri was born in the 1950s, the doctor warned her parents not to get "too attached." They should, the doctor advised, put her in a "facility." Geri's parents scoffed at the idea. This was their little girl, and she would have a life of fullness and joy. Geri's entire family always supported her, never making her feel that her cerebral palsy was a burden or embarrassment. She was valued and treated equally.

No, Geri did not experience anger.

As for her parents, they certainly had a reason to be angry. A careless driver had nearly killed both mother and baby. And the punishment was nowhere near what was deserved. But rather than dwell on their anger, Geri's parents focused on love—the love of their sweet little girl, her sister, her brothers, and each other.

TANYA

Once Tanya accepted that Nicole was dead, allegedly murdered by her abusive ex-husband, her head was filled with a red rage that overtook every cell in her body. The anger was unrelenting and all-consuming. Though she knew that such long-sustained anger probably wasn't healthy for her, she nevertheless embraced it. The anger helped her get through the first months after Nicole's murder and sustained her as she sat in the courtroom, day after day, at the murderer's pretrial hearing. Yet, she would be damned if she ever let that monster see her cry.

JC

After his conviction for murder, 17-year-old JC's emotions ran the gamut from confusion to deep sorrow to anger and back to chaos again. None of this situation made sense. What had happened to his life? How had it come to this?

As the emotions swirled around, anger came to the forefront more and more frequently. His pain turned inward and came out as rage. The root of his rage was the pain. There was pain from the betrayal of his girlfriend, the loss of the life he was supposed to have, and the thought of spending the rest of his life in prison.

At least the anger made him feel strong, temporarily, whereas the confusion and sorrow made him feel weak. JC knew where he was going and he could not afford to look weak.

LEO

Leo was angry with the fact that he had lost his eye to a picket fence. Who would not be? This meant no sports or other things that little boys liked to do. But Leo was a deep thinker, and not being able to participate in sports allowed him more time to think. He became curious about the world around him. In his spare time, he started to dismantle clocks, radios, and anything mechanical. He put all his negative energy into exploring and thinking—a skill that would serve him well.

JOE

As Joe grew up, unable to express what he was feeling over the loss of his father or even learn the truth behind why he died, he became angrier and angrier.

He was also brilliant. He excelled in all his classes and was known from a very young age as a talented poet and playwright. As young as third grade, he was writing school plays that, he found out years later, became a permanent part of the school's theater rotation.

The anger was always there, just underneath the surface. At the age of 14, he started to drink to dull the pain. He was constantly suspended from school for fighting with other kids.

Yet for all his angry outbursts, Joe was also considered charming and handsome. And like his father, Joe was extremely adept at playing a role. He was voted most popular in high school, was the star of the football team, and even won the lead role in the school play.

His firecracker temper seemed to be part of his allure—people knew you could not mess with Joe. And at the same time, Joe was unfailingly loyal. If you were his friend, there was nothing he would not do for you.

Joe was becoming just like his father.

ERICA

Erica was angry, but she did not have the luxury of expressing it. She quickly saw that anyone who showed any anger towards the Nazis would be shot on sight. So, Erica did something novel with her rage. She channeled it as energy to be remarkably polite to the Nazis. She kept a friendly smile on her face. She said, "Hello," "Good morning!" and "Thank you!" She treated them like she was their guest. It was horrible, but it kept her alive long enough to finally successfully escape and hide.

If there were a line, she would always let everyone cut in front of her. When the Nazis came in the barracks at night to take 12 people down to the river and shoot them, she smiled so that they always passed her by. Behind that smile, she was doing whatever she could to undercut or sabotage them. They were the enemy; they were evil, and she knew it. But she used her anger as a fuel to keep herself alive and cause as much damage to them as she could every chance she had.

TOM

Tom had spent years training for the 1980 Summer Olympics team. When international politics destroyed what would probably be his only chance to participate in the Olympics, he took it personally. He was angry. The problem was, he did not know where to focus his anger.

He could focus it on Russia for invading Afghanistan and then failing to withdraw by the specified deadline. He could blame President Carter, who seemed determined to keep the United States out of Moscow, no matter what effect the decision had on the hundreds of athletes who had spent their lives training to compete at this high level. He could be upset with other countries that had supported Carter's decision. He could even zero his anger on himself, if he wanted to, for giving up so much of his life for a dream that did not come true.

Tom took his anger out on everyone. It was not fair that his life was being upended by circumstances over which he had no control. It was the first time in his life that he could not change the outcome of a situation through his efforts, and he was having a hard time dealing with it.

MY STORY

Once I faced the reality that I had to have heart surgery, I was mad. I lived for summer. If I was in the hospital, that meant one thing—I would not be at the beach. That scenario was unthinkable. I let my anger rip into everyone who knew about my surgery but had kept it from me. I was mad at my parents, my brothers and sisters, and the doctors. I held onto my anger and made the classic mistake of bottling it up. Later, I did not want to discuss it with anyone. On the outside, I looked fine, but inside there was a quiet rage.

CHAPTER 4

Bargain

Unwilling to accept reality, some want to negotiate or seek a way around the trauma.

LET'S MAKE A DEAL

When dealing with trauma, "bargaining" is the act of fantasizing that things can go back to the way they were. When we are fired, we can try to bargain with our boss to give us our jobs back. When a boyfriend or girlfriend dumps us, we can try to negotiate for another chance. When a loved one is sick or dies, we can try to bargain with God to heal them or bring them back to life. Here we do not want to accept reality, so we do our best to turn back the clock or get another shot.

Like shock, denial, and anger, bargaining is yet another of nature's tools to soften the blow and let us gradually ease into our new reality. Some of the time, bargaining does not work, but maybe it will! After all, sometimes negotiation, pleading, and asking bring better results.

Life contains a series of resolved traumas and near-misses. We bargain because it's worked for us before, but not always. When it comes to people-based traumas, bargaining can be a great strategy, especially when dealing with reasonable people. This is one thing that sets the abuser apart from the non-abuser. The abuser will refuse to bargain, even when it costs them little to do so or when it may be in their best interest. Or worse, they will make a deal and then renege or gaslight, which sets up the betrayal type of trauma, possibly the worst of them all.

While negotiation can work in some situations, the fallout from the trauma requires a raw, authentic discussion that forces us to face reality directly—a process necessary to thrive. We can set forth a roadmap that allows us to navigate the path a bit more successfully. While the process is complicated and painful, we should never lose sight that this whole discussion is not about trauma; it is about healing. Surprisingly, the majority of trauma survivors eventually report having a positive change when they follow a roadmap to better mental health. This process requires authentic effort, time, and support.

Joseph Campbell, author of *The Hero's Journey* and best known for his quote, "Follow your bliss," tells us about the elements of an inspiring story. The greatest tales ever told, if you look carefully, include the most significant crises. "Act I" opens in the "ordinary world" where everything is just going along fine. Then, after an inciting incident, the characters are plunged into adventure. "Act II" dumps a massive mess in the laps of the characters we have grown to love, and we begin to doubt whether they can overcome and win the day. They fight, maneuver, fall, get up, and fight again. Finally, in "Act III," we see our heroes complete the final struggle against impossible odds, to emerge in a new world that is better and wiser for their efforts.

This is the essence of all great stories, including yours and mine.

Long-term PTSD effects can be exacerbated by how our community responds to the traumatic event. For example, soldiers who came home after World War II were given lavish parades. The community embraced them as the heroes they are. This was profoundly helpful in their recovery. On the other hand, our Vietnam War veterans were not treated correctly by our communities. This only served to amplify their trauma.

Bargaining may be a way for us to elicit a positive, caring response from our community of those close to us, so we can receive the signal that we are safe now. We are at an advantage when those around us are loving, reasonable, and stand behind us. When we do not get that, it can generate a long-term PTSD situation. Each situation is unique, and a qualified therapist can assist us in navigating our path.

Negotiation and bargaining are more social coping mechanisms. In a way, bargaining can be a type of denial or blended with denial. Bargaining can be incredibly useful sometimes, which is why we do it. Yet bargaining in an impossible situation can keep us trapped in an ongoing trauma and hide problems that need to be addressed.

A SIMPLE PRAYER

Sometimes bargaining works, and sometimes it is simply not an option. One perspective comes from the Serenity Prayer, which I heard for the first time when I attended an Alcoholics Anonymous meeting to support a relative who battles this disease. I have tremendous respect for anyone who overcomes this problem, and I am interested in what this process looks like. The Serenity Prayer was published by the theologian Reinhold Niebuhr in 1951, and it is now a staple in many recovery programs:

God, grant me the serenity to accept the things I cannot change,
courage to change the things I can,
and wisdom to know the difference.

"Serenity" comes from the word serene. It means having a calm or tranquil state of mind. It shows emotional maturity and displays a sense of self-respect and quiet confidence. It occurs to me that the bargaining phase of this prayer is the "and the wisdom to know the difference."

Some bargains work out, and some do not. Bargains can start

with not knowing what can be changed. So, we have the courage to attempt to change the things we can. That is being growth-minded and adaptive.

When the bargain does not work, we discover we have to accept the things we cannot change. This only becomes dysfunctional when we continue to bargain in an impossible situation or have exhausted all reasonable avenues for change. This is circling back to denial, the opposite of acceptance. It is healthy to try to bargain. We cannot gain wisdom "to know the difference" without an attempt.

TRAUMA-INDUCED ILLNESS

Navigating our medical care and taking care of trauma-related disorders are as essential as any other healthcare need. Medical experts have long known that there is a clear relationship between trauma and physical illness. Indeed, physical illness can cause shock, and that injury can cause additional physical disease. The brain and the body are part of the same system, and when one is harmed, the other is affected as well. When the usual bumps and bruises of life come along, our bodies are wonderfully adapted to cope and quickly rebound. However, trauma can overwhelm this system, causing our brains and physical health to be overloaded and to break down.

Brain research shows that, in the aftermath of a traumatic event, our brain's neurotransmitters are physiologically impacted, changing the way we process information. While this is true, it is also true that the brain damage is reversible with the proper treatments.

Trauma-related disorders are illnesses. We cannot just "get over it" any more than we get over a broken arm or heart disease. Mere willpower won't do it. Recovering from trauma requires a strategic effort that often takes significant time and the intervention of professional help. These illnesses can be recurrent or need a maintenance process. We do not take a shower and expect results forever. Likewise, we do not drop into a single trauma treatment and walk out permanently cured.

As we understand and untangle trauma, it is helpful to realize that there are six main categories: (1) situations outside of our control, such as acts of God, nature, or natural disasters where there is no perpetrator; (2) malicious acts against us where a perpetrator victimizes us; (3) our own malicious acts where we have been the perpetrator and have victimized others; (4) self-destructive behaviors where we have acted maliciously and have harmed ourselves; (5) acts of war, riots or widespread civil unrest; or (6) situations where we are not a victim, but we have witnessed the trauma of others.

It is helpful to identify the various types of trauma and untangle them so that we can see if there was a perpetrator or if we or someone else acted maliciously, and then identify the various kinds of trauma and abuse. Many erroneously believe that the only real damage is physical abuse, yet there are many types of abuse, including physical, mental, verbal, emotional, financial, sexual, spiritual, ecclesiastical, legal, and others. While we have not likely suffered from every kind, it can be valuable to be aware of the types of traumas and abuse, so that we can understand the overall landscape of trauma and accurately identify them.

NAVIGATING THE PEOPLE AROUND US

Healing from trauma is not a solo act. We are social creatures and trauma is a social issue. Trauma itself can be caused by others, either directly as the cause of a traumatic event, or in their reactions to an impersonal event. Our long-term responses to trauma are ultimately about whether or not we feel safe, and if the people around us do not reflect safety and healing, then our minds will get the message and build up defenses.

When the trauma comes from another individual, we can generalize that they are unsafe. It is worse when the trauma is caused by a group, such as our family, a company we are employed by, a religious organization, or a political faction. Of course, there are healthy and unhealthy people and groups, so looking at those dynamics is essential.

Unhealthy people and organizations can exacerbate trauma and stifle healing, and, likewise, the people around us can aid in our journey toward better mental health. We must identify which people and groups around us are healthy and which are not. A healthy person or group will always support some universal principles. Healthy relationships require honesty and complete disclosure of all commitments and costs. The healthy group practices "informed consent." Prospective members are given upfront, total, honest, and full disclosure of all relevant information.

A member of a healthy relationship or group is free to explore outside viewpoints, including opposing ideas. We are open to discuss, question, or challenge others' beliefs or behaviors. We are always free to utilize "critical thinking" skills, and different views are researched, compared, and contrasted. Any topic is safe to explore, research, and deliberate. "Groupthink" or "willful ignorance" is challenged. A clear "complaint box" protocol is in place. Disputes and questions are resolved directly and fairly and without the answers pivoting off-topic.

In healthy relationships, there is no tolerance for harmful behavior, and any abusive behavior or crime is reported to the police or other law enforcement. Victim shaming is not tolerated.

Unhealthy relationships and toxic groups operate much differently than healthy ones. Unhealthy groups create infected systems that mainly keep us trapped as a faithful lover, diligent employee, or an obedient group member. Destructive groups conceal information from those who join and warn against consulting outside or opposing sources of information.

We need emotional intelligence, or "EQ," to differentiate between healthy and unhealthy relationships. The principles of employing a brain trap are how fringe groups get you to stay, obey, and pay. They build power and authority from nothing. It is no less than mind control, brainwashing, thought control, thought reform, coercive persuasion, re-education, groupthink, or undue influence. Any of these methods of control can be traumatizing. On the other hand, healthy relationships shun all of these methods and instead are supportive of our healing.

HIGH-DEMAND GROUPS

As we bargain, negotiate and navigate the people and groups around us, we must migrate towards those that are healthy, and stay clear of those that are not. High-demand groups, sometimes called "cults," can worsen or cause deep trauma. A high-demand group has an unfair power dynamic that may use deception, undue influence, or mind-control methods to control its members. My first close-up exposure to a destructive group occurred in 1997 when I was retained to work on the Heaven's Gate cult case by the owner of the mansion where 39 people died in a mass suicide.

The cause of trauma can alter how it affects us and, therefore, how we heal. For instance, a betrayal makes us afraid of other people and can be a barrier to recovery because we must rely on other people to recover.

Sexually abused children who have safe parents, a supportive network of adults, and get treatment will often recover more quickly and with fewer long-term effects than a child without that support system. We heal from trauma if the people around us support us. It ultimately comes down to being around people and groups who are safe.

Heaven's Gate was the largest mass-suicide in the United States history and is one of history's most notorious cults. I was shocked and fascinated by what I saw inside the home, which led me to research and understand mind control and high-demand groups. As I walked from room to room and saw the carnage and remnants of their odd daily practices, I was baffled how this group of charming, highly-educated people could do such a thing. For months on end, the more I saw, the more I was in awe of the subtle yet powerful process of mind control.

Any high-demand group can create enormous amounts of trauma for their members. According to UC Berkeley's Dr. Margaret Singer, a cult is a group led by a charismatic leader who claims that, if you turn over your decision-making to them, they will reveal secret or sacred information. Ultimately, the cult leaders grow in control, wealth, and power, while the members provide money, free labor, idolization, sex, and the like. They can take the form of political, religious, polygamous, prosperity-gospel, occult, philosophical, supernatural, UFOs, health-based groups or can even be centered around pets. Cults are common and number in the thousands. They are all around us.

All cults are comprised of elitists who believe that they have advanced knowledge; are superior, smarter, and better than outsiders; and are the chosen people. They see themselves as having a higher calling in life. Cults recruit deceptively. They have a double ethic, where they tell the truth to fellow members, yet withhold information, tell half-truths or flat out lie to outsiders whom they view as unworthy, sinners, or somehow lesser humans. They flatter and "love bomb" potential members and provide information based on "trickle-truth" or "milk before meat." Their narrative seems compelling, but it is whitewashed and carefully correlated.

Cults are not democratic. Critical thinking and dissenting views are, at a minimum, frowned upon. In legal terms, they practice "undue influence" whereby people join without complete disclosure of what they are getting involved with. Legally, a group is prohibited from manipulating, coercing, or deceiving members. Pertinent information may not be withheld, ignored, or hidden. In healthy groups, members' conflicts are addressed, not evaded or skirted.

Once in, a cult member is expected to commit wholeheartedly and then recruit or proselytize others. They often soft-shun those who question and slap them with harsh labels such as "traitor," "deserter," or "apostate."

A healthy group will actively invite critical thinking. Biola University, a well-respected Christian school, actually invites atheists on campus to openly discuss and debate their points of view. While healthy religions place their adoration in God or a higher power, cult members adore their leaders. Being totalistic, there are often standards for dress, hairstyle, food, and drink. Indeed, there are rules for almost everything.

Cult members rarely see themselves as being in a cult. It is a myth that cults generate mindless robots. Cult members, like those in Heaven's Gate, are often actually intelligent, but they do everything within the mental constructs of the group. Healthy people are naturally drawn to a diverse group of friends, including those who have opposing points of view. As a simple test, if all of your close friends are a member of your group, you may want to seek help.

High-demand groups inevitably cause trauma because its members look to the group's leaders for guidance in all broad areas of life. In essence, members have turned the keys of their inner voice and identity over to the group, and this is never a recipe for success. Good people do good things, and bad people do bad things; however, a fringe group will get good people to do bad things.

While working on the Heaven's Gate case, I became immersed in how extreme groups operate. One of life's sad realities is that there are bad people who enjoy abusing or trying to control us. These abusive organizations, toxic leaders, and narcissists use a series of methods. This list is long, yet it helps us not only to identify those specific toxic behaviors to steer clear of, but it can also validate our observations.

- **Us vs. Them:** Abusers, toxic bosses, and dominating leaders divide people into two groups: those who agree with them and those who do not. People are identified as insiders or outsiders, members or non-members, citizens or foreigners. The outside world is vilified and seen as dangerous, and outsiders are looked down upon.
- **Leader Worship:** Toxic leaders are elitists, go on power trips, and isolate the group from outside influences.
- **Obedience:** Abusers demand total submission. Individuality, often in small issues such as dress or hairstyle, is unwelcome. Questioning authority is out of bounds and is met with threats, verbal abuse, or rejection. You must comply with the group's thinking or the group will reject you.
- **Verbal Abuse:** Toxic leaders often intimidate, call others names, or are just plain rude.
- **Shunning:** Leaving the group is always described as being

unthinkable. Those who do not comply are often given the silent treatment or dealt with in other passive-aggressive ways.

- **Belittling:** Toxic leaders scoff at outsiders, or even insiders, whom they deem unworthy. They laugh at, make fun of, or mock others. They look down upon and belittle those who are different or believe differently.
- **Isolation:** Toxic leaders are narcissists and snobs who often refuse to engage with others whom they view as unworthy or beneath them. While putting on airs of importance, they are insecure and desperate to the point where they will shun and cut off old friends and family outside the group. Challenging their façade is not tolerated.
- **Labeling:** Toxic leaders are fond of labels for themselves as well as outsiders. For insiders, title inflation runs rampant with the overuse of names such as "captain," "president," or "director." Outsiders are quickly dismissed by being called enemies, apostates, or deserters. This ploy helps instill obedience and fear within the group.
- **Public Image:** While most people want to show their best side in public, the abuser takes it to an extreme. There is a definite "onstage" and "backstage" performance by toxic leaders. Rigid happiness, broad grins, and big smiles are a requirement.
- **Perfectionism:** To control the group, toxic leaders demand an impossible level of performance that leaves members exhausted. Your best is never good enough. Members are given standards that are impossible to reach and leave them feeling defeated.
- **Secrecy**: The abuser does not fully disclose information but withholds relevant facts from all except their select inner circle.
- **No Reporting:** Abusers believe that they must answer to

a higher law of which they are the sole judge. Crimes or allegations of crimes are not reported to the police or other law enforcement authorities. They conceal and cover up domestic violence, sexual abuse, child abuse, financial scams, and other crimes.

- **Keep You Too Busy to Think:** For the toxic leader, letting the members think on their own is dangerous. After all, if we can stop and think about our situation logically, we might figure out how insane it is.
- **Keep You Tired:** The abuser knows that fatigue is their friend. When we are utterly exhausted, we cannot think, and we certainly cannot run away. Doing anything positive requires energy, and that is not there. By the leaders consuming all our discretionary time and money, we are kept on edge.
- **Put Loyalty Over Honesty:** Abusers love to create opportunities to foster loyalty. They do this by challenging us to invest our energy and openly state our allegiance.
- **Give Intermittent Rewards.** Continual rewards are not that great, but intermittent ones are as addictive as a Las Vegas slot machine. If we know that the lever will always produce a pellet, we will only pull the bar as often as we need. Yet if the lever only provides a pellet some of the time, we keep pushing and pushing. This principle not only works for gambling and video games, but also abusers.
- **Keep the Crises Coming.** One crisis after another not only keeps us overwhelmed, but it also makes us feel needed and essential. If a toxic leader or abuser is incompetent, there is a never-ending supply of crises and more work.
- **Keep You Believing in the Insanity:** If we quit believing, we will not be able to go on because we are invested in the insanity. Besides, a commitment is a commitment, and

keeping them is honorable. We see no way out. The stress and panic seem normal. We are caught in a trap. It is tough to admit we are a sucker, so we look around and smile.

- **Erosion of Our Inner Voice:** Ultimately, abusers are not interested in what we think. They want to tell us what to believe, how to feel, what to say, and how to behave. In the process, we lose our sense of direction and slowly die inside. They take our authority and steal our joy.

Author Carolyn Spring observed, "By blaming the victim, society can turn a blind eye. It doesn't need to acknowledge the scale of abuse, the extent of the trauma, the vast arena of suffering for such a vast number of people."

As we bargain with others in our healing, we must know what healthy and unhealthy people and groups look like. A sketchy group or an abusive relationship will lack proper boundaries, be judgmental, pretend to be the keepers of truth, and call for perfectionism. Yet these types tend to use mental gymnastics, desperate explanations that are motivated by deep insecurity. Members are not allowed to go off-menu. On the other hand, healthy people and groups will support your journey, foster real conversations, point to our inner voice, and have real connections.

Healthy homes, schools, churches, businesses, and groups do not attempt to turn others into miniature versions of themselves. Healthy people support everyone in what they want to do—as long as it does not hurt anyone. If we push our perspective on others, it can backfire; however, we will never experience the "backfire effect" when we point ourselves and others to one's inner voice.

Our Stories of Bargaining

DEBBIE

Immediately after the suicide, Debbie was too injured to ask anyone for help. Her heart was shattered.

The lead pastors at her church sent her a brief note offering support. But, surprisingly, no one called. Church members did not reach out to Debbie or her children, even though their family had been extremely involved in the church for more than four decades. To Debbie, the church leaders' lack of engagement made it seem as if they were embarrassed that her husband had died by suicide. They did not know about his double life. She could not tolerate any more shame.

Debbie wanted to give the pastors the benefit of the doubt. Perhaps, she reasoned, they did not know how to help or what to do, so that was why they did nothing at all. Debbie reached out to the pastors, not once but twice, offering to meet with them. She needed their help navigating her way through the wreckage left by her husband's death.

But for whatever reason, the church leaders did not make any effort to meet with her. They didn't have the time—busy schedules, they explained. *Busy schedules?* Debbie thought. No, that was not it. Debbie soon realized what was happening—she and her children had been shunned by their church home.

JOHN

John bargained with God to save the life of his little girl. He negotiated with the military to clean up the contamination, but they just packed up and left. He and his neighbors were simply stuck sitting on a radioactive island.

SUSAN

When Susan first discovered that the City of Los Angeles employees caused the landslide, she was angry—but she also assumed that the City would take responsibility, begin the cleanup and reimburse them for damages to their home. She thought that it would be a simple process of talking to them, and they would fix everything. After all, she was a taxpayer. Plus, all her life, she had more or less operated on the belief that during emergencies, and this situation was indeed an emergency, there were government systems in place designed to help people.

She was shocked to learn that she was wrong. There was no one at the City who was willing to assist her at all. There was no caring building inspector to tell her what she needed to do to get her home back in livable shape. The City flat-out refused to help her, even when confronted with direct evidence that they caused the landslide in the first place. Their response was to stonewall her.

As time went on, Susan started losing sleep—at first a few hours, then, she would lay awake the entire night. She was perpetually exhausted. She developed a pain in the pit of her stomach that never entirely went away. Her muscles were always tense, and her jaw ached from clenching it all day long, even in her sleep.

Peter, her husband, was also feeling the stress. They were both visiting chiropractors to just get through the injuries and pain from it all. She had no idea how they were going to survive the devastation.

Susan kept calling. She kept trying to bargain with the City, even offering to shoulder some of the costs. But the bargaining went nowhere. The City dodged her at every turn. She realized she would have to sue the City of Los Angeles. And that was not going to be easy. In the meantime, the mortgage and the property taxes still had to be paid.

They went ahead and did sue the City. It took an entire year until she and Peter were able to schedule a deposition with the City. In the meantime, they suffered from chronic fatigue caused by the overwhelming fear of what would happen to their home—and their lives.

SHAD

Shad and his girlfriend had decided to leave Alabama and go to California where they would "join the hippies," as Shad puts it, in protest against the Vietnam war. Although he had been a captain in the Army and served a tour of duty in South Vietnam, the horrific experience of losing 35 soldiers in a single night had severely traumatized him. Now, seeing that the war was still going on, Shad was angry. He felt that joining the protests would give him a platform to share his anger with the world.

On the way to San Francisco, Shad decided to see an old friend from the Army who was living in Los Angeles and attending grad school at USC. Shad's friend mentioned that one of the top psychiatrists in the world, Dr. Philip May, a schizophrenia expert, would be speaking that night about the experiences of soldiers in the war. He invited Shad to come along.

Shad didn't want to go. He did not want to hear anyone justify the war. Shad's friend assured him that wasn't the case—and offered to buy him a beer afterward if he would go.

Shad and his buddy attended the speech. Afterward, Shad's friend finagled an introduction to Dr. May who was, at that time, the head of UCLA's Neuropsychological Institute and acting director of the VA hospital in West Los Angeles. The moment Dr. May met Shad, he was taken with the young man's confidence and convictions. He was also impressed to learn that Shad was both a social worker and a veteran.

Dr. May felt that Vietnam veterans were not getting the services they needed but didn't know how to reach vets more successfully. He offered Shad a job on the spot and said, "Come work for me at the VA and evaluate the situation and help us understand how we can best serve the Vietnam vets who have served this country."

At first, Shad declined. He wanted to go to San Francisco, not work for the VA. But Dr. May persisted. Shad agreed to try it out temporarily.

GERI

Though Geri was deeply loved by her family and always felt valued, she could not help, at times, wishing she was like the other children. She managed to do many of the activities that other children did, but always had her special way of doing them, which set her apart, and garnered the stares and sometimes ridicule from her playmates. Even when she went swimming in the ocean, on many occasions, a lifeguard would come after her with an inner tube to save her from drowning. He failed to recognize that Geri was never drowning; she just had her own way of swimming due to cerebral palsy.

Sometimes, when she was alone, Geri would play her version of "tennis." The family lived directly next to what was then the newly constructed 57 Freeway in Fullerton. The concrete wall by the freeway was right behind her house. She spent hours throwing balls against that concrete wall and hitting them with her tennis racquet, pretending she was Billie Jean King.

While she played at this sport many afternoons after school, she created a fantasy world where she did not have cerebral palsy at all—nope, she was a famous tennis player. Geri started to practice what is called "creative visualization." She imagined life as she wished it to be.

Back in the 1970s, when Geri was a young girl, just the perfect age to develop crushes, a young singer named David Cassidy burst on the scene. The handsome, clear-eyed David Cassidy became an instant icon—and the object of Geri's long-distance affection. She even had had a Partridge Family lunch box and carried a photo of him in her wallet. As she threw the ball against the concrete wall, she imagined one day meeting the burgeoning rock star.

JC

Before the trial and his ultimate conviction, JC tried to tell the police and his attorneys his side of the story, but they would not listen. They thought they knew what had happened. They had made up their minds about him. He tried telling them that he would gladly accept his punishment for the robbery—but it was not fair to charge him with murder since he hadn't even been there.

JC wanted to talk to his girlfriend's father, the husband of the woman who had been killed, and explain what had happened to set it all straight for him. But the police would not allow him to make any contact with the victim's husband.

Seeing that law enforcement did not want to listen to him, JC started bargaining with God. *Please, God,* he prayed, *get me out of this. I will do anything. Just help me get out of this.* But it seemed like God, too, had turned away.

LEO

Leo went to church to bargain with God, but the church treasurer took off with all the money. He figured that if this was the way Christians operated, he wanted nothing to do with them.

JOE

When Joe was in his late teens, he started running with a rough crowd. He was attracted to the danger and was defiantly proud to be following in his father's footsteps. "My dad was not a bad guy," Joe told himself. He was just misunderstood.

Ray Taylor, a New York City police detective, took a particular interest in Joe when he learned that Joe had been arrested for a petty crime. Ray, it turned out, was the lead detective in Joe's dad's murder. He had interviewed Joe's family immediately after the killing. Ray remembered Joe as a sad, lost, little boy.

Ray took Joe aside and told him that if he continued to hang out with "those guys" that he was going to end up in prison—or worse. He suggested Joe get out of New York for a while.

Surprising everyone, even himself, Joe moved out to California when he was 18 years old. He made a bargain with himself. He would start over and make a fresh start. He would leave his old life behind.

ERICA

Erica could not believe that Nazis had taken over Budapest, but she bargained at every chance she had to clean the soldier's shoes, run errands, or help in any way. She did this to spend another day alive.

TOM

Tom had a hard time accepting that all his years of training were for naught. He talked to his coach and pleaded with him to call up the chain of command and get President Carter to reinstate the Olympics. After all, his coach was highly connected. Surely, he knew someone who knew someone who knew someone who could talk sense into the President.

His coach assured him that the entire Olympic committee was doing everything it could to manage the situation on behalf of the athletes. There were proposals out there to move the Olympics to somewhere other than Moscow. There were potential plans for America to hold its own Olympics with only countries that had also boycotted the Moscow Games. There were suggestions that President Carter could rescind his decision and still save face. None of them panned out.

Tom suggested that he go to the Olympics anyway as an individual. "After all," Tom said, "some athletes in the United Kingdom and France were doing that very thing, since their governments allowed each athlete to make their own decisions." Tom's coach had to carefully explain that the United States' boycott included every single athlete from every team. He would not be going to Moscow, no matter what.

MY STORY

I was unwilling to accept reality. I wanted to negotiate or seek a way around the trauma. My dad confirmed that I needed to have heart surgery. I spent the balance of the day being mad. All I got from my brothers and sisters was kind of "whatever dude" looks, and I was told to "deal with it."

So, I took it to a higher power. That night I tried to make a bargain with God himself. I told God, "Look, you can do anything. If you fix this heart thing, I promise I will be cool and never do anything wrong. Just fix my heart for me." Well, God said, "No."

At my next doctor's appointment, I tried bargaining with the doctors. Their answers were clear. "Nope." So, I bargained even harder with anyone who would listen, but apparently, a ten-year-old did not have enough chips on the table.

CHAPTER 5

Depression

A profound feeling of utter hopelessness and despair occurs that represses our soul.

FEELING BLUE

I WILL NEVER FORGET THE DAY in 1995 when I was having lunch with Denise Brown, the sister of Nicole Brown Simpson, who was murdered along with her friend, Ron Goldman, at her home in Los Angeles in 1994. Her husband, professional football player and actor, OJ Simpson, was accused but later acquitted of the murders. Denise told me something I had never heard before. She explained how physical wounds heal in weeks, but emotional wounds do not. They can linger for months, years, decades, or even a lifetime. I had never thought of it that way, and her comments were stunning. She completely altered my thinking. Ever since that day, I have looked at the emotional impacts of those I meet at disaster sites, not just the physical impacts.

Of all the initial steps of processing trauma, depression often hurts the most, is the longest-lasting, and is of the most concern. With depression, we turn inward and want to withdraw from others. We feel sad, lonely, apathetic, and hopeless. In this condition, we are no longer lashing out in anger or shouting in denial. We have given up on the failed bargains. We feel defeated, become sullen, or isolate. We have no interest in interacting with others, and the comfort we seek feels empty and pointless. In a state of depression, we can experience panic attacks and feel overwhelmed with grief. Often, the pain is so severe that we try to find ways to deaden it. Or, for some of us, we may feel nothing and try to find ways to end the numbness.

Nature provides the fight-flight-freeze responses to trauma, but, in some situations, we may feel overwhelmed. Some researchers believe that depression results from a position where we can no longer fight or flee, so we freeze, submit, and give up. It is a form of self-preservation from a dangerous confrontation. Depression can be a type of learned helplessness, an unhealthy behavior that can be carried throughout life.

Indeed, depression tops the list of trauma-related conditions and has both mental and physical effects. It can result from being harassed, oppressed, bullied, overpowered, intimidated, shunned, or shamed. Other stressors include a lack of prenatal care, maternal depression in infancy, as well as childhood or adolescent losses. We can have a genetic predisposition to depression that leaves us vulnerable to a chronic type of ongoing trauma or an acute, one-time episode.

According to the World Health Organization, depression affects more than 300 million people worldwide. In even the best of circumstances, it is reasonable to experience occasional lows. However, depression is different as it impedes our ability to function normally at home, school, or work. Depression can cause extreme feelings of sadness that may last far beyond healthy grieving.

"Functional depression" is where we become great at "going through the motions" even while depressed or anxious. A lot of depressed people are overlooked. They might show up to work with a smile on their face and then melt into the couch or go into hyper-production as soon as they get home.

Think of an injured animal. It will rush to its den, curl up in the dark, and give the wound time to heal. Depression may force us to rest and give ourselves space and time to heal. This view can help because we are not adding to the layers of stress with the idea of how terrible we are for being depressed. Depression becomes a matter of fact rather than a fight to maintain some moral standard of high productivity or pretending to be cheerful.

Dr. Kübler-Ross identified depression as a frequent product of trauma. However, it may be caused by other events as well. According to Harvard Medical School, depression can also be caused by an early loss, medical problems, nerve-cell miscommunication, genes, and chronic stress. While depression is often expected in the aftermath of trauma, it usually recedes in time. If it does not, it is particularly important to seek professional help, as chronic depression is both serious and can be treatable.

There is no shame in depression. It can even be expected with some stressors and traumas, and there are benefits to depression. It may feel like an enemy, but like all natural reactions, it is here to help us. Society should update the narrative around depression. We do this by listening to the messages it is sending. As depression is readily treatable with professional help, the only problem is when we do not seek that assistance.

GAS PEDALS AND BRAKES

In ordinary life, the brain encodes neurological pathways to process, store, or dispose of our thoughts and emotions. Our bodies continually communicate using chemical and electrical impulses. All day long, our mind is processing. It tells us to look here, read this, pay attention to that, forget this, and remember that. The body encodes information, sends it down the pathway, processes it, stores it, or disposes of it. Life, family, school, and business move on with our thoughts and memories mostly cohesive and intact. Under normal, day-to-day circumstances, we function just fine.

During a traumatic event, our eyes and ears send sensory information to the amygdala, an area of the brain that contributes to

H.A.L.T.

H.A.L.T. is a simple, powerful tool to practice self-care. When we feel irritated, anxious, or depressed, it could be that we are Hungry, Angry, Lonely, or Tired. This is a signal to H.A.L.T. and assess our situation.

Hungry

If we do not eat well, we get grumpy. Avoid junk food, drink plenty of water, and take time for good meals and snacks.

Angry

When we fell angry, avoid acting irrationally. Pause, and take a time out. Find a quiet space to take some deep breaths, and stay in control.

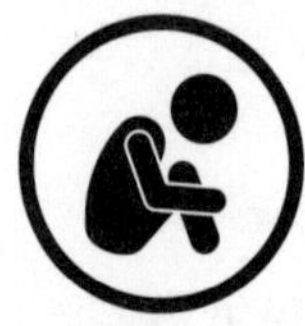

Lonely

Isolation can lead to depression or anxiety. Reach out to family or friends or join a club, church, or other positive support group.

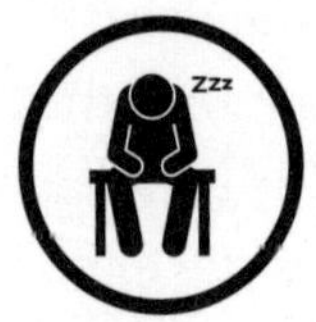

Tired

Fatigue makes us irritable. Take regular breaks, do deep breathing exercises, and get enough sleep.

emotional processing. The amygdala interprets the data and instantly sends a distress signal to the hypothalamus, the brain's trauma command center. This signal is communicated to the rest of our body through the autonomic nervous system which controls involuntary functions such as breathing, blood pressure, and heart rate.

The autonomic nervous system has two components: the sympathetic and the parasympathetic nervous systems. The sympathetic nervous system functions like a gas pedal in a car and is what triggers the fight-flight-freeze response. The parasympathetic nervous system acts like a brake. It promotes calm and rest once the stress is over.

After the amygdala sends the distress signal, the hypothalamus control center activates the sympathetic nervous system by sending messages through the autonomic nerves to the adrenal glands. These glands pump adrenaline into our bloodstream causing our heart to beat faster, blood pressure to go up, sweat to increase and breath to quicken. As extra oxygen is sent to the brain, our sight, hearing, and other responses become sharper. The adrenaline also releases glucose into our bloodstream for more energy. We hyperventilate, and our muscles tense up.

These changes happen almost instantly. Indeed, the body is so efficient that the amygdala and hypothalamus act before the brain's visual centers have even had a chance to process what is happening. This is how a person can jump out of the path of an oncoming car before even thinking about it.

When the initial surge of epinephrine subsides, the hypothalamus activates the second component of the stress response system, known as the HPA axis. This network consists of the hypothalamus, the pituitary gland, and the adrenal glands.

The HPA axis relies on a series of hormonal signals to keep the sympathetic nervous system, or the "gas pedal," pressed down. If the brain continues to perceive danger, the hypothalamus produces a corticotropin-releasing hormone which travels to the pituitary gland and triggers the release of hormones. This travels to the adrenal glands and prompts them to release cortisol. Thus, the body stays revved up and on high alert.

When the threat passes, cortisol levels fall. The parasympathetic nervous system, or the brakes, dampens the stress response. Yet, when we are unable to control extreme stress or undergo chronic low-level stress, the HPA axis remains activated, much like a motor that is idling too high even though the car is not going anywhere. After a while, this wears us down and harms our mental and physical health.

If we have persistent episodes, epinephrine surges can damage blood vessels and arteries, increase our blood pressure, and raise the risk of heart attacks and strokes. Elevated cortisol levels may help to replenish the body's depleted energy and lead to fat tissue and weight gain. Cortisol increases our appetite so that we will eat more in an attempt to generate extra energy. We "eat our feelings" which increases the storage of unused nutrients as fat. This is the body's way to get and retain high levels of drive to deal with a threat, but as there is no remaining threat, this can lead to a multitude of health problems.

Stressors, such as traffic jams, work pressure, or family problems, keep coming, and triggering reminders of past traumas can make us continuously feel in a state of danger. The repeated activation of the stress response when there is no immediate threat can take a toll on the body. The real trauma may have occurred months or years ago, yet the cycle continues.

Re-experiencing stress, even well after the event, wears us down physically and emotionally. Left unchecked, we get irritable, tired, and exhausted, and it continually feeds the depression. Society, on the other hand, pushes the "happiness trap," which is to think that life is about dodging the bad stuff. Ideally, we lounge in luxury and grab everything we want. We wallow in excess. This is not a real solution, and the cycle of depression continues.

Our society promotes a "no pain, no gain" attitude. We have a sense that stress is something we just have to expect and accept. It's as if stress is okay because the brain is somehow immune to health issues. We can damage it as much as we want and talk ourselves out of the pain. "It is all in your head" is synonymous with imaginary problems that do not "really exist." Yet it does exist.

The brain uses real electrical energy that must come from somewhere. It can sustain real emotional damage. Extreme stress is not something we have to put up with. We are perfectly within our rights to eliminate those sources of stress in our lives. At times, we are groomed or conditioned by bad actors to believe the opposite so they can take advantage of us. If we learn that lesson early on, many of society's stress-induced problems would be sharply reduced. We need to permit ourselves to say, "No, that makes me feel bad, and stress is a sign of potential harm. I do not have to accept that."

SELF-MEDICATION

While we will focus on fresh approaches to dealing with depression or anxiety, we must acknowledge a spectrum of unhealthy choices that attempt to numb the pain. Emotional pain truly hurts. While struggling with intense pain, there are both healthy and unhealthy options to offer relief and to help elevate our mood.

All of this said, we want to avoid harsh judgment, as coping mechanisms can have value. For example, crutches are okay while our leg is healing. Drinking to the point of immobility has its apparent problems, but if it prevents us from attempting suicide, this is the better alternative. The key to coping is awareness. We can ask ourselves, "Are there alternatives that get us closer to our goal while causing less harm?" "Can we plan a course toward that goal?" Awareness, self-care, and gentle progress are the key.

Depression and anxiety can lead to a host of issues. We usually wind up with feelings of irritability, unsafety, distrust in others, and hypervigilance. We can also become overly controlling, engage in risky or obsessive behaviors, have difficulty concentrating, feel unlikable or unlovable, experience disordered eating, and utter hopelessness or despair.

Self-medication occurs when we attempt to suppress or withdraw from an uncomfortable reality or trauma. We try to leave it behind and escape to a place of pleasure, mystery, and even indulgence. This is understandable because life is tough, trauma hurts, and we want the suffering to stop.

Many people self-medicate because they don't have access to mental health care, so simply saying "get help" is not always useful advice. We may experience a level of pain so strong that no amount of healthy behavior can soothe us. Our "healthy" outlets themselves become triggers because they enable us to endure the pain longer. Therapy is out of reach or not working fast enough. Higher doses of prescribed medications come with their side effects.

The things we once judged, we use. The problems seem overwhelming, so some of us turn to alcohol. The problem is that alcohol creates even more depression. We may be too anxious to eat, but when we use marijuana, food suddenly tastes good again. It can also help us sleep and stave off the nightmares.

There is a distorted reality in which we come to expect constant pain, sudden chaos, and cruelty, as well as people using us for sex, erasing our identity and replacing it with what they want us to be, and making us believe we are useless and unlovable. Those things are not real either, but we come to expect them. Heavy self-medication gives us some peace in that painful version of unreality.

Deciding what is healthy is relative to the circumstance, and it is about a reiterative cycle of nonjudgmental awareness. Ask, "Is this still healthy? Are there better ways to do this? Am I ready to do it in a better way? If I'm not, that is okay too, and I'll just become aware of it for now." This mode of thinking can relieve some of the high-pressure badgering we do to ourselves.

Left unchecked, this can develop into a highly complex rationalization of why we are still self-medicating. We can become more aware of that and change when we are ready. The point is to hold back on the destructive self-judgments and practice some self-care.

The key is to understand that there are both healthy and unhealthy ways to address the pain. The harmful approach is to self-medicate, which dulls or masks the pain, while the healthy plan is to practice self-care where we take legitimate steps to face our reality and heal. Sometimes, we need to dull the pain. It's best to deal with the pain at a tolerable Level 5 but difficult when it is Level 11 because those who go above that level can die. We might focus more on the harmful side effects of some self-medication and be aware of the costs and benefits.

Our language can help keep us down or help us move forward. If we say, "I *am* depressed," it can become our identity. Instead, if we say, "I *feel* depressed," that has a different meaning. It's easier to let go of a feeling than an identity.

DIRECT SELF-MEDICATION

When it comes to dealing with depression, there are two types of self-medication—*direct* and *indirect*.

Direct self-medication is an extension of the denial phase. It chemically alters our mind and body directly through abuse of one or more substances, such as drinking excessive alcohol, popping pills, snorting cocaine, or shooting drugs into our veins. Substances disrupt the functions of our brain's frontal cortex, the decision-making center where risks and benefits are analyzed and willpower is activated. Examples of direct self-medication include consuming harmful levels of:

- Alcohol
- Caffeine
- Illegal drugs
- Inhalants
- Nicotine
- Over-the-counter medications
- Prescription drugs
- Salt
- Sugar

These substances alter our blood flow and trigger the pleasure centers of our brains. They create cravings for more which my cardiologist calls the "potato chip effect," where we cannot eat just one and end up eating the whole bag! Reinforcement makes us repeat the behavior as it rewards us for unearned pleasure. These substances disrupt the brain's frontal lobe function, which is the "thinking layer." They will eventually damage our dopamine, serotonin, and oxytocin pathways in the midbrain, which are the "action layers." Direct self-medication can alter our neurochemical pathways and figuratively "fry" our brain.

Over time, excess self-medication will damage the brain's frontal lobe, which controls our sense of reason and self-control. At that point, we experience a distorted sense of reality in which we undervalue risks and overvalue their potential rewards. We fail to learn from repeated errors caused by our poor choices.

I am not suggesting that unearned pleasure is always wrong. This brings up society's idea of a "cheap thrill." I grew up in Southern California, and there were endless trips to Disneyland and other theme parks. They are fun! There is a value in pleasure, and likewise, the idea of having to "earn" pleasure is problematic. Abusive thinking tells us to put our nose to the grindstone and suffer our whole lives without complaint. It's okay to have fun.

INDIRECT SELF-MEDICATION

Indirect self-medication occurs through *destructive behaviors or unhealthy actions* that trigger changes in the brain's neurochemistry. In other words, rather than drinking or popping pills, our behavior causes an indirect chemical response to give us the high that we crave. Examples of indirect self-medication include cutting or disordered eating such as binging, starvation, or purging. They can also include otherwise enjoyable, normal, or healthy behaviors that are taken to obsessive, compulsive, or excessive extremes:

- Anger
- Exercise or sports
- Gambling
- Hand washing
- Hobbies
- Humor and sarcasm
- Politics
- Religion
- Sex
- Shopping
- Sleep
- Social media
- Thrill-seeking
- Video games
- Work
- Fighting
- Chaos
- Self-harm
- Socializing

No matter how we self-medicate, the brain releases various cocktails of drugs into our bloodstream and nerve impulses. Some people who indirectly self-medicate look down upon those who directly self-medicate. They may think, "Well, I might work too much, but at least I am not an alcoholic." This thinking is both flawed and hypocritical. Any type of self-medication, taken to excess, can be dangerous and destructive. Adrenaline is released during sports, fits of anger, or high-risk activities. Endorphins come out through exercise, eating disorders, religious rituals, sexual activities, work, or gambling. Serotonin is released by eating. Dopamine comes when we anticipate an outcome or get an intermittent reward, such as making a sale or winning at gambling. Oxytocin is delivered when we feel "in love" or during sexual activities. Hormones, neurotransmitters, and endorphins are generally good, but we just want to maintain an awareness if they are coming from constructive or destructive activities.

The issue is that, whether directly or indirectly, self-medication is a continual denial and dodging of the underlying stress and often creates adverse outcomes that cause a wave of secondary stress, which only compounds the trauma. While they create some temporary relief, they ultimately increase guilt, anxiety, and depression. Furthermore, they often aggravate the injury with drunk driving arrests, sexually transmitted diseases, unwanted pregnancies, lost jobs, broken relationships, bankruptcies, or other serious issues.

The most destructive of behaviors are suicidal thoughts that are focused upon eliminating the pain once and for all. Anyone who is talking about having feelings of hopelessness and thinking of suicide can be at risk. There is hope for those who have these feelings, and the first step is to reach out for support. Many people have felt this way and are standing by to help us transition to a healthy emotional state. There are many free resources listed at the beginning of this book.

DEPRESSION AND GRIEF

The feeling of loss occurs when we feel cheated or deprived of something or someone important to us. Grief is a profound sense of anguish and pain that results from that loss. These are normal emotions at times of intense sorrow. Grief may come from the loss of a loved one, a job, a pet, a friend, or missed opportunity. There are also intangible losses, such as loss of self-image, identity, faith, dreams and expectations, betrayal, or disillusionment. While "intangible," they are no less painful.

While feelings of loss and grief are healthy, some people can get stuck in heartache or try to avoid the pain and suppress those negative feelings. Either of these paths can lead to the effects of lingering trauma because both obsessive and suppressive thinking can rewire our brain's chemistry and neurology.

Some try so hard to "hold it together" that they gloss over the harsh reality and consequences of what has occurred. Obsessive and unprocessed grief can also result in emotional or physical problems, and these, in turn, can lead to self-medication or addictions. When dealing with pain, it is essential to understand that grieving is normal. Going to a quiet, private spot and processing our grief can be the right thing to do. It is okay to feel sad, lonely, and heartbroken after a significant loss.

Some feel bad for feeling bad. This is unproductive. No healthy person is happy all the time. If we do not take the time to explore the hurt, we will not heal. The problem comes if we get stuck there. When this happens, we can go from having normal grief to experiencing the trauma that we need to address.

When feeling grief, it is perfectly normal to have periods of depression, anger, loneliness, emptiness, lack of interest in daily life, and loss of appetite. Depressed feelings are reasonable, and it is also essential to know that there are both productive and unproductive ways of dealing with them. To process sad feelings beneficially, we should first accept that all feelings, even the uncomfortable ones, are healthy. We should not hold back on crying, grieving, and talking about the loss. If we have been victimized in a crime, we should report that crime when it is safe.

Depression physically hurts. Recovery from depression is a balancing act, and that is why professional help or even medications are often needed. It can take months or even years for a full recovery because of the opposing forces at play. Depression can create a feedback loop leading us to counterproductive behaviors that make us more depressed.

To heal, we need to eat a healthy diet, but we have no appetite or we binge. We need sound sleep, yet we struggle with insomnia. We need to exercise, but we are too sad to get out of bed. We need to socialize and build healthy relationships, but we do not want to talk to anyone. We need to be grateful and positive, but we want to isolate and withdraw. A professional therapist understands this landscape and can coach and guide us to make real progress. This slow progression injects small doses of positivity and hope, gradually reverses the cycle of the feedback loop, and builds a foundation for eventual recovery. Setbacks are inevitable, but they are not the end of the world. They can be managed.

It is okay not to be okay. The five reactions of shock, denial, anger, bargaining, and depression are experienced to one degree or another as we navigate through our traumas. These are each a normal and even a necessary phase; however, if possible, we want to avoid getting stuck in any of them as we can remain in the "dive" stage and thereby never heal. Healing means that we respect that process but also take action to keep moving forward gradually from the "dive" stage and get into a fight to "survive."

Depression can shut us down. If we rearrange the word "DEPRESSION," we get, "I PRESSED ON." Depression is a necessary point on the journey, but it is never meant to be our final destination. It is all right to visit here for a while, but eventually, we need to push forward. Albert Einstein said, "Life is like riding a bicycle. To keep your balance, we must keep moving."

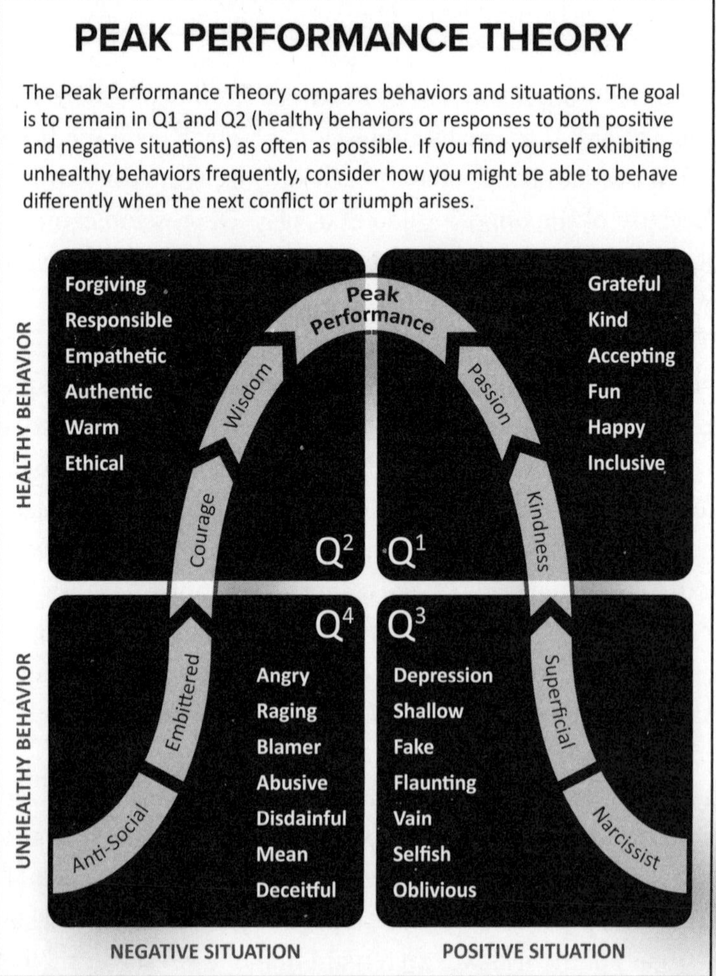
PEAK PERFORMANCE THEORY
The Peak Performance Theory compares behaviors and situations. The goal is to remain in Q1 and Q2 (healthy behaviors or responses to both positive and negative situations) as often as possible. If you find yourself exhibiting unhealthy behaviors frequently, consider how you might be able to behave differently when the next conflict or triumph arises.
HEALTHY BEHAVIOR
UNHEALTHY BEHAVIOR
Forgiving
Responsible
Empathetic
Authentic
Warm
Ethical
Peak Performance
Grateful
Kind
Accepting
Fun
Happy
Inclusive
Wisdom
Passion
Courage
Kindness
Q2
Q1
Q4
Q3
Embittered
Superficial
Angry
Raging
Blamer
Abusive
Disdainful
Mean
Deceitful
Depression
Shallow
Fake
Flaunting
Vain
Selfish
Oblivious
Anti-Social
Narcissist
NEGATIVE SITUATION
POSITIVE SITUATION

Our Stories of Depression

DEBBIE

Debbie lost her husband to suicide—horrific enough. Then she learned of his secret life. Even worse. And she soon discovered her savings were in ruins. Her church largely abandoned her. It was too much.

Just walking into her home was overwhelmingly lonely. And yet, despite all her husband had done, all the ways he had betrayed her, she missed him terribly. She missed the person she thought he was. She was heartbroken on every level. She cried frequently. It seemed like she would never recover. There came the point where she felt utterly decimated, and the feeling immobilized her.

JOHN

John felt the deep grief and pain that only a parent could feel at the loss of a child. When he thought of his little girl who died from the fallout caused by nearby nuclear testing, he would go out to a quiet place on the island, stare at the ocean, and cry. He would then walk to the cemetery and sit by her headstone to be close to her.

SUSAN

Susan was a doer. She always had been, at least until now. This was the most catastrophic thing that had ever happened to her. For a time—especially as she reached out for help from the authorities and found stonewalling instead—she became deeply depressed. It wasn't like her.

She made call after call to find someone to help her. However, once she figured out that the landslide was the fault of the City of Los Angeles, she tried to get the City to do the right thing.

Making calls was not the only thing she did. She also started looking for financial assistance. Her house was uninhabitable, but the bank kept sending mortgage statements, and Los Angeles County kept sending tax bills. It did not matter that her home was destroyed.

The government and insurance companies, whom she had always assumed would meet their obligations in a time of need, ultimately failed her. Her desperation grew.

SHAD

In 1971, Vietnam vet and social worker Shad attended an event that featured the head of UCLA's Neuropsychological Institute, Dr. Philip May, as its keynote speaker. Dr. May was also acting director of the Veterans Administration hospital in West Los Angeles.

Once Dr. May met Shad, he offered him a job with the Veterans Administration. Shad was tasked with figuring out how to best reach the returning Vietnam vets.

At the time, Vietnam vets were coming home by the thousands. But unlike the soldiers who returned home from other wars, these vets were not greeted as heroes. Instead, they were often shunned—or worse— shamed. And they were often in emotional turmoil caused by what they had seen and, sometimes, what they had done during the war. The situation was so bleak that, upon landing back in the United States, many returning soldiers went into the airport terminal bathrooms and threw their uniforms in the waste bins.

VA mental professionals at the time did not know how to treat combat-related stress, nor could they provide any guidance for reintegration into civilian society. Shad, having experienced the horrors of war, understood how to connect with veterans. He not only understood their depression, but he was also living it.

GERI

Geri, born with cerebral palsy, was bused to special schools up until high school, so she dealt with a lot of isolation after school and on weekends. For the most part, she was on her own at these times and did not develop the normal skills of making friends. She was outgoing and longed for companionship, but because she was bused so far away to school, children didn't understand her and never knocked on her door to ask her to play. Gloria made it a point to include Geri when she had plans with friends, but Geri generally entertained herself.

Although she was self-contained for the most part, she was nevertheless a human being, and humans are social creatures that long to connect with others. By the time she was a teenager, even Gloria could not fill the gaping hole of loneliness. Geri never had boyfriends, went to prom or football games, or was invited to parties. The isolation and loneliness did plunge Geri into a depression on occasion, and it was at these times that her disability also became a stark reminder that she was different. However, with a resilience that was partly from her upbringing and partly her natural temperament, Geri was usually able to overcome the negativity.

As a college freshman, though, Geri experienced a deep depression that threatened to derail her. Because she spent the first 15 years in special education, she was not up to speed academically. Even though she tried to catch up in high school, she could not fill all the gaps developmentally.

TANYA

Tanya fought depression and anxiety since she was a young adult, triggered by the shocking and heartbreaking loss of four friends in high school and then the hit-and-run death of her best friend when they were both just 20. With Nicole's murder five years later, it was nearly too much to withstand.

Fortunately, Tanya's mom, dad, sisters, and brother were all close, and supported each other. When Tanya's emotions overwhelmed her, she was comforted by one of her siblings or her parents. And, in turn, when one of her family members sank into depression, she was the one to provide the comfort they so desperately needed.

Five years later, when Tanya's dear friend Troy died in a terrible, avoidable accident, Tanya sank into the darkest depression of her life. Losing Troy, who was like a brother to her, crushed her spirit in a way that rivaled what she had felt in the immediate aftermath of her sister's murder.

Her mother recognized that Tanya was sinking into the same depression she had when Nicole died. She encouraged Tanya to see Troy's family. One month later, she did. She was still in the depths of despair, so Tanya was surprised to find that Troy's family had found peace after his death. They missed him but firmly believed that God had taken him for a reason, and it was not their place to question God.

Tanya, on the other hand, was furious with God for taking so many friends. She could not understand how Troy's family could accept Troy's loss with such equanimity.

JC

JC was sentenced to 25 years to life. JC had very little hope of serving anything less than his full sentence. At the time, California's governor was a man named George Deukmejian, who rose to power in part by pledging that prisoners would serve every day of their sentence. No time off for good behavior. There would be no exceptions for any reason. And what if you were just 17, a kid still in high school? It did not matter. It just *was*.

JC was deeply depressed. In the space of 12 months, the life he envisioned was utterly destroyed. He was looking at possibly spending his whole life behind bars. Alone in his cell at night, JC was overcome with sadness for everything lost, including the victim's life. He cried, wishing that somehow, someway, the pain would all come to an end. JC was in a living hell.

LEO

Leo had lost his eye to a picket fence, but farm life did not allow him much time to think about it. There were chores to do. Leo simply worked through his depression.

JOE

Joe had good intentions to stay in California and start a new life. Perhaps he would try to become an actor in the movies or on television, but something happened that changed everything.

For years, John Gotti had been building his reputation as a powerful Mafia figure. The media became obsessed with him, covering his life and exploits in newspapers across the country.

It was in one of these stories that Joe finally learned the truth that had been eluding him for years, the fact he had suspected but had never been able to believe. John Gotti had killed his father, and, yes, had become a "made man." And Gotti had, it seemed, been richly rewarded. He had money, power, a beautiful woman at his side, and had reached antihero status in households across America.

Joe fell into a deep depression. His father had been brutally murdered. He had grown up without a dad. Yet Gotti only served two years for the crime, which was four years less than Joe's dad had received for his armed robbery conviction. It was not fair. It was just wrong.

In the haze of anger and depression, Joe decided there was only one way to make things right. Joe decided he was going to retaliate and kill John Gotti. He left his California dreams behind and moved back to New York City. His heart was seething with rage, hate, and revenge.

ERICA

Erica would spend days on end hiding in Budapest's dark basements and crevasses, dodging the Nazis. There was no radio, television, or internet. There was not even a book. This gave her endless hours to think, grieve, wonder, and pray. She would cry herself to sleep every night, but she woke up happy to know she had lived another day.

TOM

After realizing that he would not be going to the Olympics under any circumstances, Tom sank into a deep depression. What had it all been for? He thought of the times when friends had invited him out to the movies or a party, and he had turned them down because he thought the time was better spent practicing his shot put technique. He thought of the girlfriend who had broken up with him because he didn't have time to see her since every spare moment was spent practicing for his Olympic dreams. He remembered the times he had cried with frustration when he just couldn't get the shot as far as he wanted to, no matter how hard he tried.

He felt betrayed and used as a pawn by influential leaders who abused their authority. After all, the Olympics were a time for people to set aside their differences and get together to compete in the games.

Without the Olympics as his "north star," Tom was lost. He started working out even harder than before, pushing his body further and further, risking injury. He no longer did it for Olympic aspirations but to relieve the sadness and pain.

MY STORY

After learning I had to have open-heart surgery, my ten-year-old mind was starting to understand that I had a severe problem. At Acacia Elementary School, we had a thing called the "grand tour" where we raced around all the trees at the playground's outer perimeter. Frequently, I was towards the back of the pack because I just could not catch my breath. Yet on some occasions, I made it to the middle of the pack. A few times I even made it near the front. Due to poor blood circulation, the pain in my legs eventually became so intense that I could not even finish the race.

What hurt even more than my legs was the embarrassment of all the kids looking at me and wondering, "What is wrong with him?" Nobody said anything, but I knew. This was my introduction to facing the fact that emotional pain was worse than physical pain. While typically a happy kid, I became sad and even depressed that year. This was a bigger deal than just missing out on the beach; my body was damaged and so was my young soul.

As the time for my heart surgery grew closer and more certain, it got me down. I still remember the day when I stood at the lunch table looking at hundreds of kids playing on the playground and wondering to myself, "Out of all these hundreds of kids, why am I the only one going to spend the summer in the hospital?" I was mad at God, my family, the doctors, and everything else. It was not fair; it was not right. Though surrounded by hundreds of kids and lots of friends, I felt alone.

SECTION 2

Survive Stage | We Get Back Up

HAVING BEEN KNOCKED DOWN, now is the time to stand back up. We are cautious and avoidant of abusing unhealthy self-medication, and we strive to take good care of ourselves. We declare our status as a survivor. We regain our footing. By facing our trauma and uncomfortable emotions, we get to a point where they no longer sting quite as much. We can start using our trauma to our advantage. Indeed, we use the energy from our pain as fuel to see our inner worth and reclaim our power:

- **Confront:** Here, we "sit in the fire," identify, express, and even embrace the pain head-on.
- **Sort Out:** We untangle guilt (wrongdoing) from shame (circumstances). Understanding this difference is a significant key to our progress.
- **Experiment:** It can be enjoyable as we begin to test new life skills and treatments. We practice self-care, self-grace, and unconditional love for ourselves and those who are close to us.
- **Acceptance:** As we develop our character to hold ourselves and others accountable, we continue to heal.

- **Mindfulness:** This is an essential skill to survive. "Grounding" and deep-breathing exercises connect us to our inner voice and bring energy and transformation.

CHAPTER 6

Confront

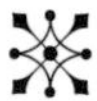

We cannot bury our feelings and heal. It is not possible. The world is full of people who have tried to ignore their past traumas, and the results are miserable. We must do something smarter.

SIT IN THE FIRE

PEOPLE ARE A LOT LIKE TEA. We do not know how strong we are until we are dropped into some hot water.

"Sitting in the fire" means that we dive into the hot water and go deep into the hurt that we have suffered. We don't put on a happy face; we do not run away from the ugliness or embarrassment. We do not hug or pat anyone on the back. We express our raw grief, hurt, and pain. We do not throw our hurts in the trash. We face them and begin to use hurts as the high-octane fuel that they are.

I have sat in the fire several times, but two occasions stand out. The first was in 1995 when I was sitting at the kitchen table with Nicole Brown Simpson's family. The "Trial of the Century" was in full swing, and the whole world was watching. To millions, it was a carnival and an entertainment bonanza.

Yet behind the scenes, it was anything but a circus. I sat at the kitchen table with Judy, Lou, Denise, and Tanya Brown, the parents and sisters of Nicole. This sweet family was in pain. I saw the raw agony in each of their eyes.

They lost their daughter and sister to a brutal murder, and the man we believed to be responsible was bouncing around on the television, acting like a clown, and basking in the attention. His attorneys were strutting about enjoying their new celebrity status. The media had created a full-blown production around the whole event while those closest to Nicole suffered.

Our conversation started with some small talk, but soon the real issues came up. Denise is usually a kind, calm person, but she went into somewhat of a rage. She had every right to be pissed.

Denise said one of the most powerful and profound things I have ever heard. It was as if a light bulb went off in her head. "Ya know, I'm going to take all this rage, go and study everything about domestic violence, and meet with all the experts out there. Then, I'm going to take all this anger and energy and use it to educate and help battered women!" She was resolute. She was intensely focused. She was strong. In a miraculous moment, I saw someone who was beaten, broken, and bruised take her power back.

Decades later, I still feel the profound energy I witnessed. Indeed, she did go on and help educate countless women and gave them the information and courage to get out of abusive relationships. I have personally seen many come up and thank her profusely. Spousal abuse is an ugly topic that most had avoided altogether. As a direct result of Denise's efforts, the problem is discussed far more often around the world.

The second time I sat in a fire was at the other end of the spectrum. This time I was sitting on a cheap, plastic chair in San Quentin State Prison. An inmate was presenting his "crime impact statement" to the group where I was volunteering. While I can never discuss any details that I hear within those meetings, I can say that this inmate went into vivid detail about the day he committed a murder. There is a story behind every person you meet, and it may surprise you.

This man, dressed in a blue smock and prison-issued orange slippers, broke down sobbing as he spoke about getting up in the morning of what he referred to as "the worst day of my life." He described walking up to a man and killing him. He broke down over the daily guilt for what he had done, the brutal end to another human's life, the unspeakable grief of the victim's family, and the never-ending shame of his family. He had strutted into prison with a macho persona, faking his innocence. That day, he faced his actions head-on and took complete responsibility for the immeasurable damage he had caused. He was deeply hurting. Nobody handed him a tissue, patted him on the back, or said, "It's all right, man." Everyone just let him sit, sob, and feel the full measure of his pain.

As one who witnessed both events, I did something right. I sat there, shut up, and listened. I did not do anything but listen. I heard each word, and many of those words stung and pierced deeply. As I sat there, my heart went out to them. I felt a small measure of their suffering. In all these many years since, I have honored their trust by never repeating any personal details. A designated person of trust must be someone who keeps a confidence.

This is sitting in the fire.

Malcolm X said, "To have once been a criminal is no disgrace. To remain a criminal is the disgrace." What I saw was a change of heart. This man had been a criminal, but now, there was an undeniable, deep, and spiritual transformation.

Though these two situations seem to be polar opposites, one with a murder victim's family and the other with a murderer, there was a remarkable similarity. Sitting in the fire opened the door to authentic healing for both a victim's family and a perpetrator. Sitting in the fire unlocks the potential for what lies ahead.

It is tough, but it is worth it. Sitting in the fire reveals a great secret: we must feel our pain to heal, but those past pains can amplify our present joys.

Many people go day after day, year after year, and even decades without having a real conversation. The goal is to support others in what they choose to do—as long as it does not harm anyone—and to allow ourselves the same freedom. Keep your eyes on the prize, which is to have open, honest conversations with ourselves and others about the things that truly matter.

DISSECTING TRAUMA

One thing that surprised me when I started going into prisons, jails, and homeless shelters was how often childhood trauma came up. Child abuse is the single largest problem in society. It is responsible for 50 percent of depression, 66 percent of alcoholism, and 75 percent of suicide, intravenous drug use, and domestic violence. If child abuse ended, workplace productivity would go up, and incarceration would go down dramatically. It became clear that if we want a better world, the starting place is to protect every child from anything that threatens their healthy development.

The "judgment center" of the brain, the cerebral cortex, develops from birth to about age 21 to 26. Damage to the cerebral cortex by abuse can impact the ability to focus and make sound judgments in adulthood.

In my volunteer work in San Quentin, the vast majority of the inmates were involved in underage drinking or drug abuse or suffered from covert or overt child abuse. Overt abuse is raw, physical assault, while covert abuse is mental and twists our emotions. But they both cause harm. *Unresolved trauma, particularly childhood trauma, is easily the most massive problem facing humankind.* Homelessness, alcoholism, drug addiction, violent crime, anger addiction, teenage pregnancy, extreme politics and religion, depression, disease, and suicide are often secondary symptoms of the underlying issue of unresolved childhood trauma.

It is a no-brainer. Every child deserves protection from any form of abuse. Every ethical and healthy organization that has interactions with children will embrace the established child-safety protocols. It is time for every individual and organizational abuser to be called out and held responsible for the damage they do. All abuse should be reported to the police or law-enforcement agencies. The perpetrators should be named. It is a crime.

There are movements to protect children that call for an end of all forms of child abuse. People are waking up, and the world is getting better. We've seen measurable progress with religious freedom, labor rights, women's rights, racial equality, and LGBQT rights—yet there is more to do, especially for the children. Every kid has a right to grow up safely. It is time that responsible adults step up and stop the epidemic of child abuse.

Making a continual effort to unpack and understand the mechanics of trauma is fundamental to cultivating healing. The word "trauma" is derived from the Greek word meaning wound or injury. Leading psychiatrist, Dr. Bessel van der Kolk, describes the problem: "A trauma is when your biology is assaulted in such a way that you might not be able to reset yourself."

Emotional or psychological trauma changes the brain's neurochemistry and can impact rational thinking or memory to the point of disrupting normal life. The damage is not imagined; it is real and can be scientifically observed and measured. These neurological issues interfere with normal brain functions. In turn, the traumatized person may have difficulty performing routine tasks at school, work, or home.

Traumatic issues are real and have the power to make us bitter or better. It is common to want to suppress our feelings and dodge all conversations about them. Indeed, we want to avoid even thinking about the matter. When we attempt to bury our feelings, they become like a volcano. On the surface it looks like a beautiful and majestic mountain. Yet under the surface, the pressure keeps building and building. Once triggered, it erupts with terrible consequences. Once, I visited Mt. Saint Helens, and learned the force of the volcano knocked down trees for 17 miles when it erupted. That is the power of pent up energy. Holding our emotions inside will also ultimately backfire and explode.

A far healthier approach is to "sit in the fire," speak the unspeakable, and honestly face our emotions. This relieves the pressure. Confronting the issues is the process where we identify, embrace, and talk about the pain head-on. It is always better to cultivate a complete emotional awareness of what has happened and how we genuinely feel about it. This is not a task for the timid, as it requires work, vulnerability, and great effort. And it takes courage. *We must let it out and feel the full extent of the pain before we can move on.*

Our traumas, even years later, can generate remarkably strong emotions. The objective of healing is to face these emotions and modulate them directly. In other words, we exert a modifying influence on them. By modulating our feelings, we process the situation, and over time, we deflate their intensity. By facing and acknowledging our uncomfortable emotions, we get to a point where they no longer sting. Our traumas can then no longer shock us or cause us to become angry or depressed. We do not numb our emotions with harmful drugs, alcohol, or fringe religions but instead authentically begin to face them. As we do this, the bite and intensity do subside. Our emotional wounds will begin to heal.

There are various approaches to *modulating* our emotions and, thereby, dialing back their intensity. Healing employs several techniques including support from others, meditation and prayer, professional therapy, and new activities, habits, and lifestyles. It is essential to find activities that fit our individual needs and interests.

We can *seek support* from others with whom we can honestly and safely share our situation. As we heal, we will need to rely upon others who are authentically caring, stable, secure, and able to help bring us perspective.

- We can utilize one or more proven *self-regulation* techniques. Self-regulation techniques were discovered in ancient times, with practices such as relaxation and meditation. Biofeedback is a more modern practice.
- We can engage in *active problem-solving*. We can take

practical steps to deal with any ongoing problems related to the trauma.

- Simply relaxing with *enjoyable and productive activities* such as hobbies like gardening, playing a game, working on a puzzle, or crafting that focuses our attention outward to enjoyable activities.
- Combining relaxation with *exercise* has proven effective for stress management. To heal trauma, work with the body. It is not all just in our heads.

In some cases, treatment by a licensed professional therapist may need to be sought. When we express our innermost feelings, we must be selective in whom we confide.

An abuser always appears strong and mighty until they are exposed. Abusers do not ever want to face the damage they do, and they want their victims to be quiet. When their victims speak up and confront them, their power is undermined, and they retreat, get angry, or laugh uncontrollably—anything but face the damage they have done. They are masters at slapping superficial labels on their victims such as "bitter," "nut job," "idiot," "apostate," "butt-hurt," or some other personal ad hominem attack. They do this to further abuse and "shame and tame" their victims while shifting attention from themselves and their actions.

Regardless of the type of abuse, toxic people and organizations will not validate our trauma. By shaming or blaming victims and bystanders, the so-called abusers can comfortably ignore accountability. By blaming the victim, they never have to face the trauma or the vast amount of damage they have caused. In toxic groups, the victim is often coerced to "just forgive and forget."

Whistleblower syndrome is a phenomenon where the group blames the person who reported the abuse rather than the abuser. This is all nonsense. All crimes of abuse should be reported to the police or other law enforcement personnel. When abuse happens in any of its forms, we must be strong and confront it wherever it is safe to do so. If we cannot go to law enforcement, we can get away to shelter or other safety. We must push aside all the excuses and gaslighting. When we break the cycle of abuse, we take back our authority. When we confront the abuse and do something to protect ourselves, we reclaim our inner voice and our internal power.

ABUSE

Abuse occurs when a more powerful party manipulates, violates, or harms a party with less power. It is ugly, and it brings an experience of profound betrayal to its victims. Often, the abuser is the exact person who should be caring for and protecting their victims. There is a full menu of abuse including domestic violence, sexual abuse, elder abuse, and institutional abuse at work, in a cult, or in fringe political or religious belief systems. Sexual abuse occurs when a powerful person forces themselves onto another through various means without consent. Child sexual abuse involves an older person forcing themselves on someone too young to consent. Ecclesiastical abuse comes from spiritual leaders who abuse their authority.

If you question if you were abused, you should consult a professional and discuss your situation and the topic of "power dynamics." In essence, every human has the right to not be physically touched without permission and treated with respect. We all have the right to be fully informed before making any commitment. We have the right to consent. We have the right to be told the truth. All healthy people and organizations provide full disclosure. If we are not given all the information or given misleading information or feel as if we cannot say "no" because we may lose our livelihood or safety, that is not proper consent. It is abuse.

Abusers take advantage of the fact that it is always easier to say "yes" and step into something, than to get out. Those who have traumatic relationships often give up their authority to toxic people or organizations. Victims can surrender their inner voice and give up too much of themselves.

RESTORATIVE JUSTICE

I am a volunteer in the Victim Offender Education Group program at San Quentin State Prison. It is a secular program that seeks to rehabilitate incarcerated men. I am certified to facilitate group discussions.

Commonly, I am asked, "What do you teach them?" I have no answer. I don't teach anything. I say very little, but I am a great listener as I know its healing effects. I have been directly challenged as to why I would want to spend my time helping those who have committed horrible crimes. After all, as many say, "Aren't these criminals animals who deserve to rot in a cell?"

Restorative justice is a shift in prisoners' thinking from denial or rationalization of their harmful behavior to confronting the issues and holding themselves fully responsible and accountable for the impact of their crimes and actions. It is a profound philosophy that is based on non-violent practices. It is a social movement that entirely shifts away from the old, authoritarian, Western ways of thinking about justice and punishment.

Rather than focusing on traditional Western forms of punishment, we seek to repair harm. It is rooted in indigenous philosophies from the Inuit in the Yukon, the Maori in New Zealand, and others. In those societies, the teenagers were getting into trouble and going to jail where things got worse. The tribal elders tried another approach. Rather than send the youth off into the justice system, they sat down and listened to these offenders. They began to spend time with, teach, and mentor the youth. They talked about their cultural roots. They backed off on judgment and turned up empathy. Things got far better. Recidivism dropped dramatically.

Here, we focus on healing and invite both the victims and offenders to the conversation.

According to the Insight Prison Project, the current social science research demonstrates that schools which adopt restorative justice instead of punitive disciplinary processes—where they talk about issues among students, teachers, families, and administrators—are more likely to reduce the number of students suspended and expelled, breaking the school-to-prison pipeline. A 2009 study by UC Berkeley's Henderson Center for Social Justice on the impact of restorative justice at Cole Middle School in West Oakland demonstrated an 87 percent drop in the suspension rate, improved academic outcomes, reduced teacher attrition rates, and eliminated physical fighting altogether.

The traditional justice system makes the state the victim and places the actual victims in a secondary, passive role. The primary goal is not to heal, but rather to retaliate and punish. When the sentence is served, the inmate can be released more angered, damaged, and violent than before.

There is a better way. First, the actual victims are given a voice and are allowed to be heard and to heal. Victims are respected, empowered, and supported as are the offenders. Both the victims and offenders are treated respectfully so that they can find meaning from their experience. The offenders work month after month to shed the veneer of machismo, false denials, and face the damage head-on that they have done to others, the community, their families, and themselves.

Susan Sharpe summarizes the principles of restorative justice in her book, *Restorative Justice: A Vision for Healing and Change.* Restorative justice reflects a belief that justice should, to the highest degree possible, do five things:

- Invite full participation and consensus
- Heal what has been broken
- Seek full and direct accountability
- Reunite what has been divided
- Strengthen the community and prevent further harm

Going into a prison for the first time was a pivotal point in my life. My entire mental framework was shattered. I expected to see men who were angry and dangerous. Instead, it was like walking into a calming, Buddhist monastery. They were warm, welcoming, and kind. I talked about this with the executive director of the program, Billie Mizell, who quietly replied, “Human life is a miracle, and human transformation may be even more miraculous.”

To my skeptical friends, I would ask a question: “It is a reality that many murderers and rapists will be paroled. Do you want them released with the mindset that they had when they entered prison? Or do you want them released genuinely reformed and equipped with a mental skillset to process the stresses of life productively, peacefully, and honorably?”

I believe that everyone is redeemable. I have seen it. Furthermore, this program is now in dozens of prisons and jails, and hundreds of incarcerated men have been through the program. Hundreds have been paroled over the years, and yet I have not seen a single program graduate revert back to a life of crime.

Vulnerability and self-expression, with the right people, generates trust and intimacy. Almost magically, they help the other party to change their behavior by their own choice. Self-expression is transformational. Vulnerability is powerful. They reveal our authentic inner strength. They transition us from pretending to be strong to having genuine strength and confidence.

Challenges are what make life interesting. Overcoming them is what makes life meaningful. Caroline Myss once shared, “We are not meant to stay wounded. We are supposed to move through our tragedies and challenges and help each other move through the many painful episodes of our lives. By remaining stuck in the power of our wounds, we block our own transformation. We overlook the greater gifts inherent in our wounds—the strength to overcome them and the lessons that we are meant to receive through them. Wounds are the means through which we enter the hearts of other people. They are meant to teach us to become compassionate and wise.”

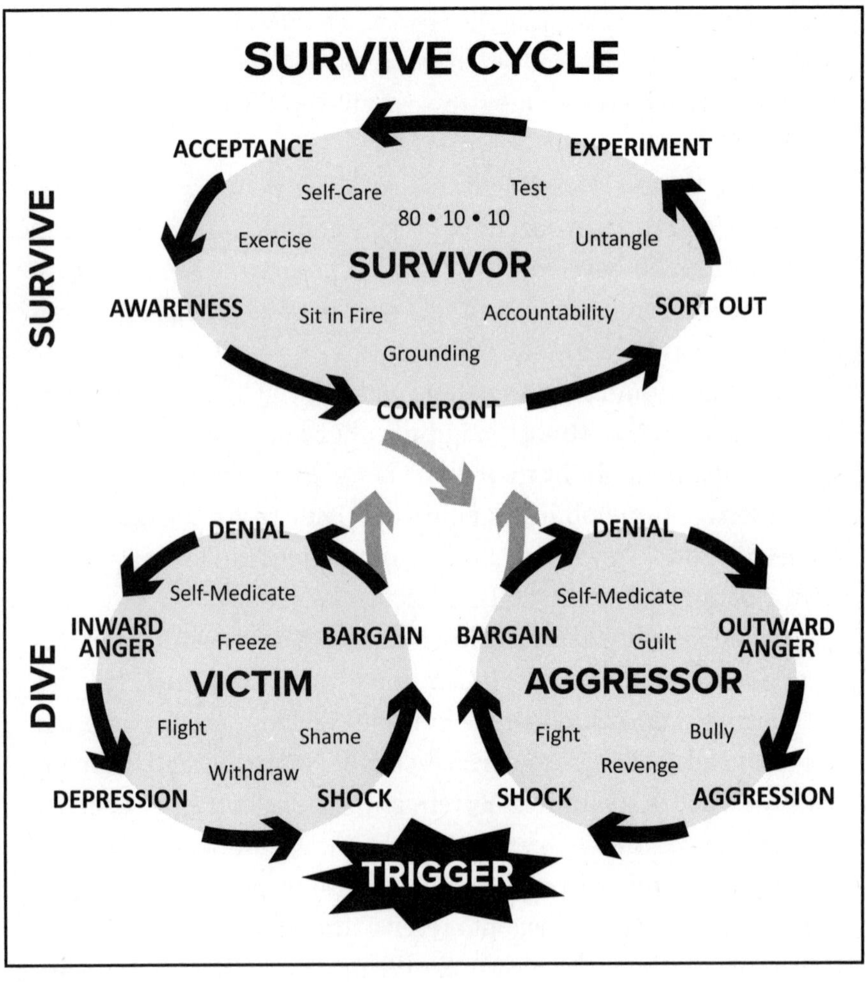
SURVIVE CYCLE
SURVIVE
ACCEPTANCE
EXPERIMENT
Self-Care
Test
80 • 10 • 10
Exercise
Untangle
SURVIVOR
AWARENESS
Sit in Fire
Accountability
SORT OUT
Grounding
CONFRONT
DIVE
DENIAL
Self-Medicate
INWARD ANGER
Freeze
BARGAIN
VICTIM
Flight
Shame
Withdraw
DEPRESSION
SHOCK
DENIAL
Self-Medicate
BARGAIN
Guilt
OUTWARD ANGER
AGGRESSOR
Fight
Bully
Revenge
SHOCK
AGGRESSION
TRIGGER

Our Stories of Confrontation

DEBBIE

When her husband died by suicide, Debbie was dropped into the "deep end of the pool." The manner of his death was difficult enough; then, she was forced to confront the fact that her husband had led a secret, decadent life that she knew nothing about.

She also had to confront the fact that her church, where they had raised their children, volunteered for years, and developed a second family, was not there for them when she and her children needed them.

It was an ugly situation, and part of her wanted to avoid even thinking about it. But she knew she needed to face the situation directly. Once she allowed herself to truly confront the circumstances she was facing, the healing process began.

Two weeks after her husband died, Debbie pulled her kids together for a talk. It was time for a change, she explained. Nine months later, Debbie sold the family home with her children's blessing. It was time for a fresh start.

JOHN

John was a humble local islander and thought he was no match against the United States military that had used his island as part of the nuclear weapons program. Yet he did. Fueled by the sadness he had for the loss of his little girl, he and his neighbors got together and decided to confront the US government directly.

SUSAN

As time went on, Susan and her husband began to shift their perspective. They were confronted by the idea that—perhaps—the catastrophe was a blessing in disguise.

For years she had daydreamed about "possibilities," but her life was comfortable. Maybe too comfortable. She hadn't wanted to risk making any big changes. But now, life was anything but "comfortable." They were still alternating their living situation between friends' homes, and the lawsuit against the city was moving along at the speed of molasses.

Now, there was nothing to lose and nothing to risk.

Susan began to focus on the future. As she and her husband started to talk through what they were going to do, they began to focus on what they would like to create. In so doing, they were able to develop a new vision for their lives.

For years, Susan had wanted to build a spiritual retreat center but had never pursued the idea. Her husband had dreams of his own—he wanted to have a ranch, a large ranch, where he could build a "Western town" that film companies could use for their Western-themed television shows and movies. After all, that was his business—supplying Western props for films. Why not a whole background?

So, Susan and Peter started to explore possibilities. Every weekend they drove around looking for land on which to build their dreams. Property was expensive, though, and they were not sure they could find something affordable that would meet both of their needs. But it did not hurt to dream, right?

SHAD

Shad's decision to work for the VA hospital on a trial basis forced him to look at how bad the situation was for returning vets. Over 325,000 Vietnam vets were in Los Angeles County at that time, a larger population than the city he had grown up in. But there was a glimmer of hope. Perhaps this would be the most important decision he ever made. Having a purpose, especially one so pressing, where he could genuinely help others, gave him a new hope for his future.

With Dr. May's support, Shad was given carte blanche to evaluate the VA hospital and work in the community where veterans lived or hung out. He started a series of "rap groups" consisting of himself and a handful of Vietnam vets. Shad hunted them out, going to places Vietnam vets would be to just "rap," or talk, with them. It was a lingo that worked.

To find out why they were not using the VA Hospital in Los Angeles, he started talking to vets in Venice Beach, then went out to the Canyons, and from there onto the streets of LA. He had let his hair grow out and sported a heavy mustache. Combined with his "uniform" of well-worn jeans and tattered t-shirts, Shad no longer resembled the Army officer he had once been. And that was just fine with Shad. His new look made the men he approached more comfortable. He was one of them.

In Shad's rap groups, vets would confront the issues they were all facing, rather than dodging or numbing them. Soon he had several rap group volunteers who helped seek out vets in churches, community centers, homeless shelters, free clinics, bars, parks, and stores—wherever they thought the veterans might be.

The rap groups worked. Finally, these vets were able to connect with others like them who genuinely understood their experience. Shad and the rap group volunteers were able to convince many of the vets they engaged with to come check out the VA and get the support they needed. Helping these men helped Shad with his own readjustment.

A month turned into a year, and then several years.

The more Shad spoke with the Vietnam vets, the more he noticed a range of behaviors and symptoms that many of them shared. Some were homeless. Others were stressed and unable to cope with the world they found themselves in. Many were depressed and angry. They disliked crowds, had trouble sleeping, and could not control their emotions.

Shad had experienced these same emotions himself during the year he returned home. He had been able to confront them by channeling energy into the work he did for the VA, but these men did not have that outlet.

As he wrote in an article for *Brainline,* an online resource for information about brain injury and PTSD, he shared, "Those were dark times, shadowed by what we had seen and done in the war. Some vets brought all that horror home, reliving it episode by episode, riding that long escalator down into despair and chronic homelessness."

GERI

Geri was born physically disabled. As a child, she had to confront the reality that she was not like other children.

Her parents could have shielded her from the world. They could have kept her in the house, away from the cruelty that people with disabilities often face. But her parents took a different path. They decided that they would treat their sweet girl precisely as they did their other children. She would have chores. She would have responsibilities. She would have an education, and she would learn to deal with whatever life threw her way.

She would learn to confront the world head-on. True to her nature, Geri didn't let the depression keep her down, though. She did what she needed to do. The world was tough enough without having a disability. Yet Geri took on each challenge with enthusiasm.

TANYA

Tanya was at home when the phone started ringing off the hook. She had just woken up and was startled and confused. She walked into her parents' bathroom where she saw her dad hitting the sink with his fist. She asked her father what had happened, although, deep in her heart, she somehow already knew—her sister was dead.

The family immediately suspected her ex-husband, OJ Simpson. Their marriage had been marred with domestic abuse, infidelity, and violent verbal threats. Nicole had finally left OJ, only to be harassed and stalked by him incessantly.

But *murder*? Had he really *murdered* her?

When they turned on the television, they saw news bulletins unfolding about the crime. Both her sister and her sister's friend, a young man named Ron Goldman who worked at a restaurant that Nicole frequented, had been brutally slain. The crime scene was horrific—the television showed the scene in full color, her sister's blood pouring down the walkway.

Tanya's mother clenched Tanya's hand tightly as they watched the news. Her mother kept repeating, "That's my kid. That's my kid." The entire family went into terrible shock.

They had to confront the idea that OJ—whom they had welcomed into their home, the father of Nicole's children, Justin and Sydney—had most likely killed her. Although they knew he had been abusive and supported her decision to leave him for that reason, they never thought it would come to *this*.

When OJ Simpson was arrested, Tanya and her family were horrified by what had happened. They wanted to run far, far away. But they faced it and attended each day of the pre-trial hearing. The more they heard, the more they realized that Nicole's abuse was much more severe than she had told them. Tanya did not know about Nicole's abuse until court. They were filled with pain knowing how greatly she had suffered. Now, not only were they faced with the loss of their beautiful Nicole, but also with the knowledge that she had hidden much of the truth about the abuse from them. They faced it all, head-on.

JC

JC wanted to confront his girlfriend for blaming him for the murder that she committed, but he knew that was an impossibility. He tried to confront law enforcement for not believing that he didn't do it. He wanted to confront the jury for finding him guilty and the judge for handing down the sentence. He imagined what he would say to all of them if only he ever got the chance.

Before being transferred to the adult prison, JC spent some time in juvenile hall. There, for the first time since he was a young teenager, JC could not hide behind stylish clothes, his charming stories, his friendly smile, weed, girls, any of it. He had to face who he was. He was alone with his thoughts. All the things he had spent his young life trying to avoid were right there in front of him.

An adult now, JC likens those weeks in juvenile hall to a journey of self-discovery. He recalls that it was like looking in a mirror and facing who you really are. JC realized that he had always taken on the characteristics of who he thought other people wanted him to be. He did not know who he was.

But he did know that he had committed a serious crime that resulted in the death of another human being. The truth was that he chose to participate in something that was horrific. His life was ruined because of it.

Or was it? As he confronted the series of bad decisions that had led to the severe consequences he was experiencing now, he realized he still had the power to make good choices. Just because he was in prison did not mean that he had to spend the rest of his life taking the wrong path. He had a responsibility to himself and his family on the outside as well. He would choose to live a good life, even in prison.

LEO

Leo faced the fact that he had a glass eye, and his boyhood hopes of sports were not going to happen. He appreciated what he did have, a curiosity about the world around him. He started to play with taking apart radios and anything electronic.

JOE

Joe returned to New York with a plan to kill John Gotti, the man who had murdered his father and destroyed his life.

Joe linked up with his cousin, and, together, they plotted their revenge. But Gotti was so well-protected that they had to plan carefully and think through every step. A few years went by. Joe's plan to kill Gotti was never far from his mind, even as he got a job, married, and settled into life in the old neighborhood.

He and his cousin continued to devise ways to kill Gotti. Finally, they settled on a plan that seemed sure to succeed. They would catch him unaware on Mulberry Street, the long thoroughfare in Manhattan that served as the heart of Little Italy. They would kill him as he emerged from a restaurant.

Joe and his cousin went out and bought two guns. The two of them got in the car to head down to Mulberry Street and do the job. As they were backing out of the driveway, Joe's wife came running out of the house, calling his name.

He stopped the car and looked at her impatiently,

"What is it?" he asked, annoyed.

His wife then uttered the only two words that would change everything. A huge smile broke out on her face. She shouted with joy, "I'm pregnant!"

In that instant, everything changed for Joe. The plan to murder John Gotti immediately left his mind, and another one took its place. He had to confront himself and ask, "What kind of person do I want to be?"

ERICA

Erica was a young woman who was alone and hiding from the Nazis. Many people wanted to avoid confronting the Nazi agenda and pretend nothing was going on.

Of course, Erica was pragmatic. She could not face them directly, and she acted with politeness and kindness to stay alive. She did, however, confront the reality that the Nazis were evil.

She cleverly looked for every opportunity to dodge the dangers, escape, and hide.

TOM

All his life, Tom had been able to control his life situation by committing himself and working hard. He wanted to shine academically, so he studied harder and got better grades. He set a goal to be the best person on the shot put team. He put in hours and hours of practice, improving a little every day. His whole life was built on the idea that if he just tried hard enough, he could overcome any obstacle.

Losing out on his Olympic dreams was the first time in his life that, no matter how hard he tried, Tom could not control the outcome. It was a painful realization.

Tom could not confront President Carter over the situation—and, even if he could, how could a 20-year-old young man change Carter's mind, if legions of coaches and politicians could not?

Tom was forced to confront his long-accepted idea that he could control everything. Knowing he could not filled him with anxiety. Did he lose his Olympic dreams? What other nasty surprise was in store for him? Would someone he loved die? Would he catch some dreaded disease? Would all his friends abandon him? Tom knew his anxieties were overblown, but the Olympic debacle had shattered the very foundation of his way of thinking. What could he do now?

Tom decided that he could either continue to be depressed and demoralized by a situation over which he had no control or he could choose to face his reality and move forward with his life in other ways.

MY STORY

Before having the heart surgery, I had a catheterization. The doctors inserted a small tube into a vein in my arm and injected dye into my bloodstream to precisely identify the extent of my problem. I was awake during the procedure. It did not hurt at all, and I was quite curious about what the doctors and nurses were doing. I peppered them with questions, which they seemed happy to answer. I asked the doctor to show me the scalpel, which he did, and I recall just how small it looked compared to what I had imagined.

After the procedure, I was wheeled into the doctor's office, and my mom and the doctor discussed what they had learned. I do not recall what they said, but something triggered me, and for the first time, I just broke down crying. I was sad right down to my core. I could not believe that this was happening to me. Surgery was coming—there was no way around it—and it was now getting very real. It was less crying and more of a deep wailing. The tears just flowed as I sobbed and sobbed. My emotions sank to a new low.

I just sat there amid the fire, sobbing. I saw the reality of what was going to happen and was forced to acknowledge it and embrace it head-on. The doctor and my mom glanced at me, but they were embarrassed and quickly looked away. I had to face this all on my own.

THE SIX HONORINGS

This roadmap was created by Ken Druck, PhD, following the death of his daughter Jenna. Dr. Druck has assisted families who lost loved ones in tragedies including 9/11, Columbine, Katrina, Sandy Hook, Boston Marathon, Las Vegas Mandalay Bay Concert, and COVID-19. Each one of these six honorings is a guideline for how to begin living courageously, heal shattered hearts, and honor our loved ones.

1. YOUR OWN SURVIVAL. The first way we honor the loss of a loved one is to slowly and gently begin to fight our way back into life. Putting best practices for self-care and healthy grieving into play allows us to learn how we can survive their death.

2. DO SOMETHING GOOD IN THEIR NAME. In doing something as simple and elegant as lighting a candle or planting a tree or as elaborate as conducting a celebration of their life or starting a non-profit organization, we show the world who they were. We express to the world that they lived and that they will continue to live on through the good deeds done in their name.

3. CULTIVATE A SPIRITUAL RELATIONSHIP. We used to be able to stop over for a quick visit, meet for lunch or pick up the phone and hear their voice. Coming to terms with the fact that we can't see or hear them again brings deep sorrow. And yet, our love for them lives on, perhaps stronger than ever, our love never dies. How and where to express this undying love leads us to cultivate a "spiritual relationship" with them.

4. EMBODY A SPECIAL QUALITY OF THEIRS. Whether it's their kindness, sense of humor, fierce determination, loyalty, or even their irreverence, choose a very special aspect of their personality and begin to embody it.

5. WRITE NEW CHAPTERS OF LIFE. This honoring is perhaps the most challenging. To the best of our ability, we try to begin living out the rest of our own lives.

6. TAKE THE HIGH ROAD. To help families torn apart in the raw grief after 9/11, Dr. Druck started a program called "Take the High Road." By treating one another with patience, kindness, respect, humility, compassion, and understanding, survivors express their love for the person who had died.

© Copyright All Rights Reserved, 1999 Ken Druck, Ph.D., Druck Enterprises, Inc. www.kendruck.org

CHAPTER 7

Sorting it Out

Shame and guilt feel a lot alike, yet they are very different and must be untangled. Guilt is over something we did wrong. Shame comes from issues over which we have no control.

GUILT AND SHAME

When I wrote the book *MeWeDoBe,* I went around the country promoting it. While I was in New York engaging in some television appearances, I had an interview on the floor of the New York Stock Exchange. As I waited to go on camera, I received two emails at about the same time. The first was from a wealth management firm in Beverly Hills asking me to speak at an event. Then I got another email that I will never forget.

The second email was from the executive director of a homeless shelter on Skid Row in Los Angeles. For those who do not know about Skid Row, it may be the bleakest place on earth. The poorest of the poor live there, and it is the most desperate area imaginable. The shelter told me that they could not afford any speaking fees, nor could they afford to buy any books, but they told me that they had a group of homeless children who needed to hear my message.

As an author, I was stunned at how my book had touched nerves from coast to coast, from the wealthiest to the poorest. I immediately told the homeless shelter to send over three dates, and I would find one that would work.

In the meantime, I was invited to meet with inmates at San Quentin. I had been volunteering at a homeless shelter in my hometown of Laguna Beach for years, so I knew what it was like spending time with society's marginalized.

Our session lasted two hours. The inmates talked about the trauma they caused to others and the trauma they experienced growing up. It was transformative. The men were calm, polite, articulate, and authentic in their quest to turn their lives around. One man came up to me and said, "I may be in prison for the rest of my life, but the rest of my life will be a good and honorable life."

I remained quiet during the meeting, mainly because I felt overwhelmed by being in prison for the first time and having all my stereotypes dismantled. I had always thought that prison inmates were ignorant, snarling, angry, and mean. I was so wrong, and in the end, I asked just one question: "Gentlemen. Thank you for allowing me to be a part of your group discussion. In two weeks, I am speaking to a group of homeless children. I imagine that they are scared and frightened, and I have been thinking about what I should say to them. I need your help—please tell me exactly what I should say so that they can beat their challenges, avoid prison, and do something with their lives."

Immediately, an inmate across from me uttered a game-changer, *"You go and tell those kids the difference between guilt and shame."*

I had to swallow my pride and say, "Sorry, I thought they were the same. I do not know the difference."

The man then taught me. He said, "Guilt and shame are not the same thing. Guilt is something I have done wrong. In my case, I committed a murder. I feel guilty, and I am in prison where I belong. Guilt can make your stomach feel sick or your head ache every moment of every day.

"Shame is very different. Shame is related to the word, 'ashamed.' As a kid, I felt ashamed that my family did not have enough money. I felt embarrassed about my dad being in prison. My family was poor, and I often went to bed with no dinner. My mom was overwhelmed, and she yelled a lot. As I got older, I covered that shame up by acting tough and macho. Deep down, I was scared, and the shame kept building up. The pressure inside me was intense.

"One day, a guy laughed at me. I exploded in rage, and I reacted by killing him.

"You go tell those kids that when they feel shame, to understand that the tough times they are going through are not their fault. Tell them to find an adult they can trust and talk to about it. A teacher, a cop, a parent, a principal, a counselor, a pastor, or anyone they can trust. Then, they need to share those thoughts with that person. By giving voice to that shame, they relieve the pressure. You cannot bottle shame inside and be successful! You have to express it! That adult may not be able to do anything about it, but talking about it relieves the pressure. That way, when someone laughs at you or something triggers you, you don't explode as I did.

"I wish someone had told me exactly what I am telling you when I was a kid. Tell them that I hope they will respond better than I did. When we feel guilty, it is about something we did. When we feel shame, it's about who we are. They are very different, so go and teach that to those homeless kids. Every kid out there needs to know this."

I have sat in the hallowed halls of universities, monasteries, churches, and shrines, but I have never been taught like I was that day by a man in a blue jumpsuit.

Indeed, I did deliver his message to the kids on Skid Row. I now talk about it every time I get the chance. Know the difference between guilt and shame, and find someone you trust to share it with. Make sure that person is emotionally mature. I once shared my shame of having heart surgery with a family member, and she just laughed and said, "Oh, that was a long time ago."

Divulging your deep personal vulnerabilities to the wrong person

GUILT VS SHAME

GUILT IS...

- A feeling when we have done something wrong (i.e. hurt someone or committed a crime).
- Healthy guilt keeps us close to our moral compass, regulates our social behavior, serves as a sign that our conscience is working properly to stop us from repeating mistakes, and involves making amends to resolve the feelings of guilt
- Toxic guilt happens when we make a mistake and are unable to overcome the negative feelings associated with the event, even when amends have been made

SHAME IS...

- A feeling about who we are, but we have done nothing wrong (i.e. "My family is poor" or "I have a medical issue")
- Protecting an idealized version of yourself
- May have deep fear of failures or shortcomings being exposed
- Individual does not want to own up to their problem and correct it
- May have a difficult time acknowledging that a problem actually exists
- Harder to overcome than guilt

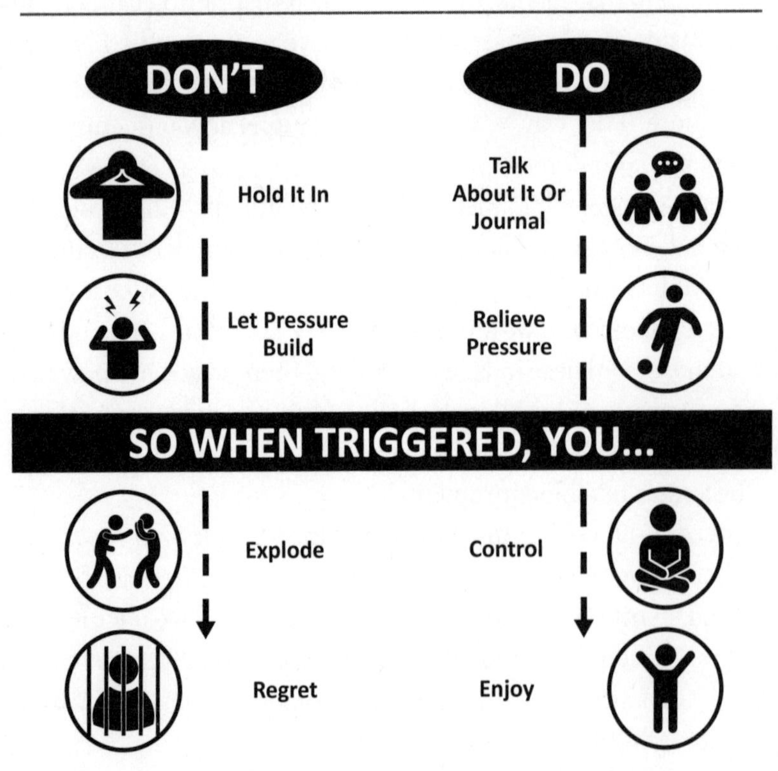
DON'T
DO
Hold It In
Talk About It Or Journal
Let Pressure Build
Relieve Pressure
SO WHEN TRIGGERED, YOU...
Explode
Control
Regret
Enjoy

can amplify the trauma. Make sure they are trustworthy. Sometimes people with good intentions think that they can soothe the pain by solving the problem. Yet this stage is not about solving. It is about feeling heard. It is about the person being a mirror for us, to listen carefully, validate our feelings, reflect back what we say, and ask thought-provoking questions. We need someone who will not judge and can simply provide a safe space to open up.

No matter what, we cannot bottle it up or else we will explode or slowly rot inside. If we bottle up our feelings, it is guaranteed that we will stay in the struggle. We can never heal from a trauma that we do not express.

UNTANGLING THE MESS

We get what we tolerate. As we untangle trauma, it is essential to understand that some things we are responsible for, and other things we are not. As this is sorted out, the responsibility for the trauma becomes clearer.

"Sorting Out" enables us to untangle the confusion about guilt, which is a sense of doing wrong, versus shame, which comes from circumstances beyond our control. Shame and guilt both feel awful, but they are very different. Shame, in all its forms, comes from issues over which we have no control, like our height, the color of our skin, or a physical or mental disability. The problem is that if shame is not addressed, it can lead us to believe that we are inadequate, worthless, or a loser. It can leave us feeling humiliated, embarrassed, or overwhelmed. It can become so painful that it feels unbearable.

Being shamed leaves a mental imprint that tells us we are beyond help and worthless. This critical inner voice cycles and recycles the messages taught to us by toxic parents, siblings, friends, peers, church leaders, or school teachers. Being told that we are ugly, selfish, too skinny, too fat, too poor, a rich brat, unworthy, inadequate, worthless, or stupid can cut like a knife. Shaming is often accompanied by shunning, where we feel rejected and cut off. In reality, some people will be critical for no legitimate reason other than to mask their issues.

Comments like, "That is a stupid question!" "What will people think?" "You look ridiculous!" "You are an idiot!" "You cannot do anything, right!" "You are not worthy" "What is wrong with you?" or "You should be ashamed of yourself!"—can leave us feeling humiliated for months or years. In response, we may have trouble making eye contact, bite our lip, stare at the ground, or have a blank expression.

Every person has the fundamental right to be valued, respected, heard, and seen, yet because of shaming, some people feel worthless. The emotional pressure builds and builds. We adopt false identities to feel important. All of this can lead to intense internal pressure. The slightest comment or the wrong look can set us off.

If we feel shame, we cannot hold it in. We need to talk about it with someone we trust, and that is why I recommend a licensed therapist. If we feel accepted for who we are by another person, it can help dissolve the shame. If we meet someone who has been shamed, we need likewise to let them know that they are loved, accepted, and valued. That striking message at San Quentin about guilt and shame taught to me by a man sentenced to prison for life was one of the most profound things I have ever heard. I learned that whatever has our shame has our power.

PHYSICAL TRAUMA

Everyone has the fundamental human right not to be touched by anyone without their permission. Physical traumas are some of the most easily identified, as they often leave physical evidence.

Any physical aggression is crossing the line and off-limits. Some examples include hitting, kicking, punching, arm twisting, pushing, beating, shoving, biting, slapping, throwing objects, shaking, pinching, choking, hair pulling, dragging, burning, cutting, stabbing, strangling, or force-feeding. Physical abuse also includes any restraint, such as blocking a doorway, grabbing when trying to leave, locking doors with no key, or tying someone up.

Any of these can be more than traumatic; they could be an

"assault" and a crime, and all crimes should be reported to law enforcement authorities.

EMOTIONAL ABUSE

We all have the fundamental human right to be told the truth and treated with respect. We all have the right to have relationships where there are no mental manipulations or mental abuse. While there can be less visible evidence of psychological abuse than physical abuse, it can be more damaging. Intimidation or verbal threats of any kind are unacceptable.

Bullying is a relatively common type of emotional abuse and could include mocking, threatening, raging, or getting "in your face." Intense staring is a form of intimidation mixed with the silent treatment, where one punishes another by ignoring them. Passive-aggressive behaviors are abusive when the perpetrator ignores and refuses to respond to their target.

A healthy person will discuss or even debate an issue, but toxic people make personal attacks. This can include labeling, name-calling, mocking, berating, and making judgmental comments. Many perpetrators are argumentative, overly competitive, sarcastic, and demanding. They frequently interrupt, talk over, withhold essential information, and interrogate. Yelling, screaming, swearing, and using threatening language are never okay.

Gaslighting is where the perpetrator lies about the past so that the victim doubts their memory, perception, and sanity. The term comes from an old movie where the husband was doing evil deeds in the attic that affected the home's gas lamps. When his wife mentioned the lamps' problems, he blamed her for her faulty memory. Perpetrators make false claims that cause doubt. They twist the facts so that the victim takes responsibility for the perpetrator's bad behavior.

One of the most damaging types of emotional abuse occurs when the abuser shares or exposes private information without consent. Breaking confidence is a sure sign of an abusive personality type.

When perpetrators are confronted, they may twist things around to blame others for their actions. Toxic people tend not to accept responsibility for their behavior and, instead, insist on an apology. Abusers refuse to take responsibility, become hostile, lie, or frequently forget promises or commitments. Rather than taking responsibility, the abuser believes that anything that goes wrong is someone else's fault. They often accuse others of being too sensitive. They may manipulate by threatening abandonment, rejection, or even death. When all else fails, they may resort to playing the victim card to gain sympathy and further control behavior.

Some types of intimidation are illegal and should be reported to law enforcement. In all cases, emotional abuse is toxic, and it cannot be tolerated.

FINANCIAL TRAUMA

Every person has the right to be paid an honest salary for honest work, take care of themselves financially, and have their basic needs met. Money is like oxygen. We take it for granted until we run out. Some financial traumas hit us directly, such as identity theft, burglary, robbery, or embezzlement. We are also financially traumatized by a sudden loss of income, such as unexpectedly being laid off or fired. Other tragedies may hit us in different ways, such as an unexpected disability or trip to the hospital, but the financial impacts are a secondary fallout. Any way it happens, financial traumas can cause panic and anxiety.

Within relationships, there are generally two types of financial traumas. The first is when one party is a shopaholic or an undisciplined spender. The other is when one is controlling all of the money. Materialism and overspending are essentially a form of self-medication to mask other unresolved traumas, yet this behavior can be traumatizing for the others that it affects. Indeed, it can be abusive to one party who attempts to keep up with another's overspending and has their finances and credit ratings damaged.

Financial traumas also include a controlling partner who blocks access to a joint checking account. They set up impossible budgets, control the paychecks, and create an unhealthy dependency for food, clothing, shelter, and other necessities. They maintain secret accounts, deplete retirement accounts without the knowledge of the other, or cancel insurance policies.

Yet another type of abuse can occur when one party interferes with the other's job. This could include calling the boss, visiting unannounced, excessive calling, insisting on having access to work emails and calendar, demanding to know details about the job. These are excessive and unprofessional behaviors that violate confidentiality.

Healthy lives and good relationships mean that we properly respect others and manage our money. We earn an appropriate income, insure against foreseeable losses, and control our spending. Anything less than this is not acceptable and can even be abusive.

ECCLESIASTICAL TRAUMA

All members of a religious organization deserve to be respected and valued. In healthy houses of worship, critical thinking and direct questioning of the doctrines and leadership are welcome. All finances should be transparent, and members should also be free to leave without shame. A healthy religious organization will provide a loving community and support each other's choices, but it will not decide what those choices are.

Ecclesiastical abuse occurs when leaders obtain positions of unaccountable authority over enthusiastic and vulnerable members. The mistake is when there is no real oversight, and the rank and file naively expect the leaders to police themselves properly. This is an environment ripe for covert and overt abuse. An example of overt abuse would be a church leader who physically or sexually assaults a member. Covert abuse is subtler but also damaging. It could be playing mind games, gaslighting, asking inappropriate personal questions, or discussing sexually explicit or embarrassing topics when alone. No church leader or member should ever be alone with our child. None of this is acceptable.

A common characteristic of ecclesiastical abuse and fringe

religions is that they damage the member's self-esteem. In one breath, we are told that we are special or "chosen" and not to beat ourselves up, and in the next breath, we are told, "Well, you are falling short, and you need to do more." This manipulation leaves us in an impossible position. We are effectively told, "You need to be perfect, and you need us to get you there."

It is a great lie when someone steals something and then sells it back to us. We are all inherently valued by God. God never created a single person that he does not love. We all have a direct channel to communicate directly with our Creator. We should never have to seek another's approval or follow another person's directives to learn God's will. Anyone who attempts to insert themselves between God and us is delusional, fraudulent, or worse.

We all inherently have a right to our inner voice and value, and we should never let anyone override our inner voice or label us as "falling short" or "unworthy." We all have worth, so no organization should ever say differently. Freedom is our right, but a toxic organization will make threats against those who dare question or leave. In any form, ecclesiastical abuse can cost our time, money, and peace of mind.

CHILD TRAUMA

Every child deserves to grow up in a safe and secure environment. Child abuse inflicts the worst trauma, as it is an act of violence against society's most defenseless people caused by adults who have a responsibility to protect them.

Child abuse is defined as causing or permitting any non-accidental harm or threat of injury to a child. It also includes communication or transaction of any kind which humiliates, shames, or frightens a child, as well as any act of omission which fails to nurture or provide for the proper upbringing of a child. A child of any age, sex, race, religion, or socioeconomic background can fall victim to child abuse and neglect.

Emotional child abuse includes verbal harm, mental harm, or any psychological maltreatment. This includes acts by, or neglect from, parents or caretakers. This can consist of yelling or screaming, using extreme or bizarre forms of punishment such as confinement in a closet, being tied to a chair, or any other threatening act. Less severe actions, but no less damaging, include name-calling, belittling, or habitual blaming.

Neglect is the failure to provide for the child's basic needs, including physical or emotional needs. Physical negligence includes not providing adequate food, clothing, housing, medical care, or responsible supervision. Educational neglect includes failure to provide appropriate schooling or a healthy social life.

Psychological abuse consists of the lack of emotional support and love, improper treatment to a child, spousal abuse, and drug and alcohol abuse, mainly when it allows the child to witness drug or alcohol abuse, sexual activity, or another inappropriate event.

Sexual abuse is any inappropriate sexual behavior with a child. It includes fondling a child's genitals, making the child fondle the adult's genitals, intercourse, incest, rape, sodomy, exhibitionism, and sexual exploitation. Commercial or other exploitation of a child refers to the child's use in work or other activities for the benefit of others. This includes, but is not limited to, child labor, child pornography, or child prostitution. Physical abuse is the infliction of any bodily injury upon a child. This may include burning, hitting, punching, shaking, kicking, beating, or otherwise harming a child.

Child abuse, in any of these forms, can have a devastating impact. Victims often live in fear, shame, and secrecy and lose trust in others. They can lie, retaliate, or be alienated from others. Their sense of self-worth and self-esteem can be damaged and, the effects can linger and hinder their psychological and social development and their ability to have healthy relationships. They can have trouble fitting into society and act in a way that does not meet social norms in school or within the community.

Victims of sexual or child abuse need to be very aware of the difference between guilt and shame. Guilt is the result of doing something wrong, and victims of sexual or child abuse did absolutely nothing wrong. Shame is very different; it means we are "ashamed" of what someone else did. Victims of child abuse have done nothing wrong. Any suggestion otherwise is nonsense.

Victims of abuse must know that the effects of a single moment of hate can devastate a lifetime; however, a moment of love can break lifetime barriers. Dr. Martin Luther King, Jr. said, "Darkness cannot drive out darkness, only light can do that. Hate cannot drive out hate. Only love can do that." As society becomes less based in fear and shame, and more based in love and healthy practices, it is more acceptable for people to talk openly about the abuse they have suffered and expose those who are responsible. This is healing for victims.

If you are the victim of child or sexual abuse, please see a reputable, licensed mental health professional. There is an army of people who can help. Furthermore, these types of abuse are often crimes and should be reported to the police or other law enforcement officials.

WELCOME TO THE CLUB

In 1890, a boy named Harland came into the world on the wrong side of town in Henryville, Indiana. His parents' strict, Christian upbringing forbade drinking, smoking, gambling, or whistling on Sundays.

When he was five, his father died. His mother got work in a tomato cannery, and the young Harland was left to look after and cook for his siblings. When he was 10, Harland began to work as a farmhand. He quit school at 13, and, by the time he was 17, he had lost four jobs.

Harland moved forward. At the age of 18, he got married and started a job as a railroad conductor, but ultimately, he failed at that job too. A year later, he became a father, but a year after that, his wife left him, taking their children with her. However, they would not divorce officially for another 36 years.

He joined the army, but that didn't pan out either. He simply did not fit in. Undaunted, he applied for law school but was rejected. He then took a job as a steam engine stoker, followed by an insurance salesman, but he failed again in both endeavors.

Harland, trying to make ends meet, took a job in a small café as a cook and dishwasher. Later, Harland ran a gas station in Corbin, Kentucky. To make ends meet, he began to cook and sell meals for weary travelers who stopped by. But when the highway junction in front of his restaurant was relocated, he lost his business.

He had failed again.

At the age of 65, he retired and applied for social security.

One day, he received his first social security check, but it did not sit right with him. It seemed to him as if the government was saying that he couldn't provide for himself. Depressed from a long string of failures, Harland decided to end his life. He sat down under a tree to write a will dividing up his meager belongings, but instead, he wrote what he wished he had accomplished with his life.

The continuous stream of failures had taken its toll.

THE SCIENCE OF HAPPY

Science reveals that happiness is determined by three key factors. While approximate, half of happiness is determined by genetics and DNA. If our biology is deficient, there are prescription drugs that can bring this into balance. Only 10% of our happiness is determined by our life circumstances. The remarkable insight from this research is that our daily habits and activities, determine 40% of our happiness. Our activities and habits are under our control. Thus, it is essential to select those that bring the most joy.

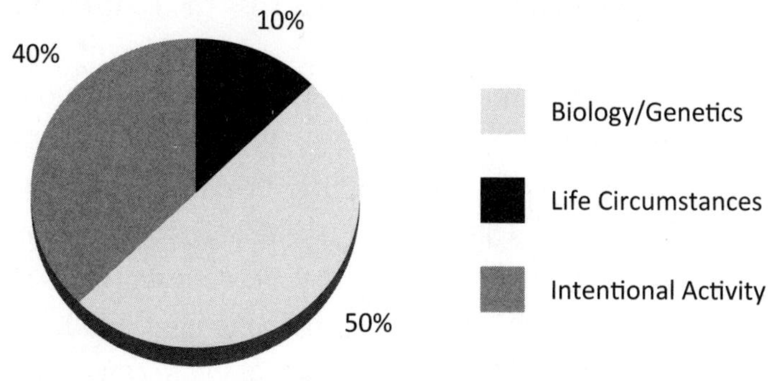

Lyubamirsky, S., Sheldon, K. M., & Schkade, D. (2005). Pursuing happiness: The architecture of sustainable change. Review of General Psychology, 9, 111-131.

The hurt that trauma causes often motivates people to do things in a way that they would never have considered before. Trauma invades our lives and cracks open our assumed reality. When we have lost it all, we may feel like there is nothing left to risk. Consequently, it can open the door to a host of new possibilities that had been lying dormant.

Harland started taking a brutal assessment of his life and then thought carefully for hours about sorting it all out. Of course, there were regrets and lots of them. As Harland wrote, he began to see that there were many things he still wanted to do. Although he had failed at a string of careers, his inner voice reminded him of his passion for cooking. Until then, cooking had just been a side thing. However, as Harland untangled his life, it occurred to him that this is what he was born to do. He could cook better than anyone he knew.

Harland forgot about his suicide plans and used some of his social security checks to buy ingredients for his favorite recipe. He fried up some chicken and went door to door, selling it to his neighbors. After a few months, Harland was encouraged by his neighbors' responses—they loved his chicken. He decided to expand his fledgling business. He began to travel around the country, convincing restaurants to let him cook chicken for their employees. If they liked it, he would sell them his "secret recipe" in exchange for a few cents on every chicken they sold. He wandered back and forth across the country, always looking for suitable restaurants.

It was a difficult life. Harland lived out of his car and ate meals from friends whenever he could.

But it worked. By 1964, he had more than 600 restaurant partners.

Soon he sold franchises of his delicious chicken recipe, and an empire exploded. At the age of 65, he was broke and wanted to end it all. Yet when he listened to his inner voice, his passion ignited, and Kentucky Fried Chicken (KFC) was born. Rather than taking his own life at 65, Colonel Sanders peacefully passed away at the age of 90 as a multi-millionaire and a well-loved icon known around the world.

When trauma hits, like it or not, we join a new club. However,

Harland is only one of the hundreds of thousands of stories of post-traumatic thriving. Each story is unique, but there is a consistent theme for each one of them, and that is precisely what we are after.

Our Stories of Sorting It Out

DEBBIE

Debbie knew that to fully heal from the trauma she experienced, she needed to be honest with her children.

Before her husband's death, their family hadn't addressed their deepest feelings, choosing instead to keep their genuine emotions close to the vest and focus only on the "positive." Debbie realized that, as a family, it was time to reveal what they were experiencing. It was the only way to move past it. It was the only way to help her children face what had happened.

Debbie shared with them all the sordid details of everything she knew. It was excruciating for them to hear. They loved their father, and it was hard to reconcile the man they knew with the one she described. But Debbie pressed on, knowing it would give them the best shot to move forward.

As a result, she found they each had their inner strength, which allowed them to go deep and take a real look at the situation. Her children challenged her with the hard questions, and she was glad to answer them.

JOHN

John not only lost his daughter to radiation poisoning from the nearby nuclear testing, but he also had to navigate a path to getting restitution from the United States government, which had conducted the tests. He had to sort out all of his options and decide to walk away or stand up and fight.

SUSAN

Susan and Peter lost their home because of an unexpected event that they had no control over. Then, they went through the stressful experience of suing one of the biggest cities in the United States.

Through it all, they did what they had to do to keep going on with their lives. Susan kept producing award-winning television shows. Peter confronted his reality and started to explore rebuilding his business in the hopes of making it more substantial and successful than ever.

Where did they get the strength to keep moving forward? Why were they able to keep pushing forward with the lawsuit despite how difficult the City made it for them? She did not know. She gives the credit to God, and she is also deeply grateful to Peter for his strength and their friends for welcoming them into their own homes with open arms.

SHAD

Shad, the Vietnam veteran, had suffered—and survived—his trauma during the war. The "rap groups" he started while working for the Veterans Administration Hospital in Los Angeles were the first of their kind in the entire country. The idea behind them was that Shad, or a veteran volunteer, would just "rap" or talk with the veterans and find out what the VA could do to help them.

Through the rap groups he led, Shad spoke with hundreds of Vietnam vets on the streets, beaches, and in the canyons of LA. Many of them were using drugs or were homeless. Shad observed that those who seemed to be most impacted by their Vietnam experience shared similar behaviors such as hypervigilance, deep suspicion, unpredictable emotions, and difficulty with relationships.

GERI

Geri had to review and sort out all of her life options. Everything, she believed, was a choice. Yes, she had cerebral palsy, which sometimes felt as though it were a cloak that she would never be able to take off. She could feel sorry for herself and withdraw, or she could stand up and walk. She chose to stand up and walk.

And on occasion, when other people reacted with uncertainty about her disability, she turned to humor to defuse their discomfort. People loved her sense of humor—her quick wit and self-deprecating humor made people laugh and feel more comfortable. She loved people and enjoyed making them laugh. Perhaps that was something to explore more in-depth.

TANYA

Tanya had so much to sort out. Her older sister was dead. She was trying to come to terms with the knowledge that she would never again share a hug, a phone call, a family holiday, or even a smile with her again.

While working through those emotions, she was also battling her anger at OJ. He had ripped her sister out of her life and radically altered the future of her family. He also damaged the lives of his own children.

And speaking of the children, Justin and Sydney, Tanya loved them immensely and wanted to support them through their grief. They were just children and really didn't understand what had happened. They moved in with Tanya's parents, and Tanya knew she needed to be there for them, even while she struggled with her loss.

Then there was her frustration and anger at the news media, which had callously turned the murder and trial into a salacious spectacle. Tanya, her parents, and her siblings were followed everywhere. The media wanted interviews with the family. It was difficult to grieve and move on because every time Tanya or another member of her family stepped outside, microphones were shoved in their faces. TV trucks with enormous satellite dishes and boom microphones camped on the main highway behind her home, congesting the street and annoying their neighbors. When they pulled out of the neighborhood, camera crews chased them just to get a shot of them leaving. When they had conversations in their home, they brought their voices down to near whispers because they were afraid those gigantic microphones aimed toward them would pick up what they were saying.

There were also practical issues facing the family. They had to manage Nicole's estate and make sure that her wishes were followed. It was an overwhelming task in the face of all the chaos that surrounded them.

JC

Shortly after arriving at the prison, JC witnessed an inmate get stabbed repeatedly over a $125 drug debt—yes, it's nearly as easy to get drugs in prison as it is in the outside world. As gunshots rang out from the prison guard's assault rifle, JC was instructed to get down onto the ground. As he lay face down in the mud, breathing heavily, stiff with fear that a bullet might find him, and chaos all around him, JC had an epiphany. He thought, *"Is this really what I want my life to be like?"* The answer was a resounding *"No!"* He may have been in prison, but he wasn't going to allow his life to be defined by violence and fear.

LEO

Leo continued working on the family farm, even though he had lost an eye. Sports were out of the picture. There was a college in town, and it offered lots of classes over a spectrum of subjects. Leo needed to sort out the best path forward for him, and that meant going to college, where he could put his mind to work.

JOE

When Joe, whose father had been killed by the mobster John Gotti, found out that his wife was pregnant, he decided to become a different man. He wanted to be the kind of father to his child that he had always wanted his father to be to him. He didn't want his child to go through the trauma of visiting him in prison—or worse, having no father at all.

Joe was blessed with a son. He focused all his energy on being the very best father he could be. He and his wife soon had another son, and life was looking better than ever.

Despite his new outlook on life, however, Joe still had to deal with his anger and depression over what had happened to his father. His internal struggle carried over into his external life, and his marriage suffered.

In 1992, after all the crime, death, and mayhem he had caused over the years, John Gotti was finally going to prison. In the preceding years, Gotti had been nicknamed "Teflon Don" for his ability to elude conviction. However, now Gotti was convicted on 13 counts, including murder and racketeering. He was sentenced to life in prison without the possibility of parole.

During the trial and conviction, John Gotti was everywhere it seemed. His name was printed in every newspaper and on the lips of every television news anchor, night after night.

Since Joe's dad had been the kill that turned Gotti into a "made man," it was impossible for Joe to escape hearing about his father's death. And invariably, when Joe's father's name was mentioned in connection with Gotti, the newspapers printed the photo of Joe's dad lying dead on the ground, blood pouring from a bullet wound.

Unable to take it anymore, Joe finally approached the editor of the local newspaper. He brought a photo of his dad with him when he was alive and asked the editor to use that image instead of the one of his father dead on the ground. The editor decided to interview Joe about what it was like to grow up knowing that John Gotti had killed his father. The next day, Joe was on the front page of the local paper, shown holding a photo of his dad.

The headline read, "My father can rest in peace."

ERICA

Erica, being chased down by the Nazis for the "crime" of being Jewish, had to sort out whom she could trust and whom she could not trust. Because the Nazis were disorganized, she had successfully escaped from them several times. She still had no idea where any of her family or her fiancé were. The Nazis may have been disorganized, but she could only count on that for a short time, as they were getting more systematic. The war was only heating up, and she needed to focus on a long-term plan.

TOM

Tom had received many college scholarship offers—full rides to top schools—but he had ignored them in favor of training for the Olympics. Now that the Olympics were no longer an option, he reached out to some of the schools that had sent him letters of interest. It turned out that all the colleges and universities who had contacted him months ago still wanted him.

For the first time in a long while, Tom began to feel excited about the future. After all, he was a world-class athlete, which meant many other opportunities were open to him.

MY STORY

The day of my heart surgery had come. My mom took me to the hospital on a Sunday afternoon. On the way out of the house, my sister thought she was funny when she said, "Well, I hope you don't come back as a vegetable."

That hurt, but it was just the beginning of the humiliation. I was checked into a small room at Loma Linda Medical Center. Everyone was friendly, and each one had a specific job to do. First, a man told me he needed to shave my genitals. I was not even sure what that meant, so he told me to drop my drawers. Since I was only 11 years old, his job was pretty easy. Then came a guy who had a hose and a bucket, and he was there to clean out my bowels. I laid on my side on a plastic sheet while that hose went up to my rectum. I had no idea that my intestines were so long. That hose was pushed in further and further. Having my mom there to watch was even more demeaning.

I just felt disgusting, gross, and dirty. A parade of people kept coming in to give me pills to swallow, inject medications into my arm and butt, and explore every inch of my skinny, shaking body. I wondered, as many who are in the middle of a traumatic experience do, just what had I done wrong to deserve this? I felt the shame of it all.

Nobody had prepared me for any of this. When they were all finished, I just laid there thinking, "What just happened to me?" There was a lot to sort out.

CHAPTER 8

Experiment

Those who heal experiment with self-care and new life skills.

LET'S EXPLORE

THE EXPERIMENT STAGE is about self-discovery. Of all the stages, this can be the most exciting and fun as we go on this adventure. Here we understand that the road to recovery is about establishing a game plan for a fulfilling life. In talking with thousands of people who have successfully navigated through their traumas, there are innumerable potential solutions. It is exciting to explore and find the ones that work for us.

We are all different, and trauma is not a competitive sport. One person's trauma from divorce may be another's great relief. One's natural disaster may result in a shrug of the shoulder and an insurance claim, while for another, it may devastate their entire core and sense of home. Yet, eventually, everyone will have to step into the role of being truly traumatized.

Because trauma itself is raw and ugly, it can bring out negative emotions. When we are in that state, it does not take much to tear down things around us. Deconstruction is cheap and easy, while, on the other hand, construction takes authentic work and effort. Decades of investment in a home can be lost to a fire in 20 minutes. A life's worth of plans built upon a significant other who turns out to be abusive can be shattered in an instant. It is easy to take good health for granted, but it can unexpectedly all go away with disability or disease. Trauma can undermine our life's story when our assumptions, hopes, and dreams are crushed.

Some people never recover, which magnifies the tragedy.

When trauma does occur, rudely and unexpectedly, it often cuts at our very foundation and disrupts our fundamental realities. Our core beliefs that the world is fair, good, just, and beautiful are shattered in a second. When our lives do become a train wreck, we ultimately have four choices:

1. Traumatize others
2. Remain traumatized
3. Heal
4. Use the energy from the trauma as fuel for doing something remarkable

Indeed, 58 to 83 percent of trauma survivors report that after ultimately healing, they experience a positive change. This research is not about those who fail in the process or return to their baseline and survive. This book is about those who not only heal, but thrive. The trauma is the fuel that takes them to an entirely new place.

Identifying the path to thriving provides a roadmap. We can then move through trauma and can move forward with more clarity. Reaching the thriving stage often requires imagination, considerable time, healing, effort, and professional support.

To be fair, although no fault of their own, some folks do not ever recover from their trauma. The injury was too great. But there is good news. Intense academic research reveals that once people navigate through the rubble, many can climb out of the hole and do just fine. Some excel even better than they would otherwise have done. Remember the saying,

"What doesn't kill you only makes you stronger." Albert Einstein stated, "Logic will take you from A to B. Imagination will take you everywhere."

As we travel this road we call trauma, let's look at some new and creative ways to think about it.

KINTSUKUROI

In Japan, there is an art form called "kintsukuroi," which means "to repair with gold." When a ceramic bowl breaks, rather than throwing it all away, an artist will not only fix it but also use gold or silver to bond the pieces together. Rather than hiding the cracks, they accent them with precious metals to reveal a new, beautiful design. In the end, it is not considered to be broken; instead, it is only seen to be different than initially envisioned. The bowl is now better, stronger, and more beautiful than before. Kintsukuroi is an attitude, a way of life that embraces our cracks, flaws, and imperfections.

Trauma can deliver the fuel to take us higher than we ever imagined. Injury is often a catalyst that brings life into better focus and brings us closer to God, a higher power, and humanity. We discover that we are more durable than we ever imagined. When we have been kicked in the teeth, betrayed by someone we have loved, taken advantage of by another, or have admitted that we have made a big mistake, we discover an inner strength we never knew we had, and we thrive.

To thrive, we might overhaul our language when the time is right. For example, words like "victim," "sucker," "abuser," and "offender" may trap a person by giving them a fixed identity and a label that becomes permanently attached. It is better to separate identities from behavior. The "victim" might better be called a "survivor," "harmed person," or "harmed party." "Offender" may be better referred to as the "responsible party" or the "person who committed the harm." A "crisis" could be called a "reconstruction" or "awakening." When you are ready, start being creative in how to relabel your trauma.

The process is a struggle. It is rinse and repeat. Yet mistakes are the price we all pay for a full life. Abraham Maslow, an American

STRESS REDUCTION

Stress is measured on a continuum from 0 to 10. When stress levels are between 0 and 4, we are using our brain's frontal lobe and are able to solve problems. Between a 7 and 10, our brains no longer think rationally. The following stress reduction techniques can help you to relax and prevent your emotional brain from reacting in a way you might later regret.

STRESS LEVEL

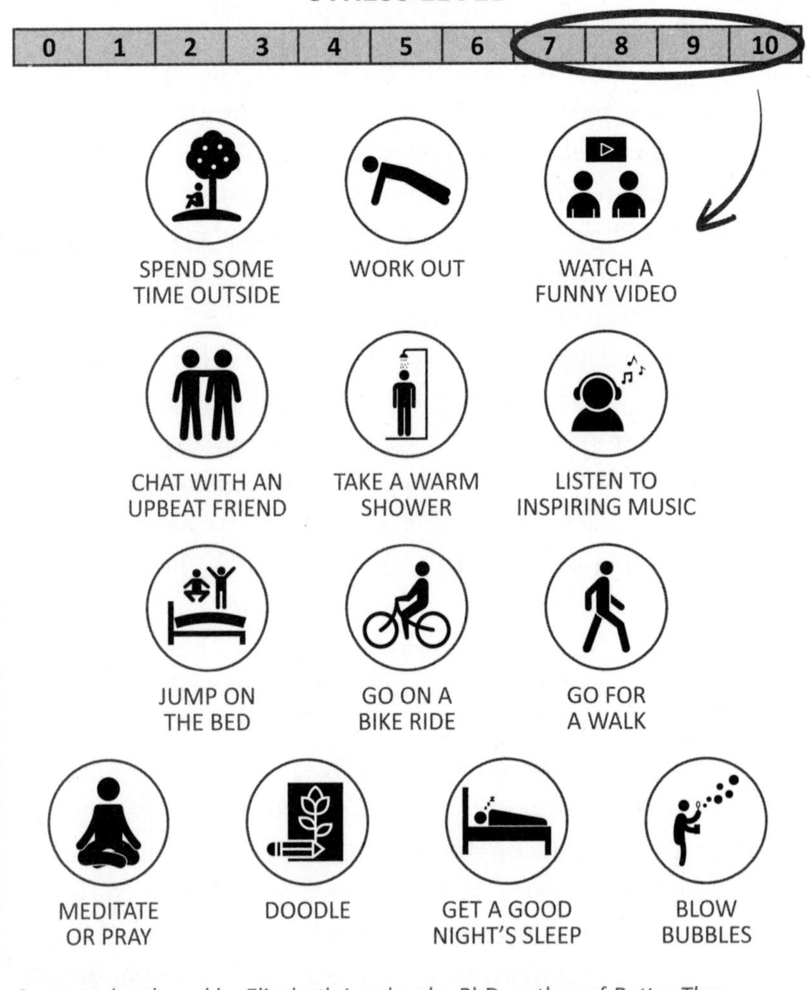
0
1
2
3
4
5
6
7
8
9
10
SPEND SOME TIME OUTSIDE
WORK OUT
WATCH A FUNNY VIDEO
CHAT WITH AN UPBEAT FRIEND
TAKE A WARM SHOWER
LISTEN TO INSPIRING MUSIC
JUMP ON THE BED
GO ON A BIKE RIDE
GO FOR A WALK
MEDITATE OR PRAY
DOODLE
GET A GOOD NIGHT'S SLEEP
BLOW BUBBLES

Concept developed by Elizabeth Lombardo, PhD, author of *Better Than Perfect: 7 Steps to Crush Your Inner Critic and Create a Life You Love*. www. ElizabethLombardo.com. Used with permission.

psychologist, noted that the most important learning experiences in human life are tragedies, deaths, and other traumas that force people to take new perspectives. We test new life skills and treatments by experimenting and learning how to practice self-care and love. We are most like the universe or our Creator when we are creative. Make time for an adventure.

GET GROUNDED

One day, I was on a small plane that made a connection from Phoenix to South Dakota. As I sat down in my airline seat, I heard a voice say, "Hey, are you Randall?" I looked up and said, "Yeah. Sean?" Sean and I had been colleagues about 15 years before, and we had not seen each other since. But there he was, seated right next to me.

It was exciting to see Sean. He is a dynamic, intelligent, thoughtful guy who has a gift for creativity. Of course, we caught up on what we had both been up to.

Then Sean looked at me and said, "You know, Randall, you will not believe it, but I have been to prison." This came as a surprise, and I replied, "Wow. So, tell me about it!" Sean then told me about how he joined a board of directors for the Insight Prison Project, a non-profit group that reaches out to both victims and offenders and helps them heal from their trauma. I listened intently as Sean told me about going into San Quentin and the mind-blowing stories of life transformations.

Sean could see on my face how interested I was, and he said, "Hey if you want to go to prison too, I can get you in!" The whole thing seemed fascinating, so I said, "Jesus taught that we should visit those in prison, and I have never done that, so I am in." I promptly submitted my paperwork and was approved by the San Quentin warden to go inside.

One of my most profound lessons came the first time I went inside a prison as a volunteer. Just getting inside was an ordeal. First, I had to fill out a lengthy application and submit it to the warden. I found it ironic that I had to pass a criminal background check to get into prison. When I was first scheduled to go, our trip was abruptly postponed because there had been an escape attempt, and the prison went into lockdown.

After several more weeks, the day finally came when I was allowed inside. I met a colleague in downtown San Francisco, and we drove over the Golden Gate Bridge to the prison. I was told not to wear anything blue or red, as those were gang colors. This left me few options, so I wore khaki trousers and a white polo shirt. I was not allowed to bring in a cell phone or any personal belongings except for my driver's license. We met by the guard office where my ID was checked against prison records. Then we walked down a very long, concrete walkway towards the prison itself.

There, another guard checked my ID a second time, searched me, and put an invisible stamp on my wrist that could be viewed only under ultraviolet light. Then, I was escorted into a steel cage where the door was locked behind me and, for a third time, a guard checked my ID. When we passed this barrier, the steel door on the other side was unlocked, and we went into a small holding area where we finally swung open an old, massive iron door.

Suddenly, we stood in the prison courtyard. As we walked across the concrete, I looked to my left and saw a large building that housed California's death row. We veered to the right and into a small room with cinderblock walls and plastic chairs. Then, in came the inmates, all dressed in blue pants and smocks, similar to what doctors wear. They smiled and seemed happy to see us, and, being new, I introduced myself. They all went out of their way to make me feel at ease. The chairs were arranged in a circle, and I took a seat. I had no idea what to expect.

After I received a brief welcome, we closed our eyes. We went through a meditation exercise here called "grounding" to avoid any perceived conflicts related to religion. I cannot explain the feeling I had when I realized that I was grounding for the first time, sitting between two men convicted of murder; however, these men were so docile and kind.

Over my entire life I never heard much about meditation, nor did

I have any real interest in it. That all changed that morning. I did not know it was coming. I was already uncomfortable just being there, but in combination with grounding, the experience felt surreal.

The process was simple, more of a focused breathing exercise. All we did was sit comfortably in our chairs, close our eyes, take a few deep breaths, wiggle our toes, feel our knees, feel the pressure of the chair underneath us, wiggle our fingers, relax the muscles in our face, listen to our breathing, and open our eyes again. This is one of the most common and basic forms of grounding, simply becoming aware of internal sensations such as breaths, aches or pains, or heart rates.

When I first began volunteering at San Quentin, I was startled to learn how much the inmates practiced and enjoyed grounding as they worked to transform their lives. For virtually every prisoner I met, it was a daily practice. It is something a person can do anywhere that costs nothing and offers considerable benefits.

I learned that grounding or meditation was a foundational part of a comprehensive program that took convicted felons and created a profound change of heart. Looking back, my first encounters with grounding were stunning because I started to make the connection between this practice and the calmness of the men in the room. The experience was so profound that I found myself repeating it when I got home.

MEDITATION, HARVARD STYLE

One day, my cardiologist told me about a Harvard neuroscientist, Dr. Sarah W. Lazar, who learned about meditation by accident. Dr. Lazar had injured herself while training for the Boston Marathon. Her physical therapist told her to do stretching exercises, so Dr. Lazar took up yoga.

Dr. Lazar told reporter Melanie Curtin, "The yoga teacher made all sorts of claims that yoga would increase your compassion and open your heart, and I would think, 'Yeah, yeah, yeah, I'm here to stretch.' But I started noticing that I was calmer. I was better able to handle more difficult situations. I was more compassionate and open-hearted and able to see things from others' points of view."

Her curiosity piqued from this experience, Dr. Lazar researched the scientific literature on grounding or meditation and found evidence that the practice reduces a host of problems, such as anxiety, depression, and stress. It also improves the overall quality of life. Intrigued by both her own experience and the academic literature, Dr. Lazar began doing neuroscience research at Harvard Medical Center using brain scans.

Dr. Lazar compared people who had meditated for years with others who did not meditate at all. The study showed that those who meditated had increased gray matter in several regions of their brains, including the areas responsible for decision-making, auditory senses, and memory. In a stunning discovery, the neurological team found that 50-year-old people who meditated had the same amount of gray matter as those who were 25!

In another study, Dr. Lazar put people who had never meditated into an eight-week program. In only two months, the brain scans showed a measurable thickening in several regions of the brain responsible for learning, memory, emotions, and empathy. Their brains also revealed shrinking of the areas associated with stress, anxiety, fear, and aggression.

I now have a six-inch-thick binder containing scientific studies published on the topic of grounding and meditation. Hundreds of university studies from schools such as Harvard, Stanford, Brown, Yale, UCLA, and Vanderbilt provide verifiable and reproducible studies that demonstrate its effectiveness. Meditation has a host of verifiable benefits. These include cognitive thinking skills, mental health, workplace performance, relationships, and overall well-being. It also measurably reduces chronic pain, mind-wandering, fearful memories, PTSD, and symptoms related to childhood adversity. Meditation and mindfulness also improve character and ethical behavior.

Mindfulness, or the mind-body connection, simply means being present in the moment or changing our focus of awareness on the present. We are not thinking about the regrets of the past or the anxiety over tomorrow; our minds are in the here and now. This means that we do not dwell on times outside of our current control but rather maintain a clear focus on what is happening and suspend concerns about whatever has happened or might happen. We take life one day at a time. In a mindful state, we function in sync intellectually, spiritually, and emotionally. Furthermore, it means that we are aware of our physical state—our body and our breathing. We are motivated to deliberately pause before reacting to situations in terms of what we say, think, feel, or do.

The process of critical s*elf-reflection* involves us carefully slowing down and evaluating our situation and the events and circumstances that got us here. By intentionally focusing and taking time to reflect on an event, many things can happen. We can differentiate between the event and our *interpretation* of the event and evaluate what went wrong and what went right. For example, if we were in a car crash, the event could be all the actual logistics of what happened, but our interpretation could be filled with the emotions. Perhaps a wrong turn caused the accident, but we were fortunate to get excellent medical care.

We can reflect upon how much control we have over a situation and all our possible choices and outcomes. We can note the difference between acting out or simply walking away. From this evaluation, we can see how to respond better going forward. We can use the experience to generate growth that otherwise might not have been.

While the effects are powerful, meditation is deceptively simple. We mainly focus on our breath. Some add mantras to their reflection, such as thinking of the word "so" while inhaling and "hum" while exhaling. Some use audio-guided meditations or create visualizations to expel unwanted energy or to focus on an abstract concept, such as compassion. Blank-mind mediation is another form where we dismiss all thoughts from our minds. Some sit, some stand, some walk, and some perform yoga poses or exercise forms as in tai chi or qigong.

Generally, it takes 5 to 30 minutes a day to see results, but some suggest it only takes six deep breaths to get the benefits of grounding. It may be better to have two shorter sessions, one in the morning and the other in the evening, rather than one long one. It is best not to meditate right after exercising and to be sitting rather than lying down. Several apps can help develop this habit.

The most significant benefits come when we meditate daily, even for a few minutes. By eliminating distractions and being mindful of "now," we connect with our inner voice. If a distracting sound or thought comes to mind, we don't judge it but gently observe it without judgment or bring our minds back to our breathing.

Meditation lays the cornerstone for transformation. While simple, it resets our brain waves, letting the calming effects ripple out to fill our entire day. It offsets what eastern civilizations call "monkey mind" or what Westerners call "anxiety."

When I was facing another round of heart surgery, my cardiologist explained how brain waves work and prescribed 10 minutes of meditation a day, every day. I just sat comfortably, closed my eyes, and focused on my breathing. It was easy, and my blood pressure dropped considerably. As demonstrated from the cells in San Quentin to the great hall of Harvard Medical School, meditation is shown to heal broken hearts.

For many who are healing and in transformation, grounding, combined with prayer, is a vital component. As faith is a personal journey, prayer looks different to different people. However, prayer and grounding are two different things. Grounding is focused breathing and an effort to listen to our inner voice, while prayer is not focused on breathing but, instead, communicating with God or a higher power. How that is combined is a personal choice.

Almost without exception, every thriver I know has a ritual of some kind, often in the early morning. They meditate, but they may also pray, stretch, read something inspirational, have a good coffee, or plan out their day. They may journal or write "thank you" cards. This is a time to contemplate. As Mark Twain once said, "The two most important days in your life are the day you are born and the day you find out why." We may shift focus and say that we are not humans having spiritual experiences; we are spiritual beings having human experiences. Whatever it looks like to you, this "daily quiet time" helps us identify and focus on our "why" in life.

We all want to climb a mountain. Meditation and our morning rituals allow us to connect with our inner voice so that we end up climbing the right mountain.

PHYSICAL EXERCISE

There are hundreds of medical studies that demonstrate a link between exercise and mental health. In 2018, Dr. Ralitza Gueorguieva of Yale, along with her colleagues, published one of the most extensive studies analyzing the responses of 1.2 million adults who participated in a Centers for Disease Control and Prevention (CDC) survey. The peer-reviewed research found that for those who exercise, the number of poor mental health days dropped by more than 40 percent.

Exercise alters how the brain functions to improve mood and lower depression, stress, anxiety, and emotional concerns. Researchers concluded that three to five 45-minute exercise sessions a week delivered optimal mental health benefits. On the other hand, it is possible to exercise excessively and cause harm, just as it can be harmful to do anything in excess. Researchers speculate over-exercising relates to obsessive behavior, causes exhaustion, and lowers one's mood. These issues are best discussed with your medical doctor.

I have a fantastic cardiologist, and when I was facing high blood pressure problems, her first step was to prescribe medication, meditation, a low-salt diet, and aerobic exercise.

When she handed me the list, I quickly boasted that I had walked five miles that morning! She just looked at me and shook her head sadly. She said, "I'd rather you run for 10 minutes than walk for an hour. A heart needs ten minutes of aerobic exercise a day to stay healthy, and do not tell me that with your busy schedule, you do not have ten minutes a day!"

Honestly, I had not run in decades. The first time I did, it was not pretty. I hated it so much that I marked the specific spot on the sidewalk that I could stop the very moment that I hit my ten-minute mark. I did it day after day. When I traveled, I put my running shoes into my luggage, went to the little hotel gym, and got on the treadmill for 10 minutes and not a second longer. I did it day after day because I was trying to avoid having heart surgery.

Then, a small miracle happened. One day when I got to my spot on the sidewalk, I felt so good that I spotted a stop sign down the street and ran to it. I was shocked when I used my car's odometer and found out I had run a total of 1.2 miles. I thought, "Well, if I can run 1.2 miles, maybe I can run 2.1 miles." So I did. I started running and walking my entire five-mile loop.

Then, a bigger miracle happened. One day, I ran the entire five-mile loop, and the next day, I ran 10 miles. I was now a runner, something I never expected to be at the age of 60. I still do it, and I love it.

Physical exercise can stop, and even reverse, the effects of stress. Running, jogging, taking a brisk walk, practicing yoga, tai chi, or qigong all combine deep breathing and fluid movements that bring mental focus and induce calm. To heal, we must look in the mirror and care for our physical appearance. As we exercise, even moderately, our glow and energy will return.

Trauma is not just all in our heads; it affects us in real and measurable physical ways. Be aware of your body, breathing, and sweaty palms, as it is all interconnected. To heal, we must learn how to relax both mind and body and know that when we exercise our body, we are also exercising our soul.

THERAPEUTIC AND MEDICAL TREATMENTS

Take control. The emotional pain from trauma is real. Stay calm and take it slow. Explore, experiment, and consider your options. Fortunately, there are wonderful treatments available in the areas of both mental health therapy and the field of medicine.

In the field of psychology, there are many therapeutic remedies such as cognitive behavioral therapy, dialectical behavior therapy, exposure therapy, cognitive processing therapy, eye movement desensitization and reprocessing, prolonged exposure therapy, hypnosis, and others. Biofeedback uses probes to monitor our body functions, such as heart rate, muscle tension, breathing, perspiration, temperature, and blood pressure. It also shows us how our thoughts connect with our body. Neurofeedback is similar but uses sensors to monitor our brain's activity. Be sure to discuss all of the options and possible treatments with a licensed health care professional whose goals are to improve symptoms, teach coping skills, and restore self-esteem.

We may or may not need medications, but if we do, exercise could possibly eliminate the need or reduce the dosage. There is no shame in medically supervised medications, as prescription drugs can stabilize our emotions, elevate our optimism, and help us feel normal again. Some can help stabilize our reactions enough to limit nightmares and flashbacks. Various prescription drugs adjust our brain chemistry and control for depression, fear, psychosis, or anxiety. Doctors often start with medications that balance our neurotransmitters, such as serotonin or norepinephrine (SSRIs and SNRIs). Doctors may also prescribe "off label" medications, meaning that the manufacturer did not ask the FDA to review drug studies for the use he or she is prescribing. These may include antidepressants, monoamine oxidase inhibitors, antipsychotics or second-generation antipsychotics, beta-blockers, benzodiazepines, or others. Drugs may not eliminate all of the symptoms but can make them less intense and more manageable. If we use prescription drugs, they may help us stabilize our emotions, but they do not cure trauma. For example, Prozac increases serotonin levels and suppresses the emotional pain. Yet the underlying trauma remains.

Through research, new medicines are being developed daily, but they should never be taken without a prescription. Medications often need to be recalibrated to obtain optimal dosages and may have severe or unpleasant side effects. The hope is to find medicines that solve more issues than they create. A drug doesn't have to make you feel spaced out or like a zombie and should not create unpleasant side effects that lead to more significant problems. Work with your doctor to find the proper medication and dosage for you.

As we move forward, we try a variety of new things. We can attack our symptoms with medical treatments, but therapy, grounding, meditation, self-compassion, and self-care attack the trauma. Some try yoga, meditation apps, relief balms, CBD oils, or lotions that can be applied to your face. Some find it easier to connect with an animal before connecting with a person. Some simply go fishing when they feel stressed. Some get involved in theater and express their inner traumas through outward roles. Others create music that expresses their feelings. We can structure an internal map, sometimes called "mind maps," where we diagram our lives and experiences.

The point is to test and explore our options, take action, and create space from the things that trigger us. Rest is always important. Our best requires rest. We cannot keep "charging" without "recharging." Balance is also good. On a trip to India, I learned a Tibetan proverb, "The secret to living is to eat half, walk double, laugh triple, and love without measure." I cheat a lot on the eating, but trying out a variety of self-care techniques is essential in a harsh world.

As we experiment, the idea is to fill up our lives with healthy stuff. For years I taught a life skills class at our community's homeless shelter. I told the homeless men and women that I could not care less about their vices and bad habits. The hundreds of homeless people I have met do not want a handout. They simply want to take back their power and be able to take care of themselves. I do not want to waste a minute talking about their vices. I tell them about the "full glass theory" and that life is like a 24-ounce glass, just like we have 24 hours in a day. I tell them to simply start filling their glasses with new, fresh, and healthy habits. I ask them to take a walk on the beach, go to the library and read a book, sit on a rock and meditate or pray, or eat an apple instead of the piles of cookies that come in every day. I tell them to try out new habits, knowing that the old bad habits will be displaced and eventually go away as we do this.

Trauma can tell us what we are against, but to move forward, we must identify what we are for. We define the life we want and then use the fuel from the trauma to go for it. Those who wish to beat the odds push through the tough times, and to reach the top, we must appreciate the sheer force of daily habits and practices. Face the truth and be quick to break negative habits while adopting new ones. A great secret is that the human brain sees real and imagined images the same, so we must choose positive thoughts, actions, and habits. Over time, and with relentless persistence, these new daily rituals, practices, and habits add up and create a whole new life.

TRAUMA TREATMENT ALTERNATIVES

"Containment" is a term used by mental health professionals to describe activities that help manage trauma, including daily habits or routines, social support, self-regulation, and life structure. We must spend time building containment before going too deep into processing trauma. We eat a bite of the pie, not the whole pie at once. We can write thoughts down and then put the paper away, knowing that we will address it when ready. We can write lists of what we want to accomplish or of what we expect of others. The simple act of writing things down can be healing as we memorialize all the stuff floating around in our heads. We can later use those lists and work through the items one at a time. We can work at our own rate. Everything is appropriately contained so that the process is somewhat compartmentalized. Trauma is messy, and this is more realistic than shoving the whole pie down at once.

If you can name it, you can tame it. In other words, we are better off if we can communicate to ourselves, our therapist, or our trusted person what emotions our trauma is causing. Trauma treatment inherently presents a dilemma as there is a need to discuss and process trauma, yet this can activate traumatic memories and PTSD. To process trauma, we must deliberately think and talk about it, yet this must be balanced with containment and self-care. Therapists can be vital because they can monitor and moderate the process, creating progress at a healthy pace.

Severe traumas should always include a trauma therapist. Here we form an alliance and a relationship with a therapist that must be founded upon trust and acceptance. We should have an active collaboration and a sense of shared goals.

Having attachment or relationship issues can make it challenging to connect with a therapist at first. However, as we do, we learn how to express ourselves, listen, trust, confide in others, resolve conflicts, and ultimately build a good relationship. In turn, this can serve as a model or bridge to building other healthy relationships.

As one suffering from trauma, you have full permission to interview your potential therapists and choose for yourself. You are not obligated to stay with the first therapist you see. If it doesn't feel right, you can keep looking. If you choose to move on, all qualified therapists are trained not to take it personally.

A key aspect of understanding trauma is understanding that our bodies cannot tell the difference between physical and emotional danger. Our brains respond with the same fight-flight-or freeze responses. In any of these situations, our minds react as if we are in imminent physical danger, which in turn yields physical symptoms.

Regardless if our trauma is physical or emotional, we must address the physical fallout to heal. We need to address the body's responses and calm the hormonal and electrical reactions. When we are struggling with healing from our traumas, we must remind ourselves that our bodies are doing exactly what they are supposed to do. They are protecting us. We need some help processing and recalibrating nature's emergency alert system.

Ultimately, we want to walk through the triggers and memories and know that they are in the past and we are no longer in danger. Working with a qualified therapist, we can process the trauma so that it becomes what it needs to be and no longer remains a part of our story that we need to avoid.

Many techniques can calm our bodies and minds. Breathing is at the top of the list. This is not just a whim, fad, or theory. Deep, diaphragmatic breathing techniques are remarkably effective as they signal to our bodies that we are no longer in danger. In other words, breathing can reverse the damage, rewire our neurological responses, and heal past traumas. Knowing this, instituting a deep breathing habit in our daily lives is possibly the single most crucial technique in healing from our wounds. Today there are many meditation apps for our smartphones.

As we work through this, we must build our appreciation for being in the present through our "mindfulness." As we progress, we will discuss several coping mechanisms. It is not practical to do all of them, so consider those that may work for you. There are a host of possibilities in dealing with stress, anxiety, and trauma. Ultimately, we need to experiment and find what is right for us.

PULLEY PULLEY

In 2007, I visited Kenya and Tanzania with my son, Steven. We loved seeing all the African wildlife, such as, lions, elephants, zebras, and giraffes. One day, we drove through a long stretch of southern Kenya. I looked to my left, and Mt. Kilimanjaro came into view. It was majestic. Mt. Kilimanjaro broke through the clouds and rose above the horizon as the dominating feature, the looming masterpiece of rock taking up what seemed like an impossible place in the sky. I thought to myself, "Someday, I would like to conquer that."

As I stared, our guide mentioned that it was the tallest mountain on the African continent and the tallest non-technical climb in the world. It was kind of a whim, but the idea was there where it quietly grew.

That opportunity came in 2019 when my buddy, Sam, was spending the weekend at our house. He told me that he was going to climb Mt. Kilimanjaro and invited me to go with him. Having done no homework and with only this old, romantic notion in mind, I quickly said, "Sure!" Now I was on the hook.

As I started my climb, there were lots of people milling around at the trailhead. In front of us was a thick rain forest. Out of nowhere, an older local man came up to me and whispered something that haunted me during the entire trek. He said, "Remember, this is not a physical thing. This is all mental. In Africa, we have a phrase, 'pulley, pulley.' It means, 'Just take it easy, go real, real slow.' You will make it if you remember 'pulley, pulley.'"

As I started the climb, I realized what a fool I had been. I was in way over my head. There I was, 60 years old, and just six months earlier, a heart surgeon had told me that I needed surgery. Besides, I'm not a mountain climber. I beat myself up mentally telling myself that I could not do it. The terrain was steep. At times it was damp and cold, and at other times, it was too hot. Many places look like Mars. The altitude made our heads spin.

I woke up, every day, freezing in a damp sleeping bag. On days when we climbed up the face of thousand-foot cliffs, it sure seemed physical to me. But something told me that he was right. I just mentally focused and must have said "pulley, pulley" a thousand times.

The biggest battles are those between our ears. Our internal struggles are the fiercest. As my buddies and I climbed the mountain, we saw scores of young people descending in defeat. We saw others coming down in stretchers. We were told that many young people do not follow the locals' advice, arrogantly charge up the mountain too aggressively, and burn out.

But we just kept plodding forward, "pulley, pulley." We took it real, real slow, and cut ourselves a lot of slack. As we hit an altitude above 12,000 feet, we were literally taking baby steps because of our lack of oxygen, but we just kept going, "pulley, pulley." Slow. Slow. Slow.

As we work our way up the mountain of recovery toward the summit of thriving, just take it a step at a time. Just go slow and remember, "pulley, pulley." As you experiment, take it slow, and do not feel pressured to do what does not work. "Experimentation" is precisely that. Take what you like, and leave the rest. Permit yourself not to eat the whole pie. Be open and give something a try, but allow yourself to decide what is beneficial and what is unhelpful. Good therapists use the word "curiosity" a lot. Experimentation is an exercise in curiosity and exploration. We have the choice to approach otherwise tricky issues with a sense of "curiosity" instead of dread.

STRESS vs. CALM

Our bodies are wired with two separate nervous systems, called the parasympathetic (calm) and sympathetic (stress) systems. We have the ability to switch "on" and "off" with our simple choices. The "calm" activities are medically proven to switch the body from "stress" to "calm." Remember that these activities flip the switch "on" for "calm" feelings, but they do not address the underlying issues. However, we can make better decisions in a calm state.

CALM

Parasympathetic Nervous System

Deep Breathing: Taking in long, deep breaths, and exhaling slowly—such as in grounding, meditation, or yoga exercises—flips on the "calm" parasympathetic nervous system

Laughter: Watching funny videos, telling jokes, or comedy clubs are outstanding for flipping on the "calm" switch

Bio Rhythms: Listening to your body telling you when you are hungry, angry, lonely or tired—and taking action—brings "calm"

Socializing: Getting together with people we enjoy brings "calm"

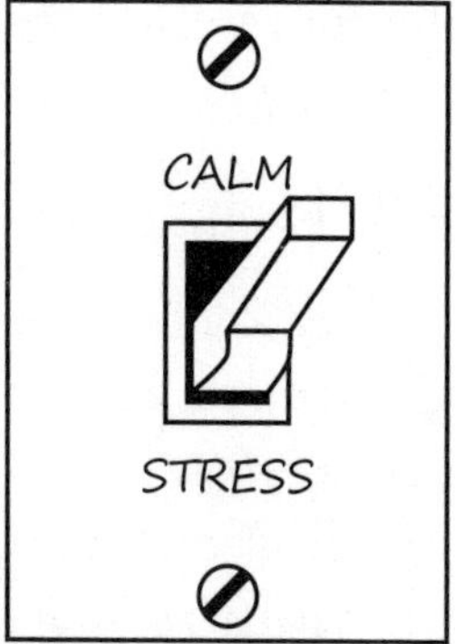

STRESS

Sympathetic Nervous System

Trauma: Any trauma can flip on the "stress" reactions, where adrenaline is pumped though our veins and we have the "fight-fight-freeze" reaction

Horror Movies: Watching any frightening movie will switch on the "stress" switch

Procrastination: Putting off essential tasks will increase "stress" levels

Arguments: Picking an argument will flip on the "stress" switch

Rigid thinking does not work well here. Of course, explore other options besides what we are discussing here. There is a world of therapies, religious practices, advice, self-help, vitamin plans, and so forth. The reason why there are so many is that some things work for some people but not for everyone. Permitting ourselves to explore can be empowering and freeing.

Progress is an iterative process. Healing, growth, and self-improvement are a similar process. We make small attempts where we will both succeed and stumble. Then we take the lessons and try again or try something new. As the shampoo bottle instructs, first rinse, then repeat.

This is what some mean when they say life is not a destination. It is a journey. There is no single day when we finally graduate from trauma. There will always be new layers to uncover and new levels of understanding and growth. The experimental phase is where we are alive and engaged in life. This is where we practice self-leadership.

You rinse and repeat until you find the solutions that connect with you.

ADVERSE CHILDHOOD EXPERIENCES

Harvard researcher Dr. Andrea Roberts notes a connection between adulthood problems and three or more childhood traumas, called "adverse childhood experiences" (ACEs). Children have no control over the people who harm or neglect them. These unprocessed ACEs remain in our memories somewhat as shrapnel within our own mental war zone. Often, the toxic people who caused the trauma condition us to believe the problem isn't the abuse itself but is instead our reactions to their abuse. This is a lie. The damage is real. It can take only seconds to hurt a child but years to heal.

While we might look fit and healthy, our inner, unprocessed ACEs are an invisible wound that weakens our immune systems and manifests as an illness or addiction. These include sleeping disorders, anxiety, substance abuse, memory loss, or chronic pain. For example, approximately 90 percent of those who have eating disorders or are incarcerated have experienced childhood sexual abuse.

Many within the medical community are coming to terms with the connection between ACEs and physical illnesses and addictions. Indeed, some physicians believe that the term "addiction" should be replaced with "ritualized compulsive comfort-seeking." Daniel Sumrok, MD, has stated that addictions are a normal response to childhood traumas, just like bleeding is a normal response to being stabbed. As such, addictions should be normalized, not criminalized or classified as "sin." When we treat people with addictions with respect, we are setting the stage for getting at the real problems and healing. Blame and shame do not work. Better-trained medical doctors know this landscape, listen carefully, prescribe group therapy, and integrate ACE science into their practices.

This is not about becoming a perfect human being. It is about discarding some of the myths we have come to believe. Rohit Barman said, "Both empaths and narcissists suffer from early developmental trauma. The difference is that narcissists are essentially weak and succumb to selfishness and hate, whilst empaths rise above their torturous past and continue to be there for humanity." When we realize that addictions, or "ritualized compulsive comfort-seeking" are normal reactions to our unresolved childhood traumas, we can pop our head up out of the water, catch our breath, and get the proper help we need.

Our Stories of Experimenting

DEBBIE

When Debbie's husband died, she discovered something unexpected—some of the people who came to her rescue were people whom, before the suicide, she barely knew.

It was an eye-opening experience for her. Naturally, when her husband died, she expected her church community to rally around her; however, they had not. Instead, they left them go adrift. But soon enough, other people stepped forward to fill the gap.

One couple, in particular, became like family to her. They visited almost daily and supported her through the worst of times. They sat next to her while she spent hours scrolling through the computer, looking for more evidence of his secret life. They held her when she cried. They took her out to dinner and parties. They made sure she had an invitation to every event they did. In their company, Debbie learned to laugh again.

Debbie also found an excellent therapist to help her—and one for her children as well. Just as important, Debbie continued her education. She was close to earning her therapy license. She could not let this situation throw her off her life plan.

Debbie resumed her internship. She found the experience

cathartic. As she helped other people, she realized she was helping herself.

Debbie also fully embraced her love for remodeling. She had a creative eye for design and the ability to visualize how a home might look if a wall were removed, a window was added there, or a ceiling was raised by a foot or so. She bought a fixer-upper in a nearby city and devoted her spare time to remaking it to match her vision. Once it was completed, she sold the home at a tiny profit, bought another, and repeated. She found pure enjoyment in remodeling homes. The process allowed her to express herself creatively while making a home more beautiful and livable for the family who would buy it.

And even as she flexed her creative muscle by buying, renovating, and selling homes, she continued to work toward her therapy license. In time, she reached her goal. Life had begun anew.

JOHN

John started on a novice law degree and explored all his options to hold the US military responsible for detonating a nuclear bomb that left his daughter dead. He took a boat into the city and talked to government officials. He started reading legal books. He started going out fishing again with his friends. John and his family had been knocked down cold with the loss of their daughter but were going to honor her memory and get back on their feet.

SUSAN

During the aftermath of the landslide and all that entailed, Susan's stress and anxiety went off the charts. The sense of hopelessness and fear—not knowing how it was ever going to work out, the never-ending anxiety—was the worst part. She could not work through it on her own.

Always a believer, Susan turned to the Bible for comfort and guidance. She had, of course, read it before, but now, she read it differently. She looked to the Bible to help lift her out of her fear. It did. The Bible's passages, proverbs, and stories reassured her and helped her understand that no situation is permanent and that there is always, always hope.

Susan spent a great deal of time praying, as well. In addition to helping her connect with God, prayer also helped her get in touch with herself. The months after the landslide were stressful, to be sure—but they were also very introspective. She began to examine her attitudes about life. She thought about how this situation had helped her draw upon a deep well of internal strength that she wasn't aware she had.

People talk a lot about how they change after a disaster or a severe illness. That was true for Susan. Through self-reflection and prayer, Susan began to recognize what wasn't working in her life—and she began to develop a plan to fix it.

SHAD

Throughout the 1970s, Shad made incredible inroads on how to serve Vietnam veterans more fully. He immersed himself in their world. He began pioneering treatment techniques for what would later become known as post-traumatic stress disorder.

Shad found, in his research, that some employers refused to hire Vietnam vets because of their characterization in movies and television as unstable timebombs about to explode. In 1974, he worked to develop and lobby for the Vietnam Era Veterans' Readjustment Assistance Act, one of two federal laws that expressly prohibit discrimination against veterans who are returning from active service and entering the private employment sector.

In 1979, he designed and co-authored the Vet Center Outreach Program under President Carter (Public Law 96-22). There are now more than 300 Vet Centers in the nation, including Hawaii.

He began to document what he saw. This data would later form the basis for a new diagnosis—post-traumatic stress disorder. In 1980, after fighting alongside other forward-thinking mental health specialists to define the symptoms from which returning Vietnam vets suffered, the American Psychiatric Association added PTSD to the third edition of its *Diagnostic and Statistical Manual of Mental Disorders (DSM-III)*. Although controversial when first introduced, the PTSD diagnosis has filled a significant gap in psychiatric theory and practice.

GERI

Geri learned at a young age that she had the gift of humor. It drew people to her and made them feel comfortable around her. Geri's idol as a kid was Carol Burnett, and she observed how Carol had the talent to get people to laugh with her, not at her. Geri started a correspondence with Carol when she was a young teenager. To Geri's sheer delight, Carol wrote back and encouraged her always to go after her dream of becoming a comedic actress like herself. She explained that there was no guarantee that Geri would become a professional comedian, but she would never know unless she tried. Those powerful words from Burnett were just the shot in the arm Geri needed to take the journey into show business. And, as fate would have it, Geri began honing her craft on amateur nights at The Comedy Store in Hollywood. She was scared but knew she had to find the courage to take her life to another level.

TANYA

Tanya had suffered so many losses in her short life. By the time she was 30, she had lost eight friends and her sister. Another significant loss was still to come. In 2004, her fiancé, suddenly and without warning, canceled their wedding just four days before it was to take place.

Tanya had been strong and survived so much. This final loss was one too many. She could not withstand it. Shortly afterward, she attempted suicide.

She survived, thanks to the intervention of her sister, Dominique. The journey back from the suicide attempt was a long one. She spent 10 days in a hospital and then another two and a half months in an in-patient behavioral health facility. It was there that she finally had the support to begin to deal with her complex, layered trauma. Her therapists guided her as she did the difficult work of exploring her emotions and learning coping skills.

After she was released, Tanya continued with outpatient therapy. She experimented with different coping mechanisms. Cognitive-behavioral therapy proved hugely helpful. Another thing that helped was, at last, having an actual diagnosis: general anxiety disorder and major depressive disorder. This diagnosis enabled her doctors to prescribe the right medicine to help alleviate her symptoms. At last, Tanya was able to truly move forward.

JC

In California, when a person first arrives at the prison to begin serving his or her time, the Initial Classification Committee interviews each person to determine what kind of job they will have in prison. It could be in the kitchen serving food or the laundry issuing out prison clothing. JC recalls some jobs being better than others. Because of his intelligence and his record of good grades, JC requested to work in support services as a teacher's aide. The role suited him perfectly. He enjoyed helping others learn to read and understand simple math concepts.

Equally important, JC decided that he would take every class, seminar, and training that the California prison system offered. JC had always loved school. As a child, he bounced from apartment to apartment and foster home to foster home. School had been the one place he had always felt safe. His teachers always liked him, and he felt a sense of pride being seen and validated for his intelligence.

Another thing he loved about school was that school was where he knew he would get a meal. The sad fact of JC's young life was that he didn't always have enough to eat. There were peanut butter sandwiches, spaghetti, and even pizza at school, and little containers filled with Jell-O or fruit.

In prison, he found that taking classes gave him the same feeling. The prison classroom was a safe space amid a violent world. In a way, it felt like coming home.

LEO

Leo, who lost his eye as a child, had a wide range of interests. He liked woodwork and metalwork and even made some of the tools for the farm. He was curious, so at school, he would sit on the lawn and watch the men who were constructing an auditorium. The workers took notice and invited him onto the job site and showed him brick and cement work, electrical systems, framing, and plastering.

Leo experimented with everything he could find. He loved tinkering with radios and record players. He just knew that the more he explored with construction and manufacturing, the better he felt. Leo studied everything he could find to learn more.

JOE

If Joe's life were a movie, the ending scene would be a shot of the newspaper story with Joe's picture, holding up a photo of his father, under the headline: "My father can rest in peace." It would have been a sweet, tidy ending.

However, situations in real life rarely wrap up so neatly. People are human, and triumphs can be fleeting. Joe had still never dealt with the trauma of losing his father so brutally. He was still angry and filled with rage.

In an attempt to self-medicate, Joe sank into a life of drugs and alcohol. His marriage faltered, and then died. His sons grew distant. He became addicted to opioids, and before he knew it, he was deeply immersed in the criminal world. And as his old friend, Detective Ray Taylor, had warned him many years before, if he did not straighten up his life, he would be arrested.

And he was. Like his father, Joe ended up in prison. He lost everything. It was all gone—his family, the business he had built, all his money, and his self-respect.

In prison, though, Joe was able to receive therapy for the first time in his life. During one session, the therapist simply laid his hand on Joe's shoulder and asked kindly, "What's the matter?"

And Joe finally was able to cry.

ERICA

While spending long periods hiding from the Nazis, Erica would find scraps of paper and coal from the trash, and then she would draw for hours on end. She loved to create pictures of her favorite childhood memories in the mountains and the city.

TOM

Tom accepted one of the top offers and invested his energy into competing at the college level. He discovered that college-level shot put gave him an immense amount of satisfaction. He loved being part of a college team. The camaraderie was terrific. Plus, there was less pressure on Tom as a college competitor versus an Olympic contender, so he was able to loosen up a bit and have fun.

Rather than spend every spare moment at practice, Tom started going out with his new friends. He discovered he enjoyed activities like going to the movies and parties. In his previous, hyperfocused life, Tom always viewed such activities with derision. Now he realized that having fun—yes, *fun*—was an essential part of life.

MY STORY

At the age of 11, on an early Monday morning, I was matter-of-factly woken up by a group of nurses and doctors telling me that it was time for the surgery. They started injecting me all over the place and inserting IV tubes into my arms. Then, they had me scoot onto a gurney and wheeled me down the hall through double-swinging doors into a large, tiled operating room. I saw a wall full of X-rays, and when I asked whose they were, they said they were mine. I was surprised by all the people who were there. Apparently, this was a big deal.

The surgeon himself, Dr. Arnold, was busy with instruments and barking out orders, but he was kind to me. Behind his surgical mask, I could see the focus in his eyes, but I felt there was a smile for me.

Suddenly, there was a lull. Dr. Arnold asked, “Well, are you ready?” I had some wit even at that age, and I replied, “I don’t have much to do; the question is, are you ready?" He just kind of chuckled and said, "I'm going to inject this into your arm. I want you to count backward from ten to zero. He said, "Nobody ever gets to zero." I took that as a challenge and told him, "Just watch me. I'm going to do it!" I started counting, "10 ... 9 ... 8 ... 7."

The next day, I woke up in a deep, deep mental fog. I immediately asked, "Is it over? Is it over?" My parents and others kept saying, "It's all over! You did great! It's all over!" During my recovery, this happened again and again. I would wake up, ask some questions, and then pass out.

It did not feel like it was over. It felt more like it was just beginning. And I was right. My voice had a strange, high-pitched sound caused by the nerves stretching when the doctors entered my chest cavity. I was told that my voice would return in a few weeks. In the meantime, I talked like Donald Duck.

I was informed I would be in the hospital for two to four weeks. However, they later said that since my surgery went exceptionally well, I could go home sooner. One doctor said that it was the smoothest surgery he had ever seen. The plastic pieces they expected to put into my body were completely unnecessary, and they were able to make the repairs with surgical stitches alone.

From there on, it was a testing of new skills, coping with the pain, and figuring out how to get back on my feet. I spent the entire summer recovering. After weeks, my regular voice suddenly came back, and I got stronger and stronger. Yet I was shocked with the length of my scar, which stretched from under my arm all around to about the middle of my back. They had to do this to get to my heart.

Afterward, every time I took my shirt off at the beach, I had to brace myself for a barrage of stares and questions. The worst was when a girl named Karen, who was a year older than me and was one of the prettiest girls in school, invited me to her house to go swimming. She was kind of curious, but it was cool. However, I never really got over the embarrassment of it.

CHAPTER 9

Acceptance

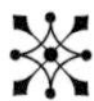

We must accept reality and have the character to hold ourselves and others accountable.

ACCOUNTABILITY

HEALING TAKES A HEAVY DOSE of humility and listening to trusted sources. Jesse Lyn Stoner, the founder of Seapoint Center for Collaborative Leadership, said, "If you are so right that you can't even listen to another point of view, you're probably wrong." Those who have suffered trauma can be in a vulnerable position. We want to consider another perspective, but also we need to be careful. It is always easy to say yes and then experience a nightmare getting out of your commitment. Navigating a trauma means being thoughtful about who we ultimately spend time with, what we accept, and what we reject.

Traumas are among the most profound challenges of life. They are ugly experiences and expose who we and those around us are. We will never know who we are until our fears, insecurities, and limits are tested. Many friends and family members may run to our aid, but we may be surprised when some of them run away and strangers rush to help. We quickly see whose love is conditional or unconditional.

As the smoke clears, our healing requires the courage and character to hold ourselves and others accountable.

Acceptance can come willingly or be our only way out when we are cornered. It can occur when our defenses are stripped away or we willingly lower our guard so we can face raw reality. David Brisbin said, "How valuable is a faith that is dependent on the maintenance of ignorance?" How valuable is anything dependent on ignorance? We need to face reality, where we begin to stabilize and start to see some hope.

On the one hand, we can only come to acceptance when we lower our defenses to face reality. Acceptance is the opposite of ignorance, which can come in many forms. Denial and other forms of ignorance, including willful ignorance, are coping mechanisms or "defenses." These have their place in the early stages of trauma, but prolonged denial is a barrier to acceptance.

The trauma may strip us of our dignity and sense of self-worth for a while, yet acceptance is where we show we are survivors, and we begin to take power back. We shift into a deliberate and new state of mind of self-awareness, self-care, and self-respect. As strange as it initially seems, healthy people accept and embrace their trauma. They talk about it, sometimes openly but certainly with a confidant. They face the problem almost as if it is an interesting problem or puzzle to be solved.

REBOOTING THE BRAIN

Resetting the brain's natural mechanism allows us to heal and improves the quality of our lives. These techniques address our "parasympathetic" body functions, which conserve energy as it slows the heart rate, calms and heals. The starting point is to become more aware of our breath. Slow, deep breathing helps in resetting our brain's reaction to past trauma. When we take large, deep breaths, our brain waves recalibrate to the regular, relaxed alpha and theta waves. Just using this simple technique helps reset our brain circuitry. More profound meditation can generate gamma waves associated with universal love for humanity, altruism and the higher virtues, and heal the brain from trauma. It is deceptively simple, but it works.

Trauma recovery takes time. Embracing our trauma, being aware of our breathing, and engaging in an intelligent course of action helps to stabilize our lives and allow the healing to continue.

STRESS VS. TRAUMA

Stress and trauma are related topics. Any injury may cause anxiety, but not all stress is traumatic. The primary consideration is the duration of the "stress reaction," which is that feeling of panic often accompanied by a racing heart rate and heavy breathing. A family member dropping a glass of milk during a nice dinner can cause stress; however, a few days later, that incident may be forgotten. On the other hand, if a child is lost at the mall and not found for hours, driving by that mall later could create the same stress reactions of despair and panic. Many mental health professionals believe that if this "stress reaction" lasts longer than four weeks, it may be considered trauma and result in post-traumatic stress disorder.

Both stress and trauma have similar symptoms; however, stress goes away while trauma remains. The brain is stuck in the fight-flight-freeze response and there are real physiological reactions such as high blood pressure, increased heart rate, and hormones pumped into our bloodstream that initiate the stress fight-flight-freeze reactions. These stress hormones can assault our bodies, which, over time, can lead to excess sugar levels, a compromised immune system, strokes, heart disease, and even cancer.

A wide variety of events can cause trauma; what creates trauma for one person may be different for another. Just like physical traumas, some heal quickly and successfully, while others linger or cause permanent disability. Emotional injuries are similar in some regards. A seminal study was conducted between 1995 and 1997 by the Centers for Disease Control and Kaiser, where they studied 17,000 patients to research the impact of childhood trauma on physical health. The Adverse Childhood Experiences (ACE) study revealed that the more adverse the childhood experience, the higher the susceptibility to a host of diseases in adulthood, including substance abuse, depression, heart and liver disease, the risk for intimate partner violence, early smoking, and early sexual activity and corresponding STIs. Stress responses can result in a host of problems, including depression, agitation, irritability, rage, violent outbursts, feelings of being unsafe, not trusting others, hypervigilance, overly controlling or obsessive behaviors, taking extreme risks, difficulty concentrating, feeling unlikable or lovable, eating disorders, self-mutilation, or suicidal thoughts.

ACHIEVEMENT PATHS

Many potential achievements begin with an intrigue of a situation that grows to excitement. After the "buy in," conflict and setbacks often set in. There is an inevitable critical juncture where the real level of commitment is determined and often one's character is tested. If truly committed, the individual will look at the situation more sensibly, implement a paced, day-to-day effort and over time obtain genuine achievement. If one fails at the critical juncture, then disillusionment or even hostility can set in.

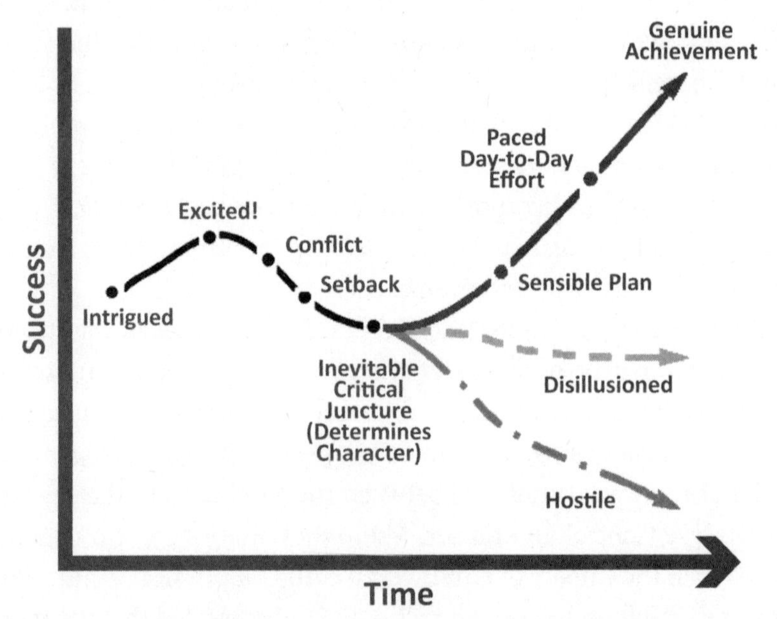

CAN WE STILL BE FRIENDS?

Trauma transports our lives and souls into an uncomfortable, embarrassing, and humiliating world, which crashes the status quo and motivates new growth. Acceptance of another's routine choices, while perhaps being different than our own, is a sign of emotional security. Accommodating others' preferences is, however, altogether different than a situation where someone choses to cross the line and be abusive.

Abusers leave a trail of destruction. Of course, they rarely take responsibility for the trauma they cause. When confronted, they are fond of saying something to the effect of, "You can leave me, but you cannot leave me alone." Once exposed, all abusers want to be left alone. Yet to heal, we must accept the reality of the situation, and that means having the courage to directly confront our abusers or any others who had a role in our trauma. In some cases, this means reporting a crime to the police or other authorities, filing a civil action, blowing the whistle at work, exposing the situation, or simply sticking up for ourselves.

Abusers are bullies with unprocessed traumas, but this is not an excuse to let them get away with it. We cannot tolerate that. We must make a choice to stand up against the abuse, or get away.

Recently, a friend invited me to attend an Alcoholics Anonymous meeting. While I am not an alcoholic, I wanted to learn about alcoholism and support him. The meeting was at a Hindu monastery, which was also a new experience.

The meeting fascinated me. The level of wisdom, authentic spirituality, and humor were astounding. One comment that stood out was from a woman who had been sober for decades. She helped another woman through the recovery process, but this other woman had relapsed and started drinking again. The sober woman did not get mad at her. She did not call her names. She did not shame, guilt-trip or lecture her, and she sure did not shun her. When she found out this woman had gone off the path, she simply asked her, "Can we still be friends?"

Acceptance does not mean we go along to get along. We can still stick up for ourselves when we need to. It means that we gently accept what is rather than deny it or shame others. This response is vividly demonstrated in healthy lives and organizations; those who take a divergent path should not be shunned. They should be unconditionally loved.

Acceptance helps us see reality clearly so that we can make the decisions and act on what is real rather than on what we wish were real. Acceptance can open the doors to new possibilities, even if they are difficult.

Our Stories of Acceptance

DEBBIE

Years passed. At last, there came a moment when Debbie simply accepted the situation for what it was. She does not recall the exact moment that it happened, but she knows that she just felt better one day. At last, she was able to move on.

When the day came for her to take her final tests to become a therapist, she had a whole team of people cheering for her. People were invested in her moving forward. After she passed the first test, she got a little tearful, remembering that she would soon know if she passed the second one.

After she passed the second test, she realized it signaled to the community that she was now an official marriage and family therapist. She had, indeed, taken a giant step forward.

So much had happened; there had been so much chaos. So much loss. So much trauma. And though Debbie still had moments of pain and a sense of extreme loss, she knew that she had made it through—and was a better person because of it.

JOHN

John lost his daughter to radiation poisoning when the US government decided to test nuclear weapons across the lagoon from where they lived. Not only that, but the land that his ancestors had lived on for hundreds of years was now contaminated.

John thought carefully about what he had to accept and what he would not accept. John was forced to accept all this and move his family to a safe place. However, John refused to accept what he could change, and he would not accept that he could never return to the islands he loved.

SUSAN

When a landslide crushed their home, Susan had to accept that nothing would be the same again. "But," she thought, "was that really a bad thing?"

Susan and her husband were handed a new chance to fulfill their dreams.

For years, they had entertained daydreams about making big changes. They had wistfully discussed "what ifs." But ultimately, they were settled into their beautiful home and a life of contentment. And at this stage in their lives, did they need to be out chasing dreams? Besides, things were fine; why take a risk at something that wasn't a guarantee?

But when their home was destroyed, their whole perspective shifted. They no longer had the beautiful home that served as the anchor to their lives. They had also discovered that they really could get through anything together—the landslide and the subsequent lawsuit against the City had proven that. Tentatively, they started to talk about all the other dreams they had put on the shelf. And they began to talk about possibilities.

"I know what debilitating grief feels like," says Susan now. "And I also know what it feels like to push through it. I had no idea that I had that energy in me. I took a dive, but it is powerful to know that we have the ability to not only survive but to thrive."

SHAD

Shad had long ago accepted that the trauma he endured in Vietnam had strengthened his life's purpose. On his first night overseeing the MASH unit, half the soldiers who came in died. It took him years, but he turned the trauma into an opportunity to help other Vietnam vets overcome their own trauma.

Shad accepted his reality and the bleak future of Vietnam War veterans. He was proud of the work that he had done with them. Now the entire world had to accept that their trauma was real, as he had been instrumental in the American Psychiatric Association's decision in 1980 to officially recognize post-traumatic stress disorder as a real disorder.

But there was still so much work to be done. The VA was trying to take over some of the programs he had founded and put their spin on it. Also, Shad learned that, on average, Vietnam vets lagged far behind their peers in many measurable benchmarks, such as homeownership and having families of their own. Many vets were dependent on drugs and alcohol to silence the memories of the war that haunted them.

In 1985, Shad started a non-profit foundation specifically to help Vietnam vets. Initially called the Vietnam Veteran Aid Foundation, its name was changed in 1991 to the National Veterans Foundation. Shad founded the organization specifically to help veterans and their families who were enduring a crisis or had a critical need for help.

GERI

Geri grew up with the physical disability of cerebral palsy; she had to accept that from birth. But she was also starting to accept the fact that, while her body was disabled, her mind was sharp as a tack. And the mind is a terrible thing to waste. Her physical disability may have set limits on some things she could do, but Geri's mind had no limits—she was free to create whatever she envisioned for herself.

Geri accepted what she could not control. She had been given extraordinary gifts that she never took for granted. She felt that she had to honor her spirituality, and she has always been aware that, in part, she is a vehicle to bring joy and inspiration into the world. Even in times when she did not feel particularly joyful, she understood that making others feel good also went a long way to making her own life more joyful.

TANYA

Each time Tanya lost someone she loved, she had to accept and come to terms with the new situation. Accepting the reality did not lessen the pain, but it did help her move forward from each loss.

When Nicole was murdered, that process was especially difficult. She had not just lost a beloved sister—she had also lost the life she lived before, the life where she had an intact family. She had also lost her innocence in a way. Murder—actual *murder*—did not happen to people like her sister or families like hers. Murder happened to someone else. Tanya had to accept that, yes, murder had impacted their family and that life would never be the same.

JC

With his court appeals exhausted, JC had to accept that enduring prison life would be a fact of life for years to come. The choice was going to be what to do with those years. He chose to educate himself. Over the years, he took self-help courses, anger management classes, and vocational training opportunities. He learned word processing, electronic repair, and how to fabricate metal. He helped keep the prison up and running as a maintenance worker.

During this time, JC also began going to church. Church was a new experience for JC. As a child and teenager, he had only gone to church sporadically.

But something had changed. It started when he was in juvenile hall, waiting to be transferred to an adult facility. One day, he heard gospel music playing over the speaker system. He had never heard anything quite so soul-stirring. He was enchanted. He started going to the church services while in juvenile hall.

In prison, he attended services more regularly. He had a friend on "the outside" who wrote him frequently. A devout woman, she ended each letter with a verse from the Bible. JC noticed this but initially did not think much of it. Over time though, the verses began to intrigue JC, and he started looking them up in the Bible to learn more. In time, he found he was reading the Bible regularly and learning more than he ever thought possible. His passion for Christ grew.

Eventually, JC was ordained as a Baptist pastor in prison and began giving sermons of his own.

LEO

One day, Leo just sat down and accepted that he had a glass eye and was nearly deaf, and that was the way it was. But he also had to realize the fact that he had one good eye and that hearing aids and lip-reading would allow him to pursue his dreams.

JOE

After he was released from prison, Joe indeed was a changed man. The change had not been caused by losing his family and all his possessions, although that was deeply painful. The change was caused by Joe finally being able to accept his father's death. The anger and the depression were gone, replaced by a heartfelt desire to be a better person and to help others.

For the last 19 years, Joe has been a drug and alcohol interventionist for teens and adults.

Over the years, he has helped thousands of people acknowledge their addiction and accept treatment. He has a 50 percent success rate in helping people overcome their issues, which is higher than the industry average. He does not advertise; all of his clients are word-of-mouth. He receives several phone calls a day, asking for help.

What makes Joe so successful as an interventionist? He jokes that he is the "junkyard dog" of intervention—he never gives up. Joe's job is to make sure that his client gets transported safely to a rehab center. He often confronts them with an ultimatum, "Look, you are going. You can go in the trunk of my car in handcuffs, or, if you co-operate, you can go on the car seat next to me." Joe is a big guy, and they always choose the seat.

On the drive, Joe shares a powerful lesson, his own story. Joe understands that at the root of nearly every drug and alcohol problem, there is deep trauma and pain. They know that he understands. They know that he accepts them for who they are, just as he accepts himself.

As he sees it, Joe's responsibility is to help people work through their trauma so that they overcome their addiction and become a better version of themself.

ERICA

Erica had to accept the fact that Hitler was a madman who had taken her entire family to the concentration camps. She had to admit that she had to hide to stay alive. But she also realized that all wars eventually end, so finally, there would be a light at the end of the tunnel.

TOM

Though Tom was happy as a college athlete, he wished, in his heart of hearts, that he had been able to go to the 1980 Olympics. He truly believed that, given a chance, he really would have brought home a gold medal.

Tom continued through college and graduated *magna cum laude*, the second-highest honor college graduates can achieve. He probably could have made *summa cum laude*, the highest status, but he had loosened up a bit on his relentless drive towards perfection and spent some of the hours he might have spent studying actually having a bit of fun with his friends.

MY STORY

In May 1977, I had one of the worst days of my life. I was at Troy High School playing tennis with my friend Kevin. We had gotten pretty good. Our high school basketball and football coaches were playing on the court next to us, and they noticed.

Right in the middle of our game, Coach walked right up to me, and he said the most devastating thing I have ever heard, “Hey, Bell. I remember when you tried out at summer camp for basketball. You were okay, and I was bummed when I found out you had dropped out. I see your athletic skills today, and I’ll tell you something. If you had stuck with it, you would have been one of my starters today.”

Coach’s comments pierced me to my very soul. At that moment, I held myself fully accountable for maintaining a lie that somehow, I was defective because of my childhood heart surgery. The problem no longer existed in my heart; it existed only in my head. I had believed a lie that I was limited. I completely blew it by not playing high school basketball, but I was determined never to let my heart surgery hold me back from anything again. Ever. I had now passed the threshold of acceptance and was ready to move forward.

CHAPTER 10

Awareness

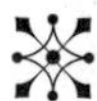

Being mindful of now and our inner strength is a big step in healing. It takes the mind off the regrets of the past and the anxiety over the future and focuses squarely on now.

OVERLOAD

THE CURSE OF THIS WORLD is the overstimulation of senses, which blocks awareness of the unseen world. Technology, social media, television, and reality shows can distract us from the reality of what is going on inside of us.

Feelings reveal themselves through sensations and reactions in our body. For example, anxiety is manifested by rapid breathing, a racing heart, or habitually clenching our jaw. We get fatigue, headaches, muscle tension, and upset stomachs. These physiological indicators are just symptoms of underlying and unresolved feelings. If left unaddressed, we continue to physically, emotionally, and spiritually spiral downward. The signs are "red flags" signaling essential issues that should not be buried but brought to the surface and addressed. If we mask them or pretend that everything is fine, these underlying feelings build up, sometimes over the years, like a volcano. Then, with the right trigger, or maybe even the wrong one, we can explode and experience a life of regret.

We can pay attention to how we feel and how our body reacts to negative emotions. We can look for correlations between our physical and emotional states. Our reactions that mask reality include distractions like excessive amounts of social media, video games, overwork, sarcasm or humor, defensiveness, overeating, or sleeping more than is needed. If we are distracting ourselves or deflecting others' honest observations, this is a clue that reveals what is going on emotionally inside us. We need to take time to listen intently to ourselves and what is going on around us. We need to go below the surface where we often disguise or sugarcoat what is going on. The more we can directly see our underlying feelings and address them, the sooner we will heal.

Because feelings can be so painful, we often do whatever we can to avoid them. Rather than taking responsibility and facing them head-on, we mask them with denial, blame, rationalization, avoidance, minimization, or even magical thinking. None of these are solutions; they are merely delay tactics and Band-Aids. While these tactics provide some temporary relief, they are not authentic solutions. As long as we blame our parents, we remain a child. We become an adult the moment that we grow up and stop blaming others. Yes, someone else may have caused our situation, but it's up to us to figure out how to move forward. To truly heal from trauma, we must not dodge or duck the problems. We must take responsibility, do the work, and face it head-on.

How we feel has a direct impact on how we behave. If we dodge our feelings, our behavior will be sketchy and unpredictable. If we are too passive and avoid confrontation, it will show in our character. If we are aggressive or macho and stave off facing our fears, we present a false face and become scary ourselves. And how we act attracts people into our inner circle who reinforce whatever pattern we are living. In turn, our superficial or toxic friends strengthen our negative behaviors, and our problems do not get solved. The trauma not only remains but also gets worse, and we are in the same repeating pattern forever.

On the other hand, if we pay attention to our feelings, acknowledge them, and take authentic steps to address them directly, we feel more genuine. In turn, we attract other trustworthy and grounded people into our inner circle. Because we have faced our feelings directly, we can clear out the negative emotions more effectively. Healing will take root, and we will begin to grow.

When we feel disrespected, we can use that energy to fuel actions that generate legitimate respect. In college, we had an exercise on negotiation skills. Out of 40 students, I did the worst. In my arrogance, I did everything wrong and got suckered. I felt embarrassed and humiliated when the professor wrote the results on the board for everyone to see. There I was, dead last.

That lousy experience stuck with me. A few years later, I had a job with the world's largest consulting firm. I went to work and studied negotiation techniques for days. I read books and attended lectures. Then I got the chance to do the exercise again with another group; however, this was not a bunch of college kids. This was a larger, sophisticated group of seasoned business executives. Now I knew the landscape. I scored first.

All I did was apply principles that work. I harnessed the energy from my humiliating experience and focused on the pure determination to compete and win. If we feel disrespected at school, we can look at our study habits. If we feel disrespected at home, we can look at everyone's healthy contributions. If we feel disrespected at work, we can develop our skills that build our career there or at another job.

As we heal, our awareness expands beyond what we have ever seen. We begin to see the problem as part of the solution. It may even become our best friend. It is pure energy. We need to see suffering as an excellent fuel to propel us and move us forward.

We build awareness and empathy by facing our uncomfortable feelings and realizing that they are merely sensations. We can focus on those sensations and how they feel in our bodies and observe the

NEGATIVE SELF WORTH

PERSONALIZE: Any feedback from or positive and negative reactions of others are always taken personally.

"IF": You believe in yourself only "if" you meet certain criteria, i.e. If "I am successful," If "I lose weight," If "I feel superior to others."

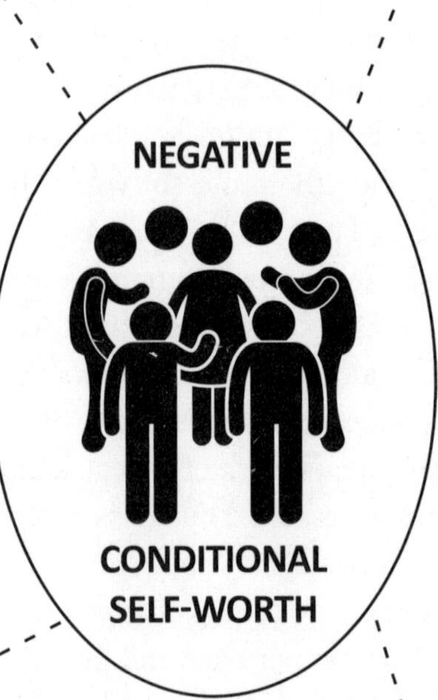

WIN-LOSE: The only way for me to win is for you to lose. Conversely, the only way for me to lose is for you to win. Another person's success makes them better than you.

OTHERS: The opinions of others are very important to your self-esteem. Without external praise, agreement, or deference, you do not feel good about yourself.

THREATENED: You believe that the success of others inhibits your own.

POSITIVE SELF WORTH

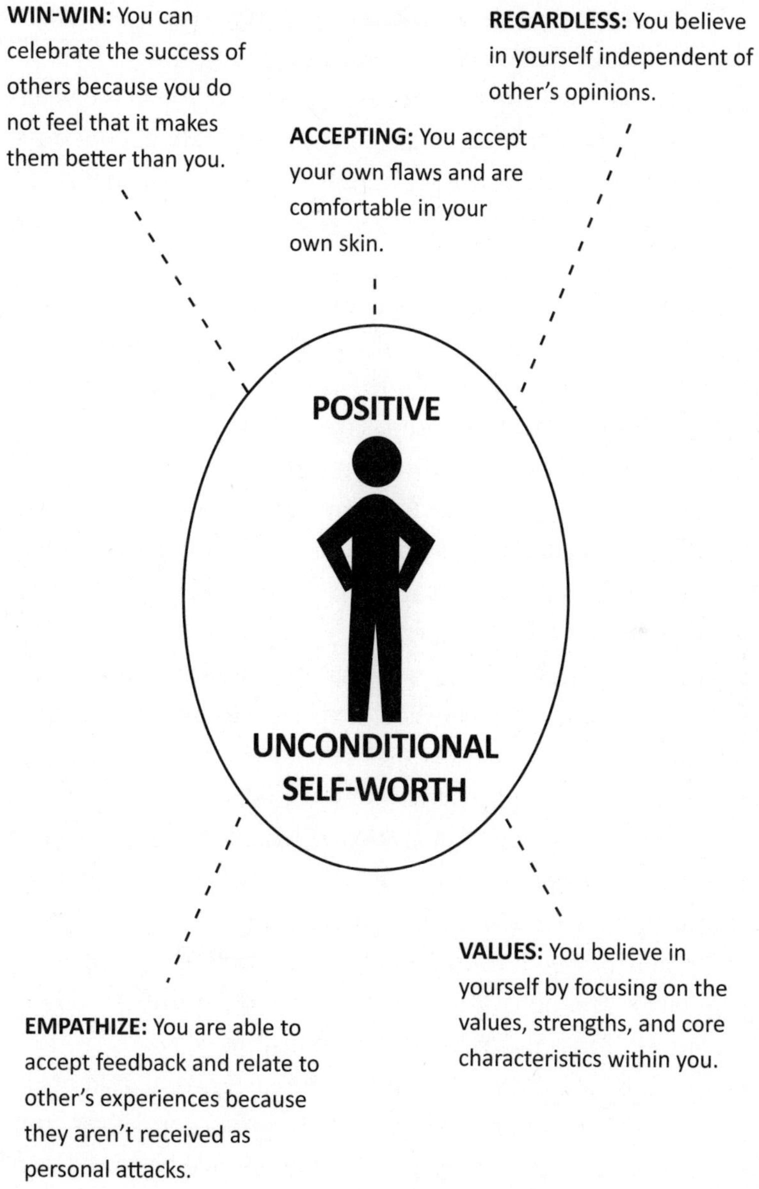

WIN-WIN: You can celebrate the success of others because you do not feel that it makes them better than you.

REGARDLESS: You believe in yourself independent of other's opinions.

ACCEPTING: You accept your own flaws and are comfortable in your own skin.

POSITIVE

UNCONDITIONAL SELF-WORTH

VALUES: You believe in yourself by focusing on the values, strengths, and core characteristics within you.

EMPATHIZE: You are able to accept feedback and relate to other's experiences because they aren't received as personal attacks.

Concept developed by Elizabeth Lombardo, PhD.

thoughts that go through our minds as if it were a movie on a screen. We do this with no judgment and by simply observing. If we practice this with real intent, just for a few minutes a day or even a week, eventually it can become a habit that we can slip in throughout the day.

Awareness starts with self-awareness. We cannot fulfill the needs of others until we fill our own. In part, awareness is about noticing if our emotional cup is full enough and learning how to keep it filled.

EMPATHY

Grounding exercises allow us to become more aware of ourselves. These practices increase our mindfulness to the "here and now" and connect us to our inner voices. Yet the full spectrum of awareness also includes awareness of the people around us.

Empathy is an awareness of the feelings of another person. When we watch the news or drive by an accident scene, empathy is that part of us that flinches or feels badly for those involved. Understanding is our ability to put ourselves in another's shoes, feel what they are feeling, and consider their perspective.

Neuroscientists have discovered that our brains have "mirror neurons" that allow us to feel others' experiences and mimic their actions. When another person smiles at us, we smile back and feel those same feelings of happiness. If someone laughs, we also start laughing. If somebody twists an ankle, we flinch in pain too. These mirror neurons allow humans to connect with others and experience the same emotions that others are experiencing. We even have these reactions when we see a beautiful picture. By building upon this biological factor and cultivating empathy, we connect with others, create intimacy, and build authentic relationships.

We lose empathy in a variety of ways. We can become cold or callused when we repress our feelings or try to protect ourselves from unfavorable circumstances or people around us. We become jaded, macho, cynical, harsh, or even aggressive. This process can begin in childhood and continue in adulthood. Eventually, we master the art of repressing it all. We draw a blank at disturbing sights and shut ourselves off from what we see in the world. We are comfortably numb.

This is not a solution. It is misery. To heal, we must work to feel. We must revisit that vulnerable, young child we once were. As we are honest with our hurts and can express them honestly to those we trust around us, we do heal. The numbness around us begins to fade. We can improve and go from living in black and white to living in color again. We not only regain our humanity but also see it in others as well.

AWARENESS OF OTHERS

"Attachment theory" is a term that psychologists and sociologists have given to the connection we have with others, particularly childhood caregivers and other close relationships. Here scientists have researched how healthy attachments occur and how poor relationships can have harmful or even traumatic effects. Attachment theory's objective is to understand the underlying reasons why some people are warm and giving while others are hostile, distant, or angry. Often, exploring childhood attachments provides insights into how to develop mature, loving relationships as an adult.

The field of attachment theory includes parent-child relationships, and also those with siblings, extended family members, friends, neighbors, teachers, and romantic partners. Often, it focuses on primary caregivers who set an example of relationship building. Overall, it is an opportunity to explore all relationships and how they formed our worldview.

In an ideal world, children have primary caregivers who model healthy relationships, creating a secure foundation for forming other relationships. The primary caregiver could be the biological parent but can be any adult role model during the formative years. He or she will be sensitive and attentive to the child's needs and set a tone for careful listening, play, and loving communication styles. In this ideal state, the caregiver is sensitive to the child and in tune with their needs. The development of the child is watched over carefully, while life's lessons are shared as age-appropriate. It creates an intelligent, intimate, thoughtful, and secure position from which to explore the world.

"Secure attachment" brings a stable foundation from which the child can form healthy relationships, be resilient, explore the world, and have an overall sense of security. The secure child sees an optimistic future, and life makes sense. Here, the caregiver responds to both the verbal and non-verbal cues of the child and builds a bond of trust and respect. There is a balance of smiles and play, chores and responsibility, as well as productive conflict resolution. At all times, the child feels safety, security, and protection.

This is the ideal situation, but, far too often, children do not have the solid, stable upbringing that they deserve. Rather than having a focused, permanent caregiver, they may be juggled between extended family members, foster care, or friends. The caregivers may be inexperienced, stressed, distracted, inattentive, or dealing with their own traumas. In some cases, caregivers may be dysfunctional or even abusive. The child may look to after-school programs, coaches, teachers, church members, or others for the role models they need. This can all lead to inconsistent, insecure, ambivalent, or even toxic attachments and relationships. The net effect can lead not only to children who are ill-equipped to function or be happy as adults but also to chronic toxicity that they carry into their new relationships, which extends the cycle of trauma. They may be insecure, reluctant, worrisome, anxious, or troubled.

Ambivalent caregivers may be inconsistent, or they may only respond to the physical needs—feeding, clothing, and so forth—while neglecting the child's emotional needs, like human love, interaction, and connection. In this world, the caregiver may be undependable, inconsistent, unresponsive, confused, or unreliable. As a result, the child may be reluctant to form close relationships.

Psychologists give the term "avoidant attachment" when caregivers physically or emotionally neglect the child or are nonresponsive to their needs. As a result, the child may feel insecure, helpless to improve their lives, or too frightened to engage with others. The world becomes a cold place where nobody cares. In adulthood, these people may avoid close or intimate relationships with others, check out emotionally, or detach from others.

"Disorganized attachment" is the term given in situations where what should be a child's "safe haven" is a frightening place. This includes enduring emotional, physical, or sexual abuse, witnessing domestic violence, or experiencing severe neglect. The child is put in the impossible position where the very caregivers he or she depends upon are the same people responsible for the trauma. He or she cannot seek refuge, nor is he or she in a place to run away from the danger. The injury from such situations can last well into adulthood and even a lifetime.

If a caregiver experienced trauma in their own life, which statistically is likely, that does not preclude them from doing a good job. Indeed, having successfully worked through their trauma can mean that they are an outstanding caregiver. Their experience and authenticity can be inspirational.

Caregivers are rarely perfect, and sometimes, their deficits bring extreme consequences. Real fallout results from a lack of authentic attachment. Children can grow up yearning for those relationships to which they were rightfully entitled. Heroin use can be like a warm mother's hug that the user never had. Alcohol can numb the chronic pain of never being listened to. A pimp or gang leader may be a counterfeit for the father figure we never had. When these people become caregivers themselves, the cycle continues.

In dealing with our traumas, there is a paradox in knowing that other people may have caused them. As a result, we may not trust others and want to retreat. However, our survival and ultimate thriving demand that we learn to trust again. It is impossible to thrive alone. We need connections with others. If we enjoyed a secure attachment as a child, we need to be grateful. If our attachment was avoidant or disorganized, we might have more work to do. Most of us are somewhere in between.

Trust is multifaceted. For example, we can trust someone with our lives, but also know not to share a secret with them because they will gossip. Trust is earned. We should start at a place of guarded trust until we get to know someone. We can trust them a little bit at a time until we see how they act with that trust. If they behave well and don't betray us with the little things, our trust can grow. Be wary of those who ask you to trust when you're not comfortable. Abusers and toxic people will manipulate and get you to trust them fully and immediately and may express hurt if you do not. They may use that hurt to pressure you into believing them. This is a big red flag that they are not trustworthy and will not treat you with respect or care.

LOOKING BACK

As adults, we now know just how tough adulthood can be, and this perspective can allow us to cut our primary caregivers some slack. Maybe we can talk to our parents or others about their views at the time. Maybe they were dealing with traumas of their own. Just as our childhood formed our outlooks, their childhoods did the same for them. In the process, our blame can turn into understanding. These insights can provide clues into both what they were dealing with as well as what formed our worldview as adults. In those areas where our childhoods were deficient, we can make deliberate efforts to fill in the gaps. As adults, we are now in a better position to take control and productively process these experiences.

Reparative measures include developing a deeper understanding of our upbringing and early childhood, providing insights into our insecurities, and developing our self-care and self-compassion abilities. We can mourn for the pain we suffered. We can cry. Grieving over the traumas we have experienced is a healthy alternative to harboring bitterness. Grief and mourning can be an expression of self-love when we allow ourselves to improve.

If we had weak attachments in our childhood, we could use that energy to fuel a desire to be responsible and diligent with our children. *We can be the ones to stop the multi-generational cycle.* We can pass on healthy attachments that result in close emotional bonds. We can provide a haven for healthy attachment and a prevailing sense of security. We can be a "home base" for which there is always a refuge from the outside world. While this attachment is developed at the earliest stages of life, *everyone craves security and affection throughout life.*

Secure attachments bring a sense of self-confidence. However, a lack of them can bring insecurities and self-doubt. Avoidant attachments often result in a strong desire to detach and take care of everything entirely by ourselves. Ambivalent attachment often results in a roller coaster of emotional storms, clinging to our caregivers while feeling anger, frustration, and resentment that leads to poor relationships in adulthood.

The need for being emotionally grounded and having healthy attachments are lifelong needs and not static. The need to receive and give care will flux and change over time. They are also intertwined with secondary caregivers, such as extended family members, siblings, grandparents, friends, teachers, counselors, co-workers, spouses, romantic partners, coaches, professionals, and even pets. As life evolves, healthy life practices allow room for change and growth.

In the survival mode, we do get back on our feet. This is a wonderful accomplishment. Yet here in the survival mode, there may be less room for full love or nurturing. To do this, we need to thrive, and that is where we are headed!

Our Stories of Awareness

DEBBIE

Debbie had attended a local church for many years with her husband and family. It had been a regular part of her life.

However, when her husband took his life, she reached out for support from her church family but did not find it.

She realized that, perhaps, the church was not where she would find the greatest support. Her friends, who had rallied around her when her life fell apart, became her "church." Unlike the people from her church, her friends didn't pretend it hadn't happened. They accepted the situation—they accepted *her.*

Over time, she added meditation and began to see her relationship with God as something more personal, rather than defined by the confines of a church.

JOHN

After losing his daughter to radiation poisoning from the nuclear testing across the lagoon, John started on a journey as an activist to take on the US Government for the trauma that they had caused. For an islander, this was a formidable task.

To keep himself grounded, he had a morning ritual of rising early, sitting down by the ocean, and quietly meditating by focusing on his breathing. It brought a calm to his mind that continued throughout the day. This brought focus and conviction into his heart and soul, which fueled him for that day.

SUSAN

Amid all the chaos surrounding her immediately after the landslide, Susan began to notice that some people went through terrible events but seemed to bounce back. Why were they able to recover so quickly? What were they doing that she was not? Susan began to pay attention to people around her who appeared to be thriving.

Susan discovered that all these people had a routine of some kind, something they did each day, that got them moving and motivated. For some, the routine started with a five-mile run. For others, it started with meditation or prayer. She noticed that these routines gave people a foundation on which to build their day.

While Susan was busy making these observations, she also started reading up on life coaching. Susan had always wanted to help others—being a life coach seemed like the perfect way to do it. And given what she had been through, she knew she could relate to trauma in a way that she had never been able to before.

Susan decided that she would become a spiritual life coach.

But before she took that step, she needed to make sure her foundation was strong. She needed a routine of her own. One of the first things she did to establish her routine was to start journaling. At first, it was challenging to find the time to journal consistently. It was a commitment. But like everything that requires dedication, she found that it was worth it.

Journaling became her way of expressing thanks for all the wonderful things in her life. Starting her morning with gratitude made her feel more happy, light, and full of hope and anticipation for what each day would bring. Journaling also helped her focus on her goal of becoming a life coach.

She didn't give up her job as a producer, though. She loved it, and it gave her meaning. But she could still be a life coach. In fact, in a way, both vocations complemented each other. As a producer, she was responsible for managing every aspect of a television show. As a life coach, she could give others the skills and tools to access and manage their lives.

SHAD

In 1985 when Shad started what would later become known as the National Veterans Foundation, it was just Shad, a handful of volunteers, and a toll-free number. The concept was based on something that Shad had learned long before—sometimes, what a vet really needs is for someone to talk to. His volunteers are vets themselves.

At first, they worked out of Shad's home. The toll-free number was available 24-hours a day, seven days a week. Shad often found himself taking on 24-hour shifts when a volunteer was not available to help with the phones. He did not mind the long hours—what mattered to him was helping people out.

However, the vets who contacted Shad and his volunteers were not always in immediate crisis. While they did get their fair share of callers who were on the verge of suicide, many more just wanted to talk. Some needed advice on finding a job. Others were upset with a personal relationship, and some wanted to talk about the challenges they faced reintegrating into society after an unpopular war. All of them wanted to speak to a live person.

The biggest challenge facing a new organization was funding. Shad had invested $10,000 of his own money to keep it going. They operated on a shoestring budget—every penny was accounted for, and no one took a salary. The money was used to pay for the phone line and various advertisements on radio, television, and the newspaper.

But, then, fate intervened again, as it had when Shad had made the fateful decision to take a job with the VA instead of travel up to San Francisco.

In 1982, Shad published a memoir of his experiences in Vietnam, *Captain for Dark Mornings,* a soldier's memoir on the psychological injuries suffered by many neglected Vietnam veterans. The book gained him nationwide acclaim, and he was known as the "Voice of the Vietnam Vet."

Keith Knudson, the former drummer of the Doobie Brothers, which had broken up in 1982, read that book, and it had a considerable impact on his life. Knudsen reached out to Shad. He wanted to help Shad fund his organization.

Knudsen reached out to the ex-members of the Doobie Brothers and asked them to reunite just one time to play a benefit concert for Shad's group. All 12 former members agreed.

On May 27, 1987, the Doobie Brothers played the Hollywood Bowl for the benefit concert. More than 19,000 people attended, and the event raised more than $300,000 for the National Veterans Foundation.

Thanks to the money raised, the foundation was able to get an office and staff. "It was," Shad says, "miraculous."

GERI

From the time she was a young girl, Geri felt that not only was she a survivor of her condition, but that she also had immense potential. She had huge dreams—it was just a matter of taking steps to make them come true. She envisioned a future where she did what very few people have ever done, with or without a disability—she would be a stand-up comedian!

Geri was keenly aware that she had an uphill battle ahead. It would be hard for people—especially those who make decisions in the entertainment world—to see past the cerebral palsy. Worse still, they might think that she was not intelligent. At times, she had found that people spoke to her slowly and carefully, as if they thought she was having difficulty understanding what they were saying.

But rather than be discouraged by these thoughts, Geri was galvanized by them. She knew she was smart. She knew she was funny. And most importantly, she knew in her heart that, if given a chance, she could win over even the most skeptical booking agent.

TANYA

Tanya struggled mightily after her sister's murder. The stress of Nicole's death, followed by a tumultuous trial and the subsequent acquittal of the man that Tanya and her family knew in their hearts committed the murder, created a void in Tanya that she felt she could never fill.

Then she met a man who, for a time, seemed to fill that void. But soon enough, the relationship became controlling and emotionally abusive. Tanya loved him, though, and thought she could change him. But after one particularly frightening interaction, Tanya realized that she was following in Nicole's footsteps.

She broke it off with him, and fortunately, he let her go. But Tanya was now aware that she tended to gravitate toward unstable relationships. This awareness helped her recognize "relationship red flags" and seek out healthier situations.

JC

JC was an angry 17-year-old when he was sent to prison. While he tried to project a macho exterior, JC longed for peace. He was also keenly observant. He noticed that some of the inmates seemed far more mellow and calmer than others. He wondered why. He soon learned that the men were participating in self-help classes. JC wanted to be part of it.

The first prison he was sent to, Salinas Valley, was a Level-4, high-security facility. The self-help classes primarily consisted of televised videos that he watched and then answered questions about. When he was transferred to Vacaville State Prison, a Level-3 facility, the offerings were much more comprehensive. JC immersed himself in education even more. And he was also recognized by the warden for his outstanding contribution to the educational department.

It was in Vacaville that JC truly started working on himself. When he was simply watching the self-help videos and filling out the questionnaires afterward, JC could still lie to himself about his real issues.

Once he started working with real volunteers, however, there was nowhere he could hide.

At Vacaville, JC became involved with the Alternative to Violence Project (AVP). The three-day, intensive workshop was designed to help inmates understand their past traumas so they could move past it to be the best version of themselves, even in prison. One of the breakout sessions was about how the inmates were disciplined by their parents. When it was JC's turn to speak, he had no words. He had to get up and go to the bathroom, where he cried because he started to realize the profound effect that his childhood played in his decision-making process, which resulted in him being in prison.

Listening to the men around him, JC realized that his childhood was not normal. The beatings, the verbal abuse, the horrific things he witnessed and experienced—he had been, his whole life, the victim of abuse. It was hard to accept, yet he realized that it was true.

JC did not leave AVP; he signed up for phase two of the program, where he learned more about his "triggers" and how to manage them. And then, JC trained as a facilitator and began to run the workshops himself. JC found that by helping other people, he was helping himself even more.

While he was still in Vacaville State Prison, JC helped found the "Long- Term Commitment Group," which helped men address the issues that they struggled with so that, when they went before the parole board, they would have a better chance of securing parole.

JC continued to work on himself and help others when he was transferred to San Quentin State Prison, a Level-2 facility. It was at San Quentin where his most dramatic change took place. A friend had encouraged JC to sign-up for a program called Victim Offenders Education Group (VOEG) offered by Insight Prison Project. This nationwide curriculum provides courses to prisoners and parolees through a process of self-transformation accomplished with an integrated curriculum specifically designed to bring about a shift in ingrained patterns of harmful and destructive behavior. This program was the missing piece for JC. After completing the program, JC was never the same.

VOEG had introduced JC to meditation—or, as they called it in prison, "grounding." He led other men in grounding exercises, which, among other benefits, have been shown to reduce stress, control anxiety, enhance self-awareness, lengthen the attention span, and help fight addictions. JC is a devoted Christian and an ordained minister.

Over time, JC became aware of who he was—and who he was becoming. He had been many things in his life—an abused little boy, a frightened adolescent, a cocky teenager, a betrayed lover, a terrified prisoner, and a man in search of meaning. He realized that human beings are always changing and that everyone has the potential to be the best version of themselves. They just have to commit themselves to that goal and follow through.

LEO

Leo lost an eye as a kid and was mostly deaf, but he felt a great passion growing inside to use his creative talents and invent instruments that could change the world.

There was no beaten path to follow, so every morning, he would pour a large, boiling bath and soak in it for nearly an hour. During that time, he would calmly meditate, focus on his inner voice, and center on his core passions.

JOE

Joe's battle with drug and alcohol addiction was rooted in his untreated trauma. It took going to prison for Joe to receive the therapy he needed to overcome his past. During treatment, Joe learned to look inward and examine his deepest feelings. He learned to understand and diffuse his triggers and be more aware of the things in life that put him at risk for falling into old habits.

ERICA

Erica's road to awareness was a matter of survival from the Nazis who were continually searching for Jews. When she was hiding, she would focus on her breathing to keep calm. She noticed how much better it made her feel, so when she started feeling scared or anxious over her missing family and fiancé, she would take some time to focus on her breathing quietly. Indeed, Erica learned to control her breathing, as she had to be quiet many times while the Nazis walked by.

TOM

In retrospect, Tom looks back on his dashed Olympic dreams with equanimity. Losing the opportunity to go to Moscow was painful, but he gained more than he lost. Before the Olympics, Tom was single-minded in his goals to the exclusion of anything and anyone else. He was overly controlling, believing that he held all the cards in life. He thought that he could shape any outcome by sheer force of will. The Olympic situation showed him that sometimes, no matter how hard you try, you do not always get what you want. Until that time, Tom always got everything he had wanted. Then reality hit him, and he had not known how to handle it.

Tom feels that, in retrospect, the situation made him a better person. He is more relaxed now, less judgmental, and more empathetic to other people's problems. He does not necessarily view losing out on his Olympic dreams as the most significant trauma of his life. Still, he does see it as a tough, upsetting situation that he ultimately had to get through to be the person he is today.

And who is that person? Tom is an extraordinarily successful business owner, happily married husband, father, grandfather, and volunteer in his local community. He is known as a steady, reliable friend and as someone to whom others can always turn in times of stress. Although he has not done competitive shot put for 30 years, he still works out regularly.

MY STORY

My emotional recovery from my heart surgery evolved gradually. While the talk with my high school coach forced me to face that I was physically 100 percent, some of my emotional insecurities remained.

I did not wake up to my strength and make a genuine

transformation until my 20s when I was working for a consulting firm in Newport Beach, California. On a whim, I applied to graduate school at UCLA. Frankly, I did not give myself high odds of being accepted, but I grew up in the John Wooden era, and he was one of my heroes. I had a deep admiration for him and UCLA generally.

UCLA was a Top 10 school in my area of interest, and at that level, my application was marginal. I received a call that said there were 10 more seats available and about 50 applicants being considered, and I was one of them. I was asked to come in for a one-on-one interview with the school's dean. I did, and I put everything I had into it.

When I heard I had been admitted, I was euphoric. It was a wake-up call to my own inner personal strength. It took years, but I finally was able to put both the physical and emotional setbacks of my heart surgery entirely behind me—or so I thought.

On March 12, 2019, I stepped onto a treadmill for a heart stress test. My cardiologist is the best, and I was in a good mood because her office overlooks the ocean. I was in decent shape; I had just run and walked for five miles that morning. Then, something startling happened. Before the test even began, my heart raced to about 150 beats per minute. I could feel a surge of stress come over me, but I had trained myself to suppress it. Outside I looked fine, but inside my cardiovascular system was going insane.

This was the first time I became aware that I suffered from PTSD. This is why throughout this book, I say, "we" and "us", because we are all in this together. I am not teaching or preaching. I am doing the research and documenting the stories of several of my friends, but I am in this thing called life, too, and I am dealing with trauma myself.

I realized that the episode was triggered by my childhood trauma from when I grew up with heart specialists and surgeons. My parents, thinking they were doing the right thing, suppressed conversations on the topic. At the age of 60, I realized that I had been in denial about my childhood trauma my entire life. Meditation, facing attachment issues with my parents, and all the other tools discussed here have helped me heal, just as they will help you.

SECTION 3

Thrive Stage | We Blast Off

WHEN TRAUMA HITS, it can either take us down a dark path or act as a catalyst for remarkable change. We see our trauma as the valuable asset that it is and use it as fuel to do some amazing things. In our post-traumatic lives, we can become stronger, happier, wiser, and more connected. We appreciate that our past traumas amplify our current joy. We propel far beyond where we were before:

- **Faith:** We ignite our passion in God, nature, or a higher power. We awaken our spiritual or existential awareness.
- **Connection:** Thriving is not a solo act. Relationships with others allow us to accept support and be supportive. This empowers us to form new ways to love and relate to others.
- **Forgiveness:** We don't want to forget our trauma, but we want to let go of the destructive bitterness and realize our new possibilities.
- **Resilience:** The ability to bounce back is within us. It gives our life meaning. This is the capacity to reframe our life, envision big dreams, and set goals with a newfound excitement for life.
- **Gratitude:** Our trauma reveals our character and can give

us a greater appreciation for life. While we may not be grateful for trauma, we can be grateful for its lessons. This experience activates our desire to serve others and make a difference in other's lives. In the end, wisdom takes our inward focus and turns it outward.

CHAPTER 11

Faith

The research is verifiable and repeatable. Faith in God, a higher power, spirituality, or existential awareness wakes up our passion not just to survive but to thrive.

A PATH TO WISDOM

RICHARD ROHR, A CATHOLIC SPIRITUAL TEACHER, sets forth thoughts in "From Naïveté to Wisdom," in which he suggests that to grow toward love, union, salvation, or enlightenment, we must move from "order" to "disorder" and, finally, to "reorder." His concepts help navigate through a trauma successfully.

In the stage of "order," we are naïve. We feel comfortable. Everything is good and has meaning. We have a seemingly God-given, unshakable, and satisfying explanation of how things are and should be. Those who try to stay here tend to avoid confusion, conflict, inconsistencies, suffering, or darkness. They do not like disorder or change. Our ego compels us to pretend our status quo is entirely right and should be good for everybody. Permanent residence in this stage tends to create naïve people and control freaks.

In the "disorder" stage, our comfortable, presumed reality is destroyed. Our perfect world is rocked. As Canadian songwriter Leonard Cohen puts it, "There is a crack in everything, that's how the light gets in." Our loved one dies, we lose a job, our children leave the church, or we lose our happiness. This stage of disorder is like the fall Adam and Eve experienced in the Garden of Eden. It is necessary if real growth is to occur. It is all uncomfortable and even ugly, so we try to dodge it and get back to the order that we feel entitled to. Permanent residence in this disordered stage tends to make people bitter, negative, cynical, angry, opinionated, and dogmatic.

For those who move beyond the "order" and "disorder" stages, the "reorder" stage becomes the new normal. Every religion, each in its way, is trying to move us to enlightenment, nirvana, heaven, salvation, or resurrection. Mature spirituality points to life on the other side of death, victory on the other side of failure, and joy on the other side of the pains of childbirth. It insists on going through—not under, over, or around. When we reorder, there is no nonstop flight. To arrive there, we must endure and learn. It is rinse and repeat. That is the hard-won secret.

As we discuss "spirituality" and "faith," they should be defined in a way accessible to everyone. This includes believers, skeptics, and people who have been traumatized by organized religion. Spirituality may or may not mean "religion." It may or may not involve a host of doctrines or dogmas. These are individual and personal decisions. The important thing is a sense of purpose, connection, and guidance by an inner voice. Spirituality is the total of a person's moral center, firmly held values, awareness, mindfulness, sense of purpose, sense of fulfillment, sense of connectivity to other beings and the universe, and interpretation of the world. It is the meaning we ascribe to everything. It encompasses our emotions, subconscious, and psyche. Everyone has some sense of spirituality when it's defined this way, whether we are aware of it or not. "Passion" is our spiritual world. However we choose to define it, passion and spirituality are deeply linked. The objective is to allow all, including believers, skeptics, and those burned by religion, to have access to their spiritual world.

We must admit that we are powerless to change the past trauma. Rohr suggests that we should hold on to what is good about the naïve order, but also include needed correctives. People who have reached this stage, like some of the Jewish prophets, might be called "radical traditionalists." They love their truth and their group enough to critique it. And they critique it enough to maintain their integrity and intelligence. These wise ones have stopped over-reacting and over-defending. This is the real objective.

The academic community began focusing on the topic of post-traumatic growth in 1996 when Dr. Richard Tedeschi and Dr. Lawrence Calhoun of the University of North Carolina developed the conceptual foundations and empirical evidence on the subject. Their studies outline five areas of growth that may emerge from a traumatic experience. One area that strongly correlates with growth is faith in God or a higher power along with spiritual or existential awareness. Their work and the work of many others have produced collective research that is verifiable and repeatable: spirituality is statistically and inseparably connected to healing from trauma. In other words, there is an enormous body of both expert and scientific research that now demonstrates the importance of faith. God and spirituality are irrefutably linked to a serious discussion of post-traumatic growth. We cannot address the topic of growth without a discussion on faith.

CASINOS AND SLOT MACHINES

My family has a small condominium in Las Vegas where we live part of the year. We take advantage of all the shows and entertainment, including the $4 movies at one of the nearby casinos.

One night, we were walking through the main floor of the casino to get to the movie theater. There were thousands of people playing the slot machines, and the casino floor was flooded with every light, buzz, and sound that stirs up the gaming business. As an observer of people, I looked over the sea of machines and noticed that there was not a single person who had a smile on their face. They all had a rather a robotic look of boredom or eager anticipation.

In the past, I just thought of gambling in terms of brain neurology, whereby the mind gets a tiny jolt of feel-good chemicals for wins and near-wins. However, on this night, I wondered what the basic, underlying emotion with gambling was. Was it "fun" or "greed" or "excitement"? Was it a mental escape? Was it merely entertainment? What is the single, dominant emotion that drives millions of people to pour onto the Las Vegas gambling floors?

After some thought, I concluded that the underlying emotion of the hardcore gambler is "hope." It is a hope that we beat the odds and cash in big. With those winnings comes the end of all misery and a new life. It is a "hope" for a brighter future. Anticipation alone is a powerful emotion, and emits a shot of dopamine, which feels good. We all want to end our problems and enjoy a brighter future, and the casinos are cashing in on that basic human drive.

I am not judging or criticizing anyone who goes to the casino for a little fun; however, our core hope should not be placed in the casinos' hands. This is an artificially manipulated environment that is deliberately engineered around the physiology of the human brain to extract as many dollars as possible. This may be amusing, but it is not authentic hope.

Authentic hope comes from a higher power. This could be God, the universe, humanity, nature, or a cause greater than ourselves.

We need to include God, or however you want to define a higher power, in our path for healing and thriving. From my point of view, God has never created a single person that he does not love, and that includes you. God gives us all a real purpose and authentic hope. When we are radically humbled, we must face our higher power, admit our predicament and shortcomings, and humbly ask for help.

FOX HOLES

Being taught to avoid talking about politics and religion has led to a lack of understanding of politics and religion. What we should teach is how to have civil conversations about politics and religion.

For many, discussions about God, faith, and spirituality are deeply personal and, sometimes, uncomfortable. Spirituality and religion can be touchy subjects. However, they are not touchy if everyone sticks to "I" statements or begins with saying, "For me...," so that pronouncements are not meant to apply to everyone. If we center ourselves around discussions of spirituality instead of how we think others should perform their spirituality, then many calm, interesting discussions can occur. We can build relationships when we talk about what works or does not work for us and avoid telling others what to do.

Emotions are strong, both with those who are believers and those who are non-believers. In some circles, there are fist-pounding declarations on the absolute certainty of a chosen religion. On the other hand, in other circles, the mention of God is frowned upon or even considered strictly taboo. One atheist went so far as to say that the universe was created from nothing, by nothing, for nothing. Still, religions themselves can be beneficial or harmful forces. Many people have had great experiences with healthy faiths, while others come from toxic and controlling organizations that have abused and taken advantage of their faithful members.

I am passionate about this work involving wide-scale renewal. I have been researching disaster recovery cases since 1986. The media has called ever since 1994 when I consulted on the OJ Simpson case, allowing me to sit down with the people behind the headlines to listen to their stories. Because people know that I respect them and keep confidences, many tend to open up. Of course, those I have discussed in this book have given permission. It is interesting how often people bring up the topic of God or a higher power as they share their journey of trials and triumphs.

The old saying goes, "There are no atheists in fox holes." Whether or not this statement is taken literally, it suggests that trauma wakes up the spiritual or religious domain in our lives when we are under fire. It is under fire when we most seek meaning. Some experience a deepening of their spiritual lives, which results in overhauling their fundamental belief system. There are many ways to feel spiritually centered, and it is up to each of us to discover what works for us. If you are Christian, you may find solace and meaning in prayer. If you are agnostic or atheist, you can consider looking to nature or towards the goodness of humanity as your higher power. Regardless of the specific method or path, I have observed that those who move into the thriving realm connect with a higher power or their inner spark in one way or another.

Denying the existence of God leads us to the remarkable conclusion that nothing produces something, dumb luck produces a fine-tuned universe, and raw chemicals magically produce self-forming, self-replicating cells with DNA more complex than the space shuttle. More fantastic is that cosmic debris randomly became conscious, self-aware, and altruistic.

While some "big questions" remain shrouded in mystery, the cumulative evidence has compelling explanatory value. When there is evidence of design, it is quite reasonable to believe in a designer. In contrast to atheism, theism provides a path for hope, justice, and the ultimate reconciliation of humanity.

A power greater than us can heal us. In the interests of full disclosure, I am a simple Christian. I accept the bits about loving God and loving our neighbors. The teachings of Jesus are easily the most profound in human history, and we measure time and dates based on his birth. Though much has been layered on over the centuries, Jesus himself taught universal truths that are difficult to argue with. The essence of Jesus' mission was to give to the needy, feed the hungry, be merciful, clothe the poor, visit those in prison, and be empathetic and understanding. He denounced hypocrisy and took naps on boats.

Jesus is cool. He hung out with society's marginalized. Jesus taught to love your (black, white, brown, gay, straight, Christian, Buddhist, Muslim, atheist) neighbor. He fought against the norm and upset the hyper-religious people. He told stories that made people think. He taught us to be humble, forgiving, and charitable. He promoted peace. With that said, the discussion here will be far broader and all-inclusive of every religious, non-religious, and spiritual practice. There are fundamental truths to being a happy, healthy human that transcend specific religious tenets. In other words, all are welcome to this dialog as we expand on how passion, faith, trust, love, charity, and other universal spiritual qualities assist us in thriving after trauma. Take time to plan, focus, strategize, worship, and reconnect to a higher power or to your spiritual center. Whatever speaks to you. If we are too busy to care for our spirits, we are too busy.

We can turn to a higher power, however we understand that. I often think that God created every person I meet just the way he wanted. I see a God who can create this vast universe, being quite capable of embracing and loving all unconditionally, and I will leave all judgment, if there is any, to God. I do not believe that God will want to see our bank balances, journals, portfolios, hobbies, positions, games, trophies, or diplomas. I believe He is going to simply ask how we treated ourselves and other people.

KEEP THE FAITH

The debate over the existence of God has raged for centuries and will likely continue for many more. Some people dodge any conversation on the topic, yet this is a fascinating subject that exposes a wide array of intelligent observations and extreme, militant diatribes. I know some people who "know" there is a God and are quite dogmatic in their belief. On the other hand, recently, I heard an atheist say that he was "100 percent sure" there was no God, which is also outrageous. The atheists I know don't agree with this dogmatic position.

A-theist simply means "not a theist." Saying that I simply lack a belief in God, is not the same as a belief there is no god. Some atheists and believers frame the argument as "Darwinism vs. Theism," but this is problematic. In his book, *On the Origin of Species,* Charles Darwin acknowledges a Creator, right down to the last chapter of the book. On top of that, the design and mathematical complexity of DNA challenge the theories of atheism.

Of course, there are more sensible conversations with those who have strong faith but do not claim to "know" all the answers. The big picture is that there are six main points of belief, with gradients in between each one:

- Extreme atheists "know" there is no God.
- Atheists believe there is no God. They are not necessarily certain there is no God, but instead, they are certain that they do not believe in God.
- Agnostics question the existence of God, although they may lean in one direction or another.
- Deists believe that a powerful Creator made the universe, but that the Creator has not dabbled in human affairs since the beginning. Deists reject revelation and turn instead to the natural world to learn about creation.
- Theists believe in God and religion. This includes most Christians, Jews, Muslims, and other faiths. However, Buddhists and Hindus believe in enlightened beings and polytheistic gods that are different from the Abrahamic faiths.
- Extreme theists don't question, but rather "know" that there is a God and that their religion is true to the exclusion of all others.

I do not find extreme positions to be compelling. One can have strong faith, and even reasonably dedicate their lives to that faith, but legitimate and fundamental questions will always remain. That is why it is called "faith."

Ultimately, the more compelling discussions center around the trio of deism, agnostics, and theism. Each of these includes a blend of evidence, faith, and questions. The adventure to understand God is fascinating, as whoever God is, He did not want us to have all the answers. The word "Israel" means "to wrestle with God." People may find themselves confused in these areas, but they may also find themselves in multiple places at one time. Yet, in the end, for me, the evidence for intelligent design is persuasive.

While the academic literature does not generally address the existence of God per se, a considerable body of research shows a statistical correlation between faith and positive benefits in life, particularly in the area of trauma recovery. This reconciles with my work in jails, prisons, and homeless shelters. Most, but not all, of those who successfully process their trauma have some type of faith. Many have also noted that old-school programs, such as Alcoholics Anonymous, founded upon a belief in a higher power, outperform the newer, strictly secular programs.

As I understand atheism, it claims that "nothing created everything." In my view, this is a difficult notion to swallow. The most persuasive evidence of God is in the simple principle that, where there is creation, there is a creator. "Nothing" could not create something. For me, it makes sense that when we have a design, there is a designer.

Many of history's greatest minds, along with my heroes, believed in a higher power. The greatest philosophers, Aristotle, Socrates, and Plato, were believers at some level. My historical heroes were believers as well, including Dr. Martin Luther King Jr., John Wooden, Abraham Lincoln, and George Washington.

I once had lunch with a celebrity who is a devout atheist. He told me, "If it involves faith, you can count me out!" I challenged his position as it seemed intellectually dishonest. We all have faith every day. Every time we drive through an intersection, we have faith that other drivers will stop at the red lights. We have faith in the pilots who fly our planes. We have faith that the sun will come up tomorrow. The notion that we can avoid all faith is not compelling. We all have faith in something.

I see God filling in the numerous, wide gaps left by science. I see God as the Creator of all nature, and thus I see God in the entirety of the universe. So, where did God come from? I do not know. The vastness of the universe and the incomprehensibility of eternity is beyond the capacity of my three-pound brain. Yet I do know that science cannot answer the simple question of where a rock came from.

As we heal from trauma, let us embrace some faith. We cannot let the extreme atheists, who bully and mock all faith, get in the way of our healing and recovery. The discussions around God require an honest examination of the evidence and humility in admitting there is much that we do not know. There is a great passion for these questions. The fact that they are difficult or impossible to answer is a testament to the beauty and magnificence of the universe, and I worship that. It can fill us with spiritual awe.

A PURPOSE AND PASSION

No single version of growth exists. It is highly personalized, and everyone has a path to wholeness. Finding your way to spirituality is part of healing and learning how to thrive. In the United States, Christianity is offered as the default spiritual path. Still, it does not speak to everyone, and some who have been traumatized through high-demand religious groups may not find solace or meaning through traditional faith. Spirituality can be found through organized religion, or it can be found through a solitary practice. True spirituality is not dictated, but it is self-directed from your inner "still small voice," which you can follow through quiet moments when you can listen to your heart and the gentle messages that come to us through God or nature.

However, some form of religious and spiritual practice is a crucial aspect of growth. We must engage our traumas and find spiritual meaning, instead of just succumbing and blending into nothing.

The term "spiritual" can be a loaded one because it is co-opted by many to exploit the vulnerabilities and trust of others for gain. Simply put, I mean spirituality is our inner sense of purpose and direction, value system, and/or our sense of connectedness to others or the universe. It is our drive, and our state of internal well-being, the total of our sense of self. It is how we decide what it all means and how we make hard decisions when there simply isn't enough rational information. It is our sense of hope and trust. These aspects can include a belief in the unseen, but that is not required to find a personal spiritual center.

Spirituality must balance a strong, centered sense of self with our sense of the beings and wider world around us. That is where a higher power comes in.

The belief in a higher power can be seen from a variety of

viewpoints. Some refer to it as God, source energy, quantum consciousness, the Akashic record, a supreme being, and an over-intelligence that is beyond time and space. The important aspect of holding the idea of a higher power is that we think of things beyond ourselves and our myopic view of our relatively tiny lives and look towards something greater. There is comfort in knowing there is a bigger picture. And there is healing that can come from surrendering to that which is greater than ourselves.

Healing from trauma is connected to our purpose and personal passion. When we tap into our purpose and direction in life, all the rest falls into place. To discover our purpose, we may have faith in deity. Passion grows from that relationship. Our inner direction and motivation are connected to how we tap into our purpose. The energy from our trauma, coupled with faith in a higher power, ignites that fuel to blast off. When we are living in sync with our divine purpose, all the pieces of life come together.

Divinity is so much larger than anyone's perspective of God. It is bigger than science. It is bigger than religion. It is an all-loving presence. Spirituality may or may not include a religious community. There are more than 4,000 religions around the world because they fill a human need to explore the mysteries of the universe and wrestle with life's most important questions. A religious group can provide enormous support during a time of trauma, yet some organized religions get in the way. A sense of community, whether religious or not, is vital as, ultimately, loneliness is more toxic than drugs.

We must look to our higher power and make a full moral assessment of ourselves. Muhammad Ali said, "A man who arrives at 50 with the same point of view he had at 20 has wasted 30 years of his life." This is why listening to our inner voice is crucial, as it reveals who we are and our real purpose. It is the finest means of establishing our moral compass, which is our benchmark for life. Roy Disney said, "It's not hard to make decisions once you know what your values are."

Of all sacred writings, by far my personal favorite is a verse spoken by Jesus in response to where to look for God's kingdom. Luke 17:20-21 says, "Neither shall they say lo here or lo there, behold the Kingdom of God is within you." In other words, to find divinity, we don't look outward; we look inward. Never turn your calling or inner voice over to someone else. Neglecting our inner voice is neglecting everything. Science is catching up with what Jesus said 2,000 years ago.

Our outer voices can be loud, shouting out to promote ego, cheap pleasures, appearances, and harsh judgments. Our external voice can scream arrogance and materialism. It is shallow and fleeting. On the other hand, our inner voice tends to be quiet, spiritual, humble, and vulnerable. It brings fulfillment through music, nature, and sacred texts. Here, we connect to our own sacred story. It is fully present. It is an awakened consciousness that is observant and loving and gives compassionate service. Here, we are present with those we meet. This inner voice may be present when we attend a mosque, church, temple, or park, and also faithfully shows up when we visit those in jails, prisons, homeless shelters, and treatment centers.

Prayer and meditation can calm anxiety. We can read inspirational works or scripture as a prayer. Music or worship are other ways to stir passion and love of life, bring the mind to the present moment, and calm anxiety. Religion is great for many, but has its limits. I am religious, but trauma recovery can be impeded by religion. Some use external religion as an excuse to avoid their inner voice. They claim they do not have to do the work because they already discussed the matter with their priest, rabbi, bishop, cleric, or pastor. That is a start, but there is still a lot more work to do.

Trauma can cause us to doubt, so we must be aware of this, build back that trust, and especially, learn to trust that which is worthy of our trust. Indeed, it is essential to look to our inner voice and not allow anyone to tell us what we should believe. We must listen to our internal spiritual center and never turn over the keys to someone else to drive our bus. We must learn to trust again—first in ourselves, and then in selected others.

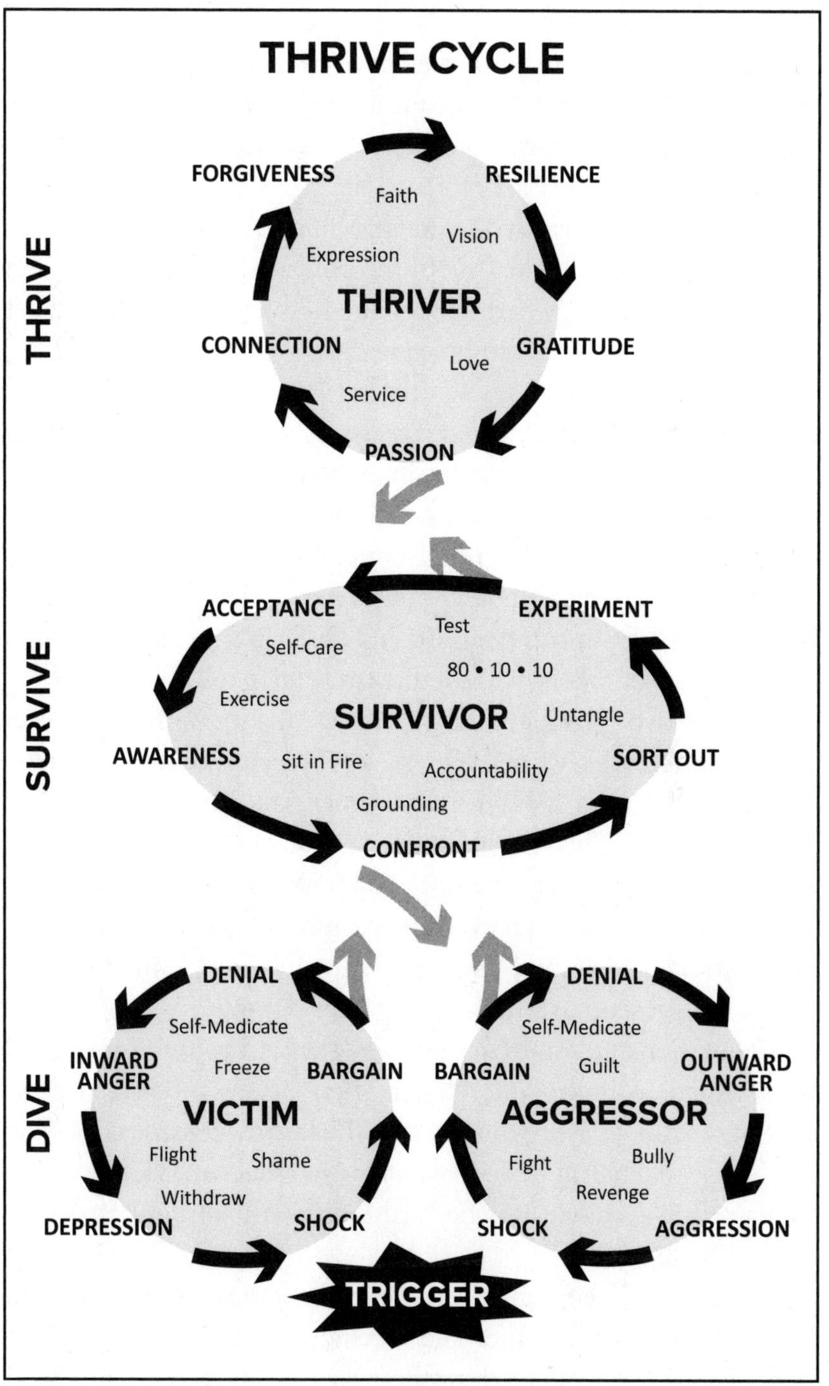
THRIVE CYCLE
THRIVE
FORGIVENESS
RESILIENCE
Faith
Vision
Expression
THRIVER
CONNECTION
GRATITUDE
Love
Service
PASSION
SURVIVE
ACCEPTANCE
EXPERIMENT
Test
Self-Care
80 • 10 • 10
Exercise
SURVIVOR
Untangle
AWARENESS
Sit in Fire
Accountability
SORT OUT
Grounding
CONFRONT
DIVE
DENIAL
Self-Medicate
INWARD ANGER
Freeze
BARGAIN
VICTIM
Flight
Shame
Withdraw
DEPRESSION
SHOCK
DENIAL
Self-Medicate
BARGAIN
Guilt
OUTWARD ANGER
AGGRESSOR
Fight
Bully
Revenge
SHOCK
AGGRESSION
TRIGGER

THE GREAT MINDS

My heart surgery physically healed nearly half a century ago. Yet my emotional healing did not come until much later when my belief in God was challenged. Ultimately, I had to confess just how ignorant I was and give the topic serious thought.

Once I was interviewed by *Rolling Stone*. At the end of the interview, the reporter asked about my philosophy of life. I had just returned from India, where I had visited Hindu temples, Buddhist monasteries, and a Muslim mosque during prayer time. I told her that Buddha had said, "Life is suffering", and I think that he had it half right. Life is suffering, *but it is also joy*. We can suppress either one. We can suppress our suffering through avoidance, denial, or self-medication. We can suppress our joy by getting too busy, working too hard, feeling undeserving, or merely neglecting those things that bring us our bliss. Buddha also taught us that our unnecessary attachments lead to suffering. To end suffering, we can end these unhealthy attachments, while letting in what is fulfilling.

The idea that "life is suffering" can also be a comfort. It gets us to stop resisting. When we feel depressed or anxious, we can surrender. When we are having a painful day, we can say, "life is suffering" or "life is struggle." This is a Buddhist's version of "this too shall pass." We accept what is, at least for now. Suppressing our suffering is unwise because it creates an internal volcano that will eat at us inside and eventually blow, and that eruption will be ugly. Suffering and joy are both essential. Suffering amplifies our joy.

Unquestionably, some have used religion as a hook to control and abuse others. A controlling religion often focuses on the shame in your past while delaying your joy into the future. Regardless of what has already happened or lies beyond today, what we do know is that we have this moment. It is far healthier to embrace our suffering and joys today.

A healthy religion will always teach us to love all humankind, including ourselves. Author and theologian Barbara Brown Taylor said, "The only clear line I draw these days is this: when my religion tries to come between my neighbor and me, I will choose my neighbor. Jesus never commanded me to love my religion." If caught in a high-demand religion, leaving it or any abusive institution will allow us to go from black-and-white thinking to color.

We can embrace both suffering and joy. We need to face our realities, express our emotions, be grateful for the wisdom and character that they build, and thank God for the adventure. Faith in God transcends the understanding of all of our tiny brains. Yet clearly, God wants us to enjoy our purpose, connect with people, be productive, and make progress. If there is an afterlife, and I believe there is, I do not think that anyone will get a theological test. Yet I do believe that we will need to address how we found meaning in our challenges and how we, ultimately, loved ourselves and others.

THE SKY

Once I was in Africa hiking, and we were camping for the night at an extreme altitude of over 15,000 feet. I got up in the middle of the night to answer nature's call. While I was stumbling back to my tent, I happened to look up. The stars and the Milky Way were blazing the brightest I had ever seen. We were far above the cloud line, and the view was spectacular. While it was freezing, I just stood there staring into the heavens. Looking up at the sky can be breathtaking and inspiring.

I once visited the site of one of humanity's worst nightmares, Auschwitz. I was there during the early spring, so there were no tourists. I will never forget walking all alone down the train tracks, through the gates and guard posts, and around the barracks, hanging gallows, disgusting mass toilets, and dungeons below ground from where the convicted men had a sneak preview of the walls where they would face the firing squads. I walked through the forest where people were forced to wait their turn to die. I stood by myself in the gas chambers and walked through the halls of ovens. Finally, I came to a pond where the ashes were disposed of.

I felt stunned by the unspeakable horror. I stood outside, alone in the forest, by that pond, and I looked up to the sky and just asked, "Why?" My visit to Auschwitz occurred over 25 years ago, yet I still feel the shock as if it were yesterday. The crimes of Hitler and his Nazis have never really been settled. Millions of victims of torture, rape, molestation, and murder have never seen justice. There are murderers walking our streets right now who got away with it. Despite all our efforts, our world is filled with unsettled scores and crimes without punishment.

Despite this, the believer's sky has hope. There are seasons with storms, but even at Auschwitz, the sky was crisp and blue. Yes, we do see the horrors, but we also see a higher power. I look up, and I see ultimate justice and mercy. In our sky, we see a Creator who gave us a free choice, and some of those choices have been horrible. But in a believer's sky, there is a God who will *only endure* the horror for a while. In a believer's sky, there is a God who will *ensure* that there will be ultimate justice for perpetrators and healing for their victims. In the believer's sky, there is some comfort and reconciliation.

We do have a purpose in life. Challenges are what make life interesting, but overcoming them is what makes life meaningful. Our comfort is less important. Our character is what is important. To heal from trauma, we need to see that beautiful sky with a sense of awe, look toward the future with a sense of hope, and fight for one another with a sense of justice. We must use our emotional and spiritual drive to bring about ultimate healing for ourselves and others.

In 1944, Corrie ten Boom was sent to the Ravensbrück concentration camp, a horror like Auschwitz, for hiding Jews from the Nazis. She suffered much, and her sister died in that camp. After the war, she set up a rehabilitation center for those who had survived. Here is what she had to say about the experience in her book, *The Hiding Place*: "Today, I know that such memories are the key not to the past, but the future. I know that the experiences of our lives when we let God use them, become the mysterious and perfect preparation for the work he will give us to do."

The secret of grief is to face it, and even embrace it. We can use the tragedies we see as fuel to motivate us to alleviate the suffering of both ourselves and others. We live in a culture that will tell you the opposite and use materialism and a host of shiny objects to distract us. Use your problems as a solution. The most magnificent works of art and literature squarely face suffering and capture it rather than whitewash it. Find your spiritual well of energy and make it a part of your recovery.

Our Stories of Faith

DEBBIE

When Debbie lost her husband and the life she thought they had together, her church left her. But Debbie never left God, not in her heart. She developed a direct relationship with God. Rather than focus on Him just once a week at church, He became a constant part of her life, a continual presence on which she could rely.

JOHN

John lost his daughter to the nuclear fallout of the nearby atomic tests, but he has a deep spiritual connection to her and his ancestors. He loves to visit the small cemetery on the island. He remains quietly committed to his simple, Christian faith and hopes that he will be reunited with his daughter in the next life.

SUSAN

For Susan, whose beautiful home was destroyed by a landslide, her faith in God and her commitment to her religious community were of paramount importance.

Susan's friends from church—her church "family"—were the first ones to step up and offer their help when her house was destroyed.

From the moment Susan called them, they were at the ready. They offered her and her husband a place to stay, brought food, and, perhaps most importantly, provided love and a listening ear when the stress of the situation just got to be too much.

God was there every moment of the ordeal as well. Susan felt His presence and leaned on Him when it seemed that everything had just gotten to be too much. Her belief in God played a significant role in her ability not only to survive but also to thrive.

Susan reminds herself of God with this acronym:

TRUE GRIT

The	**G**od
Reason	**R**esilience
Under	**I**nner drive and meaning
Everything	**T**enacity

SHAD

Shad believes that God has put him in the right place at the right time throughout his life. From meeting Dr. Philip May during a side trip on his way to San Francisco to meeting the drummer of the Doobie Brothers, who then raised $300,000 for Shad's fledgling organization, Shad has felt God's hand at work.

It was not always that way. Though raised a Catholic, Shad lost faith and belief in God in the years immediately after returning home from the Vietnam War. He couldn't believe in a God who would allow so many fine young men to die in such brutal, painful ways—and for what? Nothing!

Yet as he worked with Vietnam veterans, he started to believe in God again. He saw the progress these vets made when they had the support they needed. Shad felt God helping heal his pain by giving him so many opportunities to be of service.

Shad got to see the other side of trauma. His belief was restored and is even stronger than before.

GERI

Geri was raised Catholic and has always had a deep and abiding belief in God.

While she no longer is a practicing Catholic today, Geri has always maintained her faith. Indeed, her faith has been essential in facing the day-to-day hardships of living with a disability.

A few years ago, Geri lost her dear sister, Gloria, to cancer. Without her faith in God, Geri does not believe she could have made it through. She misses her sister daily, but she has faith that her sister is her guiding angel, and she feels profoundly connected to her. Geri knows that one day she will be reunited with her sister and family in the next life, and this provides her the comfort to move forward.

TANYA

Tanya was raised Catholic. Like many people, she only attended church on the major holidays.

After her dear friend, Troy, died in 2000 of an accidental fall, Tanya hated God and blamed Him for everything that had happened. She could not understand how a supposedly "loving God" could so cruelly end the lives of so many people she loved—her friends who had died in high school, so young and with so much life left to live; her best friend who was run over by a hit-and-run driver and left to die in the street; her amazing sister who had finally, she thought, escaped a monster and was just beginning to live life on her terms; and finally, Troy, who had struggled with addiction for years and had finally gotten sober and was planning to marry the love of his life. How could God be so vicious as to steal them all?

Tanya learned that blaming God, or anyone else, is disempowering. Troy's family helped Tanya understand that God has a reason for everything, and that if she could just allow God into her heart, she would eventually find peace. They prayed for her and prayed with her. With their faith as an example to follow, Tanya let go of her anger towards God and accepted His will.

She was re-baptized as a Christian soon after. Now, Tanya embraces all positive expressions of a higher power and God. While she is a Christian, she has a respect for all beliefs and feels that God is big enough to include all of humanity in His grace.

JC

JC is a devoted Christian and an ordained minister. Throughout his years in prison, JC grew closer to God. God has given him the strength to get through the worst of times. God put people in his life who guided him and helped him through his struggles. And most importantly, through God's grace, JC has found the forgiveness that sets him free.

LEO

God gives everyone a purpose. According to Leo, God led him to invent the electric guitar and change the world of music. While he was not religious for most of his life, this profound belief drove him to get instruments into musicians' hands. The fact that it turned into a billion-dollar company was incidental. It was never about the money. It was about doing God's will.

I have visited with Leos' widow, Mrs. Fender, in the dressing rooms of some of the world's greatest country and rock stars, and I am astounded how often God comes up in the conversation about their purpose to create music.

JOE

Joe's commitment to God came later in life. As a boy and young man, he attended a Catholic church with his mother and grandmother. He was an altar boy and even sang in the church choir. But the God he learned about in the Catholic Church seemed to be cruel and almost indifferent to human suffering. Life under this version of God looked like an endless punishment. He did not want anything to do with a God like that.

In prison, Joe believed he was introduced to the real God, one of loving guidance and consistency. Joe realized that everything he has experienced was directed by God so that he could become the person God always knew him to be.

ERICA

Erica was raised Jewish, and she maintains her belief in God despite the horrors that she faced from the Nazis. She is particularly drawn to nature and loves the sunshine, which she feels flows from God. She is often found in the outside courtyard of her senior home, reading and contemplating life.

TOM

Tom is unsure about God's existence and even leans toward being an atheist, but he does have faith in humanity. He feels compelled to keep an eye on those who are struggling and frequently steps in to assist those who are. His acts are often quiet and go unnoticed by everyone except those whom he helps.

MY STORY

The evidence for God is not only compelling but also overwhelming. When I realized that God created me with a heart problem and that was exactly how He wanted me to come into the world, my emotional healing could progress from surviving to thriving. My life was ideal in almost every other way. God wanted me to build a little character by going through the ordeal. When I realized that my heart problem was part of God's purpose, it made sense.

CHAPTER 12

Connection

To get to the thriving stage of trauma, it is essential to find a trustworthy person and talk about our innermost feelings. Until we find one, we can journal. We must accept support and form new ways to love and relate to others.

SYMPATHETIC RESONANCE

WE ARE SOCIAL CREATURES. There is a saying, "Our vibe attracts our tribe," and there is science to prove it.

General semantics is a system of linguistic philosophy in self-improvement and therapeutic programs founded in the 1920s by Polish-American Alfred Korzybski. His 1933 book *Science and Sanity* launched the concept of human behavior as an extension of language and expression. From there, thousands of studies have been conducted that show the importance of connecting with others and clearly expressing ourselves. Essentially, this science shows that there is great truth in the adage, "Birds of a feather flock together."

Furthermore, the science of harmony, vibration, and soundwaves is fascinating and has produced the concept of "sympathetic resonance." Essentially, this is a principle that says that if we send out a soundwave, it will resonate with everything that is in tune with it. For example, if you strike a tuning fork, ring a bell, or hit a note on the piano, the vibration will travel through the air to resonate with other things that are in tune with that vibration. While that second bell was never touched, it will start ringing. Other strings will start vibrating in unison. Even crystal glasses in the room can begin vibrating musically. Soundwaves set off vibrations all around them. Being aware of this interplay of harmonies is a powerful principle for all musicians.

Vibrations are all around us. Music has a vibe, but so do people, businesses, families, and organizations. They all emit a vibe that resonates with others who are in tune with that same frequency. If a group of strangers is put together in a room, before long the outgoing people who have a great sense of humor will be hanging out with each other, the introverts will be whispering together, and the toxic people will be clustered together gossiping.

We are the product of the five or six people that we spend the most time with. If we want to heal from trauma, we must get in tune with our vibe, knowing that it will attract others with a similar wavelength. Ultimately, if we want a vibe of love, healing, humility, and kindness, we cultivate that vibe within us, and others on the same frequency will be attracted to it.

We are all tuned to a frequency. There are good vibes and bad vibes. Go for the good harmonics. Healing takes humility, willingness to learn new things, and connection with people who are healthy and will support you. Morgan Freeman stated, “Correct a fool, and he will hate you. Correct a wise man, and he will appreciate you.”

There is no such thing as a self-made person. There are always those who believed in you, taught you, lifted you, and gave you what you needed to start. Our relationships with others constitute an essential cornerstone of life.

Healing involves communication. We need the courage to face deeper truths and expose our most authentic selves. Keeping things inside works for a while, but to heal, we must be able to communicate.

Even when we say nothing, we are delivering a message. We can communicate verbally and through our actions, body language, tone of voice, or facial expressions.

Humanity is dominated by verbal communication, so it is vital to choose our words mindfully. When our communication style does not match others, it can hurt feelings, initiate conflict, or create misunderstandings. We must be mindful of others' cues and have empathy for where they are coming from. A "throwaway" comment of no consequence to us may be deeply meaningful or hurtful to another. Furthermore, there are many aspects of communication that go beyond the words themselves. Timing and delivery are critically important. Along with this, we should evaluate whether we are being listened to and if we are carefully listening to others.

Bad communication often stems from an undisciplined style where we eliminate filters and say whatever comes to mind. Or the converse, where we don't say what we mean, but it nevertheless comes out in our actions. Healthy communication includes a variety of deliberate tools and techniques. Gary Chapman teaches the "Five Love Languages," which describe how people connect. They are "words of affirmation," "physical touch," "quality time," "physical gifts," and "acts of service." Being aware of how we and those we love respond to these five love languages can help us better connect.

Being mindful of and understanding our true feelings is essential to effective communication. If we wish to communicate effectively with others, we must first learn to communicate with ourselves. There are *primary feelings* and *secondary feelings.* Primary feelings are on the surface, while secondary feelings are buried inside. For example, someone may primarily feel anger at his or her financial situation, but underneath have a sense of shame for growing up in poverty. To heal, we must take an honest look at both sets of feelings.

In my view, there is a trilogy of all-time environmental disasters that include Chernobyl, the Bikini Atoll, and Bhopal. Bhopal was a chemical plant leak in India that killed tens of thousands of people living in the neighborhood. After inspecting the site where the leak occurred, I sat on a hilltop overlooking the city with Ajay, a Hindu man, and we spoke for a long time. He was conversant in all major world religions. His family was hit by the Bhopal disaster, the world's worst industrial accident. For the first time, I listened to the teachings of Hinduism, the caste system, Buddhism and Muslim faiths, and their sacred books. Frankly, many of my notions and judgments were wrong. There I was, a tall, white guy from Orange County on a mountain in India, learning new ideas from a wise Hindu. It later hit me that this was very cliché! This all brought perfect clarity to what I will accomplish with the rest of my life. Everyone has a mission in life, and mine is to serve others with my non-profit, Core IQ, which teaches life skills such as time management and goal setting online at no cost.

While I have faced traumas, I am also aware that I have had a privileged life. Thankfully, I am capable of learning new things and defer to others when I think they might know more than me. I am committed to the truth to the point where I can admit I was wrong. While I have core values, I am open-minded enough to take interesting information from all over the place and incorporate it into my belief system.

Peace comes from integrity. Healing comes from honesty. The very word "integrity" comes from the word "integrated." To have integrity, our inner voice must align with our outer choices. If we ever allow others to control our inner voice, we will create a war within ourselves. Don't kill yourself for a company that can replace you within a week or a toxic partner who will hurt you when you are vulnerable. Be kind to yourself. Stay away from negative people. Such people have a problem for every solution. Don't look for someone who will solve all your problems. Look for someone who won't let you face your challenges alone.

We must connect with people to thrive. We must be a part of a tribe. In 1979, Dr. Lisa Berkman, of the Harvard School of Health Sciences, studied 7,000 people between the ages of 35 and 65. This nine-year longitudinal study concluded that people who lack any community ties are nearly three times more likely to die of medical illness than those who have active social lives. No matter how educated, talented, or cool we think we are, how we treat people tells all. It is a jungle out there, and, as the saying goes, "A lone monkey is a dead monkey."

How our community reacts to a traumatic event will utterly determine the long-term effects of the trauma. For instance, we know that sexually abused children who had a supportive and loving family and received proper professional therapy early did not suffer PTSD as often as those who did not have those resources. Traumatic stress lingers when we don't feel safe in our environment. If the people around us are not safe, we can't be safe, even if the earthquake is long over. The earthquake not only destroys our home but also reveals who is safe and who is not.

Recovery from stress is not a solo act. We need social support. Yes, we need time on our own, but we also need to play, have fun, socialize, and have intimate conversations. Our family, friends, confidants, and even casual acquaintances are all essential resources. The Buffering Theory suggests that those who enjoy close relationships fare better than those who face stress alone. The theory shows that a social support system helps buffer or shield an individual from the negative impact of stressful events, including physical, emotional, or mental illness.

MUTUAL RESPECT

Clinical psychologist and author Dr. Elizabeth Lombardo states that there are four types of communication: passive, aggressive, passive-aggressive, and assertive.

Passive means we quietly sit by and remain silent. This is fine in some situations, but if we remain passive when we should be speaking up, this can be a problem. For example, let us say we have a bully verbally attacking us. What do we do? If we remain silent, it is as if we agree with them, or what an attorney may call, "implied admission." Or we appear defeated.

Aggressive means we verbally and loudly attack another. This is usually a turn-off to whomever we are speaking with and shuts down communication. In our example of the bully, if we verbally and loudly attack the bully back and say, "Shut up you jerk!" we may shut them up for a bit or start an argument. Ultimately, this approach will spread their venom, which is precisely what they want.

Passive-aggressive means we ignore people and their concerns. We let our anger out in less visible, yet still aggressive ways. While we are quiet, this is generally considered offsetting or rude behavior. In the bully scenario, if we verbally say nothing to the bully but later make snide remarks about them to others, the bully can feel satisfied or self-righteous when he hears about it. In other words, the bully wants to excite a reaction and upset you, and, in this case, he got it.

Finally, there is *assertive* behavior, which is usually the ideal. Of these four types of communication styles, being assertive is often the best approach. We speak up, but in a reasonable way. We want to be calm. Here, we are respectful of others and ourselves and clearly communicate our positions while hoping to have a firm but healthy dialog. If we confidently respond to the bully and do not scream but instead communicate our position clearly and calmly, we can be productive. For example, we might simply respond by saying, "Well, I'm sorry you feel that way. I don't agree, but I hope you have a great day anyway!" Here we speak up, retain our power, and show emotional maturity.

When we are assertive, we are attentive to others' positions and needs while also paying attention to our own. Coming to a mutual understanding is most likely going to happen when we have assertive communication because we speak up and identify our observations and needs. If a person responds to assertive communication with aggression or passive-aggression, that is a sign they may be toxic. We ought to protect ourselves by setting boundaries or limiting contact.

Developing an assertive communication pattern is not always easy, nor does it come naturally to many people. Indeed, it may feel inappropriate, selfish, or awkward. In many family and cultural dynamics, we may have been taught to avoid conflict and stay quiet.

We are considerate of others' feelings while giving our positions and preferences a back seat. After all, we do not want to come off as being selfish or overbearing.

People with passive communication styles seem quiet on the outside, but negative feelings are brewing on the inside. People who use these styles may feel hurt and have anxiety and a low self-image under the surface. This person may seem shy, timid, and overly apologetic. They avoid expressing their real thoughts and feelings. Often, they are manipulated and taken advantage of and do not stand up for themselves.

Being assertive, on the other hand, is showing respect for ourselves and the other person. It is open and honest. It provides balance to everyone's interests, where all parties, including ourselves, are given a voice.

Clear differences also exist between being assertive and being aggressive. People with aggressive communication styles are easy to spot. They are loud, obnoxious, and generally inappropriate. Aggressive people are often arrogant; they use people as objects and try to dominate others. They also tend to be sarcastic and demeaning.

On the other hand, the tone, timing, and delivery of assertive communication are calm, respectful, and thoughtful. Being aggressive is being harsh and overbearing. It is winning at any cost. Being assertive is approached in the spirit of having character and a willingness to resolve issues.

While passivity, aggression, or passive-aggression are generally considered to be negative traits, there are exceptions. For example, if we have trouble with our temper, it may be preferable to remain passive while collecting our thoughts. Later, we can express our feelings assertively when we have our emotions under control. If someone is violent or emotionally abusive, we may have to react aggressively to protect ourselves and put ourselves out of harm's way.

Assertive communication is thoughtful, proactive, and not reactive. It reflects a high level of emotional intelligence, or EQ, and pushes through our limiting beliefs. With assertive communication, we are aware of our environment and express our feelings directly, but respectfully. We respect the boundaries of others, while also requesting others to honor our borders as well. This projects a healthy self-confidence, humility, and a positive self-image. We are aware of others' dispositions and know when to take a step back and when to step up.

When communicating our feelings to others, it is far better to use "I" statements than "you" statements. When we start a sentence with "you," it often puts others on the defensive. On the other hand, when we begin a sentence with "I," we convey our feelings about the situation or relationship. For example, if we say, "You never ..." we are likely to get into an argument or make the other person feel like they are being attacked or blamed. But, if we say, "When this situation happened, I felt...," it expresses our own needs without being judgmental. This can ultimately lead to both parties better understanding each other and result in a successful resolution of the issues.

One communication formula that might be helpful is to say, "I feel X when you Y because of Z. I would prefer it if you did A instead." For example, "I feel nauseated when you leave all the dog's stuff on the kitchen counter because it looks messy and does not seem sanitary. I prefer that you put all the dog stuff in a designated drawer or cupboard instead." Or, "I feel anxious when you don't give me a check for household expenses without my asking. I prefer that you set up an automatic, direct deposit account instead."

Words are powerful—words matter. To heal, we take care of our thoughts when we are alone and our tone and words when we are with people. Being passive, aggressive, or passive-aggressive are different types of communication, yet they all reflect something in common: the person's needs are not met, and the wounds of past traumas are not healed. The more we honestly face our issues and are pleasantly assertive, the more we will be able to move past them.

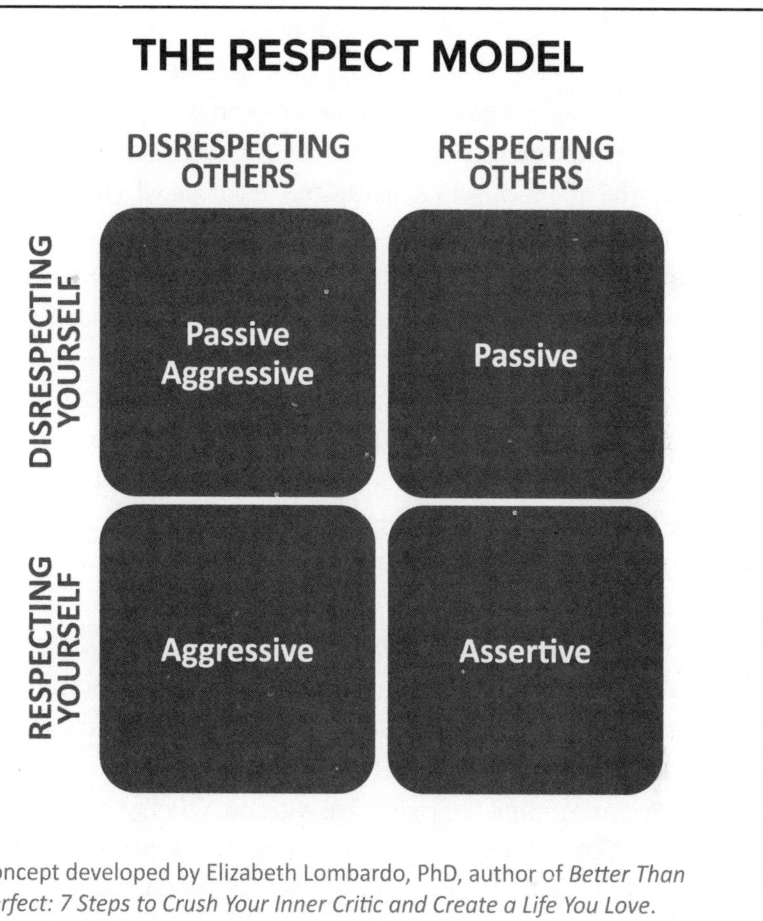

Concept developed by Elizabeth Lombardo, PhD, author of *Better Than Perfect: 7 Steps to Crush Your Inner Critic and Create a Life You Love.* www.ElizabethLombardo.com.

TOXIC VIBES

In 1967, Dr. Albert Mehrabian of UCLA carried out the most widely cited study on communication in his paper, "Decoding of Inconsistent Communication." Remarkably, he found that 55 percent of people respond to visual messages, 38 percent respond to our tone of voice, while a mere 7 percent respond to the actual words we use. In other words, to connect with others, we must pay keen attention to our appearance and body language, as well as our tone of voice.

We need to speak up and express ourselves. Dr. Martin Luther

King, Jr. said, "Our lives begin to end the day we become silent about things that matter." When trauma hits, we learn who is there for us. Some run away altogether, some drop off a casserole and leave, while others stay for the long haul. There is no question that trauma can often be a lonely, solo experience. Yet those who thrive do not entirely go at it alone.

Sometimes the crisis exposes false friendships or even a sense of betrayal. Trauma can yield a host of relational problems, including fear, rage, control issues, isolation, aggression, abuse, longing, neglect, betrayal, co-dependence, and a yearning for affection. Often, these signs and symptoms of trauma can later materialize in our relationships when we are triggered. If our world is full of chaos and we have had multiple relational train wrecks, we must make an honest assessment of the suspect who was present at each of those crime scenes—ourselves.

Yet if our wagon is hitched to a toxic person, we can be in the center of a chaos vortex, and we need distance from that person. This can be a blind spot, as we have spent so much time holding the view that the chaos is all us. Abusers are fond of pointing out our relationship history to "prove" that the issues are with us. When we have doubts, we should look for objective sources for guidance. So, it is a balance. We do need to take a look at ourselves while not dismissing the possibility that we need to get out of abusive relationships.

Here is the good news: there is healing after abuse. Even those who have endured childhood trauma can develop secure attachments in adult life. We must create a network of healthy relationships with like-minded family, friends, romantic partners, and work or school relationships. Being self-dependent does not mean that we avoid relying on others for security. It means that we can manage and take care of ourselves when we separate from toxic relationships and form healthy relationships.

Being committed to others is honorable. Honoring our commitments is a sign to others that we are loyal and dependable. However, that changes when we learn that the person or organization turns out to be toxic. A healthy person will face reality and take appropriate action. Unfortunately, many traumatized people remain comfortable, at least part of the time, because they are already maxed out, and they can't see taking on additional risk, even if doing so will free them. When challenged, they double down, not on the issue itself, but with their sense of commitment. When the choice is between honesty and loyalty, too many choose loyalty.

Loyalty has a high value for narcissists. If someone demands obedience, this is a big red flag. Loyalty is a fine quality; however, unless you are a medieval lord or a military commander, it is not something that should be demanded. Loyalty is earned, and it is up to us who deserves our loyalty. Abusers can spend a lot of time on this one and demand "support." When they say, "You do not support me," it can mean, "You do not agree with me 100 percent, and I am going to keep grinding on you until you do."

Abusers, and the groups that harbor them, always prefer that victims, witnesses, and fellow members hush up. Perpetrators and their enablers thrive in secrecy and darkness. On the other hand, healthy and well-adjusted groups foster honesty and open discussions, even on the severe and embarrassing issues. That is what mature, healthy people do. Decent people take responsibility and require that the lights be fully turned on.

LEAVING THE FOLD

We are social creatures. We gather in clubs, schools, places of worship, and businesses. One thing they all have in common is that some organizations are healthy, while others are not. Peter Enns, a biblical scholar and theologian, published some liberal views about the Bible that forced him to leave Westminster Seminary in Philadelphia. He said:

"If your present community sees your spiritual journey as a problem because you are wandering off their beach blanket, it may be time to find another community. One should never do that impulsively. But, if after a time you are sensing that you do not belong, that you are a problem to be corrected rather than a valued member of the community, maybe God is calling you elsewhere and to find for yourself that 'they' aren't so bad after all. That decision is very personal (sometimes involving whole families) and can take some courage to make, but it is worth the risk. One thing is sure: if you stay where you are without any change, the pressure to either conform or keep quiet will work in you like a slow-acting poison. And if you go too far down that road, it can be a tough haul coming back from bitterness and resentment—especially for children."

When one leaves an unhealthy club, its members often shame deserters with comments like, "They lacked commitment," "They were weak," or "You can leave, but you can't leave it alone." This is more nonsense. Abusers always want to be left alone. If a group is legitimate, it will stand up to any scrutiny and not allow toxic relationships to flourish. One person who left a toxic group said, "When I left the organization, not one person reached out. Not one friend. This is mind control. It has nothing to do with the good behavior they espouse. It has everything to do with blind obedience." We need to scare the hell out of abusers. We need to be the good people who stand up and say, "No, I am not going to let you get away with that."

When we step away from toxic people or organizations, we may panic. This root of this fear stems from our co-dependence and makes us want to return to our abuser. However, if we keep moving away, we may still experience considerable anxiety as if our whole world has crashed and burned. Questions, doubts, and depression can swirl all around us, binding us to the trauma. Some traumas are multi-generational. It ran in our families until it ran into us. That is the good news; We are here to break the cycle. Amid all that turbulence, we will discover that a clean slate is a great place to design a new life.

When we calm down and realize that we are okay now, we feel much better. We ask ourselves how we could have been so gullible. Once we are out of an abusive relationship or a toxic organization, we can see that it never made any sense in the first place. The friendship was not real. The stress is suddenly gone. None of the labels, threats, enticements, or incentives have any value. We cannot believe what we believed and did. The sense of relief is unimaginable!

While from the outside, toxic systems seem apparent, the truth is that anyone can get trapped in one. The process is typically slow and starts with a period of charm and love-bombing. Those who operate toxic systems do not fit the system to the person. They fit the person to the system through careful manipulation and control, even if it means breaking the person.

As we distance ourselves from toxicity, we develop a healthy self-image, which has two profound consequences. First, our heads are in a good place which contributes to our sense of well-being; and, second, we will naturally repel toxic people and attract same-minded people into our lives. Practicing acts of self-protection and finding secure relationships are the proven pathways out of traumatic bonding. To heal from trauma, we must first practice self-care and enjoy healthy relationships.

We can never heal from something we hold onto. Thrivers eventually push through these challenges with a heightened quest for authentic connection.

HEALTHY BOUNDARIES

Each person has an energy field around them. You are the sole gatekeeper of what can enter your space. Be aware of energy thieves, and maintain positive relationships and set healthy boundaries. For example, "Nobody can touch me or my property without my permission"or "I am not obligated to discuss topics I'm uncomfortable with."

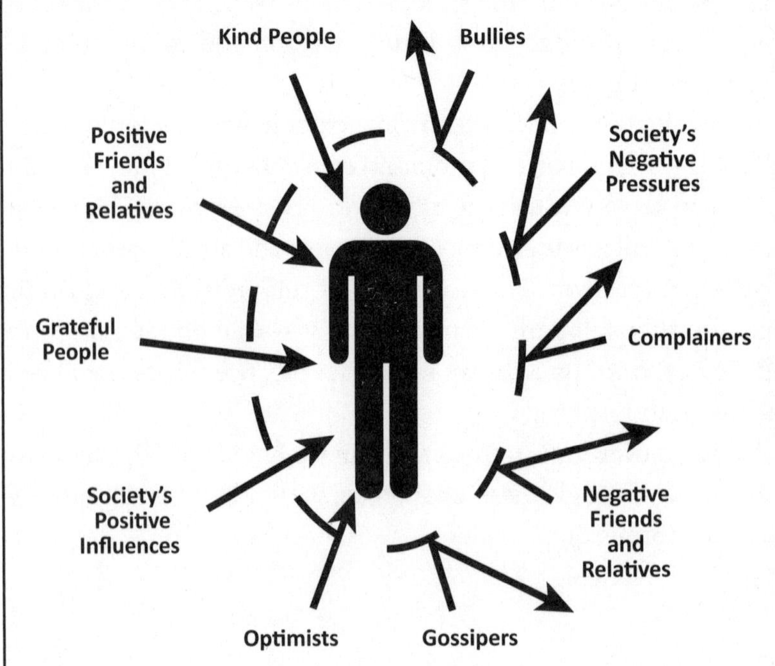

HEALTHY GROUP ETHICS

Connection means that we work well with others for our healing. One way we can connect is to join a group; however, for healing to occur, the group must be healthy. Here are several trademarks of a healthy group.

First, functional groups have full disclosure and practices of *informed consent*. Before joining, prospective members are provided upfront, complete, full, and honest disclosure of all relevant information.

In healthy organizations, critical thinking is not only allowed but also encouraged. Members utilize *critical thinking* skills, wherein they are free to question or challenge all points of view, including the group's own beliefs or behaviors. Critical thinking does not mean we are obnoxious or confrontational. It merely means that we are open to thought and discussion on a topic. Nothing is so sacred that we should not be able to point out its flaws. In my family and business, I often say, "Do not believe what I say. Research what I say!" Opposing views are investigated, compared, and contrasted. Independent sources can reveal corroborating or disconfirming information from parties with different or competing interests. Any relevant topic is safe to explore and discuss within the boundaries of appropriate timing, delivery, and good taste. *Groupthink* or *willful ignorance* is challenged. A healthy group will have a history of ethical behavior and apologizing for errors.

No quality organization will practice undue influence where its members are manipulated in any way. The group should not coerce or deceive members. Pertinent information should not be withheld, ignored, or hidden. Members are never induced to act opposite of their own free will or without adequate knowledge of the consequences.

There will be conflict in any organization, so the protocols for conflict resolution will include addressing any member's concerns. Members' disputes are resolved, not avoided or evaded. There is a clear *complaint box* protocol. Conflicts, concerns, or questions are directly addressed and discussed without pivoting off-topic and all parties have input. Any allegations of illegal behaviors are immediately reported to the police or law enforcement. Victim shaming is not tolerated.

In a healthy organization, there is a system of oversight. There should always be a fair appeal process or an independent body with the power to oversee the organization's leaders to prevent any one leader from abusing his or her power.

Finally, in healthy groups, the members may always safely exit. Members may choose to leave the group without the fear of being shunned, shamed, harassed, or hounded.

These group ethics are valid and helpful, whether the group is a club or a religious, social, political, educational, or vocational group.

Our Stories of Connection

DEBBIE

Debbie connected with those who could relate best to the trauma of losing her husband to suicide—her children.

Two weeks after her husband's death, Debbie and her children shared a profoundly cathartic experience. Fully dressed, they all got into the shower together, the shower where he had taken his life.

They turned on the water, drenching themselves. They started to sing, softly at first, and then louder. Their voices grew strong. As they sang, their eyes met. A feeling of deep love washed over them, much as the water from the showerhead washed over their bodies. They were all in this together, and they were all there to support one another for life.

JOHN

John grew up on an island in a small village. Everyone knew John and shared in the grief when his daughter died from radiation poisoning from the nearby nuclear tests on the Bikini Atoll. The villagers continually brought John and his family fish, coconuts, and taro roots. They cried with them and played games.

The entire village shared in the family's grief. The town showed love and sent the message that "we are all in this together." That spirit of unity never faltered. While John deeply missed his daughter, at least he knew he and his family were loved.

SUSAN

Susan had a close relationship with those in her church, but those relationships became even deeper as she and her husband sorted through the mess caused by the loss of their home to a landslide. Her church friends were simply there for her. They immediately gave her a place to stay, invited her for meals, and paid attention to her needs. They came through and now have a bond for life.

SHAD

In Shad's first five years working with vets at the Veterans Administration Hospital, he buried 17 of his patients. It was heartbreaking to see their pain while alive and even more heartbreaking to stand at their gravesides.

These losses impressed upon Shad the importance of uncovering someone's real issues and working towards a solution. "The sooner we get to the problems," he says, "the more success we will have."

Using the information he recorded from his experience at the VA, Shad founded the Vietnam Veterans Re-Socialization Unit at the VA Hospital. It was a groundbreaking program, and it soon gained attention nationwide. Psychiatrists, psychologists, and social workers from around the country, who had also been observing the issues with the newly returning Vietnam veterans, began to reach out to Shad for his insight.

Shad also stresses the importance of connection. That is what the National Veterans Foundation and its vet-to-vet model are all about. The National Veterans Foundation has expanded its services tremendously over 35 years. Services, delivered through the toll-free crisis information hotline and the NVF website (www.nvf.org), include job programs for returning veterans, vet-to-vet counseling, support for returning veterans, housing and medical services, education benefits, financial counseling, and workshops offering training in peer-to-peer counseling.

Though initially founded for Vietnam vets, the National Veterans Foundation welcomes any vet from any branch of the military and their families. Since 1985, more than 450,000 veterans have connected with the services the Foundation provides. Each vet is understood, valued, and assisted.

GERI

Geri's openness about her life and her willingness to put herself "out there" has made it possible to connect with many kinds of people from all walks of life. A naturally kind and empathetic person, Geri makes people comfortable. Her humor, too, is a connector—especially on stage, where she uses the challenges she has faced as a person with cerebral palsy as fodder for some of her routines. Her acceptance of her life situation encourages people to be okay with the challenges they face—and the connection they feel with her deepens.

Geri's respect for herself and her love for others comes through bright and true. She is surrounded by friends whom she loves and who love and adore her. By the time she was in college, she was hopscotching emotionally, psychosocially, and academically. If it were not for her innate intelligence and loving and supportive family and teachers who believed in her, she would not have been able to last even one year in college.

TANYA

Tanya lost her sister, Nicole, to a horrific murder. Her family was already close, and after Nicole's death, they came together even more. They would sit around the kitchen table, cry about the situation, and laugh about the great memories. Before the murder, the family was warm and welcoming to all. After the murder, they still were stronger together and took turns supporting those who were having a bad day.

JC

During his years in prison, JC made several deep connections with other people that helped him overcome the trauma of being sent to prison at such a young and vulnerable age. Perhaps the most impactful of these people was a gentleman named Claude Grimes, who served as JC's mentor the entire time of his incarceration.

Claude was JC's guardian angel in a time of darkness. Over the next two-plus decades, Claude was a consistent presence in JC's life, even when JC's family and friends on the outside slowly dropped away. Claude wrote JC letters and accepted his collect telephone calls regularly. Claude also visited him and attended multiple graduations that JC was a part of. Claude proudly sat in the audience when JC earned first his GED and then his college degree. JC was deeply grateful for Claude's friendship and mentorship.

There were times over those two decades of life behind bars that JC became profoundly depressed, and thoughts of suicide crossed his mind. He trusted Claude and could tell him everything he was feeling. "We are fighting for you on this side of the wall," Claude would say to him. "You need to fight on your side."

JC also created secure connections with many of the inmates with whom he took classes. As their time came up or they gained parole, JC stayed in touch with them, encouraging them as they started to rebuild their lives in the world beyond the walls.

LEO

While going through life with a glass eye and mostly deaf, Leo still liked people. Borrowing money against his Ford Model A, he rented a storefront on 107 South Harbor Boulevard in Fullerton, California and set up a radio and record store.

Leo's shop became a hangout for local kids, where they would go to listen to music. While not extroverted, Leo liked people, and he became friends with the local kids and his many customers.

JOE

Joe values secure connections now more than he ever has in his life. The relationships he has built over the years with therapists, friends, and clients have helped guide him. He may "walk and talk tough," as he puts it, but inside he is empathetic and driven to help others. His connections keep him grounded and focused on what is essential.

Given the path his life has taken, there have been some lost connections over the years. His two sons, now in their late 20s, grew distant from Joe after he and their mother divorced. His drug addiction and subsequent prison term pushed them even further away. And the situation grew worse due to their mother's constant negativity and anger towards Joe.

For years, Joe's sons didn't speak with him. It broke his heart, but he continued to reach out to them. His goal was to reconnect with them and build a relationship with them as adults. The good news is that his consistency is beginning to pay off. He and his sons have started communicating again. Not as often as he would like, but Joe is still grateful for the opportunity to potentially renew their connection.

ERICA

Erica hid from the Nazis by herself. She really could not trust anyone, as rewards were being paid to those who turned in the Jews. This meant long years of hiding in every little place she could find. She needed a source of food, which came in the form of eating potato skins, something she had always thought were poisonous.

One day, she was so desperate and starving that she ate some. She was shocked to see she was still alive, so they became her primary source of food for years.

When the war was over, she learned that her family had been killed in the concentration camps, so she moved to the United States to meet new people and start a new life. Erica loves people, and she attracted a wide range of friends.

TOM

Tom was shocked when President Carter's decision to boycott the 1980 Summer Olympics crushed the Olympic dream he had worked toward for years.

On a larger scale, this action changed the lives of hundreds of would-be Olympic competitors. Since Americans—and athletes from West Germany, Japan, and Kenya—were not allowed to participate in the 1980 games, the "true" winners of the gold, silver, and bronze medals will never really be known.

Before the boycott, athletes from the US were predicted to sweep in several key competitions. Instead, other potentially less-skilled athletes took home those awards. The whole mess rippled out from there. The Russians returned the favor and boycotted the 1984 Olympics. Who would have won if everyone were allowed to compete? The answer will never be known, and the 1980 and 1984 Olympics were tainted.

In any event, Tom had to move past the situation. He focused on his college athletic career. As he had in high school, Tom won awards and accolades in every college-level event he participated in. He formed tight and lifelong bonds with the other athletes on his college team along the way.

Plus, Tom was able to obtain a genuinely stellar education. He made friends in his classes and created connections through internships, and years later, those people have become valuable business contacts.

MY STORY

I never spoke about my heart surgery unless someone else brought it up. When I realized how essential it was for me to discuss it, I brought up the topic and used it to share some principles of life when I was giving keynote speeches.

My cardiologist is the first person I confided in about being triggered by the event on the treadmill that day. She told me to swing by her office anytime and stand on the treadmill to process the anxiety. I have done that, and she completely understands.

At first, it was uncomfortable to admit the whole thing, but today the stress is completely gone. Mention of my heart surgery no longer triggers or bothers me at all. I faced it, dealt with it, and it is over.

CHAPTER 13

Forgiveness

We must use the hurts of the past as fuel to grow and realize new possibilities.

FORGIVE AND FORGET? YEAH, RIGHT

ONE OF THE BIGGEST MISTAKES people make is to think they need to "forgive and forget." Are you kidding me? Who is going to forget a murder, rape, incest, or child abuse? Who is going to ignore death, war, illness, or a horrible car crash? "Forgive and forget" is likely the single most damaging statement on the topic of healing.

While it is easy to forget a small bump in the road, it is ludicrous to think one can forget sexual abuse, betrayal, genocide, or other crimes. Humanity's worst nightmares, such as the Holocaust, wars, or serial killers, may or may not be forgiven, but should not be forgotten. These horrors inflicted a high price on humanity for the lessons they taught, which are lessons to be remembered and preserved.

Often, this ridiculous advice is dished out by perpetrators who are trying to avoid accountability. If the crime is forgiven, they never have to answer to or pay the same price as their victims, and they are free to offend again. Yes, we do want to heal, and we want the memories of the trauma to pass through our minds without triggering or disabling us, but suggesting we "just forget it" is a joke. To heal, we need to dismiss these pressures to simply "move on." Perpetrators should always be held accountable.

Some in the older generation will be quick to say, "forgive and forget," "let us never speak of this again," "it is best we not talk about that," "why can't you just get over it?" or other such common sayings. These notions are harmful to our mental health. Healing is an active process. Rather than forget, we must face what has happened to us and the fact that another human being might have caused the harm, maybe even on purpose.

To start, we can find someone who is proven to be trustworthy, and preferably licensed, to help us through the trauma. Talking about it and its fallout reduces the stress it causes. It may or may not solve anything in and of itself, but it relieves that pressure and allows for healing to move forward. By talking, we establish a narrative. Telling the story may help push the memory from the brain's amygdala, which processes fear and other emotions, through to the hippocampus, which regulates our motivation, emotion, learning, and memory. In other words, and while this is a simplified explanation, talking about something can rewire our brains and shift memories from the area of the brain that gets "charged" or "triggered" to the part in control of our emotions. Talking can also clarify things for ourselves.

When working through severe trauma, finding professional help is essential. Trained and licensed mental health professionals can listen to your honest experiences, keep your information confidential, and not toss around anecdotal advice that can be damaging. A good therapist will guide you to find and follow your inner voice and trust your instincts, rather than tell you what to think. A good therapist never gives unsolicited advice and allows you to come to your own conclusions about the best course of action.

We must understand that no competent therapist, or anyone else, can make our personal decisions for us. They can provide a safe sounding board, perhaps prescribe medications when needed, and give us intelligent feedback. Ultimately, we must accept responsibility for our attitudes, relationships, actions, and goals.

I have four adult children, and I am proud of them and love each one deeply. As a dad, I give them my advice. I tell my kids that they will hear lots of comments and information from others all around them. But, ultimately, this is their life and their journey. Smart people research all sides of an issue. I ask my kids to please consider my thoughts and the thoughts of all those who love them, but, ultimately, they should listen to and follow their inner voice. The saying goes, "Follow your bliss." It is not, "Follow my bliss," or "Follow her bliss." Only your inner voice can tell you what that is.

We must find our authentic inner voice. We can listen to parents, priests, popes, pundits, prophets, and politicians, but ultimately, we must take a real look at all of this and then, determine who we are and what our purpose is. The Dalai Lama says, "There are only two days in the year that nothing can be done. One is called 'yesterday,' and the other is called 'tomorrow,' so today is the right day to love, believe, do, and mostly live." A good therapist can help you in this quest to live mindfully today.

REFRAMING OUR WORLD

Forgiveness is often a misunderstood topic. How we forgive is a profoundly personal thing. Some say we must forgive, yet some cannot forgive. Some state that forgiveness is useful or even essential. Perhaps our religious texts and teachers have instructed us to forgive. For some of us, after years have passed since the trauma, we still feel anger and resentment. Others say that we cannot heal until we forgive our perpetrators. Yet others say that we must forgive ourselves before moving forward. Some say that God has already forgiven, while others say that some acts are unforgivable. It is one thing to be told to forgive or say the words, but it is another thing to do so. Ultimately, forgiveness is an issue that we must decide for ourselves.

When traumatic events happen, it is essential to face them, go through the anger process, and express the rage that we feel.

Forgiveness never means forfeiting our legal rights, having the responsibility to report a crime, or remaining in a toxic relationship. Numbing ourselves and shutting up never results in healing. Some events cannot, and should not, be forgotten.

Forgiveness is a somewhat abstract concept, and because of that, we all experience it in different ways. Self-guided forgiveness allows us to listen to ourselves and trust ourselves. Sometimes we do not want to forgive, at least not yet. If there is still hurt, anger, or bitterness, it is there for a reason—even if we do not know what that reason is. There may be a lesson to learn by exploring those emotions as we go through life and encounter new experiences. Those feelings may be protecting us until we find replacement coping mechanisms. Or the event may have impacted us so significantly that we may just need to process it slowly. There is a difference between not being ready to forgive, which can be healthy, and holding a grudge, which is a more active feeling that causes us to obsess and take unhealthy actions. Setting boundaries is part of this, as there are people we may not ever want to speak to again. However, this may be more about protecting ourselves from their toxicity and less about punishing them or seeking revenge. If we are holding onto a hardcore, vengeful grudge, we should seek help.

Remembering a hardship is essential for many people. Simply knowing this and setting aside the bad advice to do otherwise can bring us a big step closer to healing. Some say that we cannot forgive until we feel the full measure of hurt. Forgiveness is a personal and individual experience. It is a matter of the heart and cannot be cajoled or forced. For some it comes easily and for others it takes years. Yet for some, it simply never happens. Generally, we cannot forgive until we face the pain that was caused. Premature forgiveness may be retraumatizing. Yet those who do forgive may call it a mystery, grace, or gift from God.

To truly thrive, we must be at least open to the idea of forgiveness. We must at least see the benefits and make a conscious decision of whether we are ready to forgive and what forgiveness means to us.

In other words, we can take the steps and put ourselves in a position where forgiveness is more likely to happen. Many people report that forgiveness finally came unexpectedly or at a time when they listened to their inner voice. They were intentionally practicing self-care or building the courage to face their perpetrator head-on. But we are all different. The essential point is that we are taking steps to heal and create peace amid chaos.

Not forgiving may cause us to be hypervigilant in order to protect ourselves from being revictimized. Few would dispute that forgiveness is a desirable objective, and there are some practical considerations in the process. Carefully consider what the world would look like without mercy. If you find yourself angry and bitter, talk about it with someone you can trust. Think about how resentment towards those who harmed you is causing you harm. Talk to your doctor about the long-term effects of extended stress, brooding, blame, and anger. Consider how fixating on another's bad behavior is affecting your good behavior. Think about ways to channel the anger into a constructive cause.

Merely hoping for forgiveness is a tangible step toward achieving it. Even a scant or halfhearted effort is a step in the right direction. Forgiveness often does not come all at once. At times, the word "forgiveness" is inadequate. It fails to capture the profound damage and grief we experienced and the intense work needed to overcome them. Being a victim of trauma shocks us to the core. We feel broken, violated, and dehumanized by the terrible acts. Working towards forgiveness can help us reclaim our rights to humanity.

FORGIVING OURSELVES

Everything happens for a reason. However, sometimes the reason is that we made a bad decision! In other words, sometimes we hold some level of responsibility for our trauma, and we need to own it.

Decent people want to be forgiven for the pain they have caused others. They find it difficult to move forward without obtaining forgiveness. Considering this, it is essential also to forgive ourselves.

Whenever possible, if we have hurt others, we need to apologize. In some cases, we also need to forgive ourselves. It is essential to understand that we need a healthy relationship with ourselves.

Dwelling on anger, resentment, and self-blame is damaging both physically and emotionally. If we want to love others, we must love ourselves—not in a vain way but in an authentic, self-respecting way. We can heal the hurt that is raging inside of us. Lowering our defenses makes us vulnerable, but it also opens up the possibility of healing. We must look at situations where we have harmed others as an opportunity for growth and healing.

Both forgiveness and self-forgiveness are not for the timid. They are acts of courage. When we forgive ourselves and others, we liberate ourselves, regardless of what the others do. If you feel it is the right step, commit to a process of forgiveness. Read about it, talk about it, and take real steps to make it happen.

Continuing a relationship with one who has harmed you may not be safe. However, meeting someone who has caused similar harm to another person may bring insight into your healing. Above all, turn to a higher power or your inner awareness for guidance toward forgiving yourself. Seeking a more elevated perspective will help you focus on life after the trauma and not constantly relive it. Buddha said, "In the end, only three things matter: how much you loved, how gently you lived, and how gracefully you let go of things not meant for you."

EMOTIONAL INTELLIGENCE

Forgiveness requires emotional strength. Emotional intelligence, or EQ, is essentially a person's ability to be in control of their emotions rather than letting their emotions control them. It is the ability to identify, monitor, and manage emotions. Those with high emotional intelligence understand themselves, relate well to others, and cope effectively with difficult situations and individuals.

When we are physically threatened, the brain naturally manifests one of three defenses—fight, flight, or freeze. We may physically fight back, run away from the danger, panic, appease, or shut

POST-TRAUMATIC THRIVING

In the midst of a traumatic event, we are usually faced with the fight-flight-freeze responses. In the aftermath of the trauma, triggers can result in revisiting these same realms.

In the post-trauma stage, a fourth option emerges. Specifically, we can face the situation by developing healthy self-care skills.

	Disrespect Others	Respect Others
Disrespect Yourself	Avoid, Escape **FLIGHT** Passive Aggressive, Addict	Gullible, Obey **FREEZE** Passive, Prey
Respect Yourself	Abuse, Control **FIGHT** Aggressive, Predator	Self-Care, Understand **FACE IT** Assertive, Healthy

down altogether. Our emotions work the same way. When we are threatened emotionally, we may engage in verbal combat, avoid the situation, or emotionally detach ourselves. Nature responds to any threatening situation with a quick reaction designed to save us from imminent harm.

While nature provides us ways to avoid emotional distress, this organic process can backfire. Blocking our emotions can produce severe and long-term problems. After a cooling-off period, we need to address these emotions directly and work toward complete awareness. This way, we can process the events and regulate our responses in such a way as to bring the optimal results.

Our emotions break down four ways. Being aware of all these elements allows us to regulate them more effectively.

- *Cognitive appraisals* include our intellectual knowledge, spiritual feelings, and philosophical beliefs. In other words, our general mindset, interpretation of the situation, sense of well-being, and ability to cope.
- *Physiological responses* include our heart rate, blood pressure, sweating, and overall physical reactions to cope with stressful situations. Being aware of our physical responses allows us to better regulate and deal with our emotions.
- *Adaptive actions* are our responses to think on our feet, stay, run, or respond to the accompanying body language. Merely being aware of our option to fight or flee is essential. Freezing is understandable but may not be the best choice, as we are left with no defense as we face the trauma.
- *Conscious feelings* provide information about our emotional state. Of course, trauma can result in a variety of emotions, such as rage, panic, hate, anger, hostility, fear, or anxiety. Trauma can cause us to go from an average baseline affability to extreme rage in split seconds. Our emotional response is a good stimulus that helps with

> self-preservation, and we are more prepared to use those emotions effectively if we are aware of them. If we are unaware, feelings can erupt into reactions that we might later regret. Understanding our feelings is an essential aspect of healing.

Janet Louise Stephenson said, "Authenticity requires a certain measure of vulnerability, transparency, and integrity." Those with high EQ tend to be calm and genuine people who are kind and generous. They are confident, without being egotistical, and tend not to pass judgment. They listen to what others have to say and treat a CEO with the same respect as the kid at the fast-food counter. High EQ people do not show off, are not materialistic, and are true to their word.

Ultimately, controlling and regulating our emotions is a combination of our awareness of them, coupled with understanding our options and opening up a discussion about them. Healing requires that we face our feelings and identify the trusted family member, friend, or therapist with which to discuss them.

MADDOG

When I think of EQ, I think of one of the most exceptional humans I have known. Greg Madsen, also known as the "Maddog," was a great friend for decades. Greg had incredible energy, a special love for every person and creature he ever met, a contagious smile, a great sense of humor, and a beautiful family. He just seemed to get life right.

One day, we spent hours talking in his home office, and we decided to write a leadership book together. He had some special coating on a wall that allowed us to draw our ideas all over it with dry-erase pens. This was a total Maddog thing.

Over the following weeks, we started working on the book and developing the concepts. I was so excited to research and explore this topic with him, and we got into it. A couple of weeks later came the shocking news that Maddog was diagnosed with stage four lung cancer. He had never touched a cigarette his entire life! He has always been one of the fittest, healthiest guys I have ever met. True to his nature, he fought back with everything he had.

The entire time, he worked on healing himself and had a great attitude and optimistic outlook, and I never heard him complain once, though he had every right to. He had pure class and complete dignity.

When I told Maddog about my new book concept for *MeWeDoBe,* he just went nuts. I had no idea, but behind the scenes, he went to work and got an invitation for me to give a TED talk. He became my coach throughout the entire process. The conversation caught on, and every television network profiled it. That got me in front of the media talking about the *MeWeDoBe* concepts, but it all started with Maddog working with me to get everything refined.

Remarkably, Maddog did all of this with stage four lung cancer. He spent a significant amount of time helping me get this thing off the ground. He did this kind of thing for many other people. I am sure that I am only one of the hundreds of people that think of Dog as a best friend. I am just glad that I am one of them. I love the guy and his family.

EQ is not a degree, position, calling, status, or title. EQ is doing things in a way that others instinctively want to follow. Greg Madson was one of the world's great leaders. Maddog had a beautiful wife, four beautiful kids, a beautiful home by the beach, and a great career. He was a great surfer and skier. But what made him the Maddog was a continual flow of pure love and refreshing energy to everyone around him.

Not everyone can be as stellar as Maddog, but it is a state of being we can all aspire to. When I think of people that I have known who I would like to be like, my dad, Greg Madson, and a couple of others top the list. I am glad that I took a moment to tell him directly when he was here on Earth.

The Bible makes it simple and tells us that the first great commandment is to love God, and the second is to love other people. Greg Madsen simply hit the bull's-eye. Maddog hit the jackpot of love. He nailed it. He did not manipulate; he inspired. I am grateful to God that I got to see such an epic, ideal life up close. Maddog's life gives me something to shoot for.

Maddog had an arsenal of one-liners like, "make your own fun," "choose gratitude," "do lots of one-on-one trips," "do things for people who cannot help or harm you," "love is spelled TIME," "just listen," "say yes to life," "make time an adventure," "make it epic," "live life with the end in mind," and "choose happiness."

Maddog was quick to forgive and quicker to love everyone. All I can say is that heaven must be perfect, but I am sure that the day he arrived, it became more perfect.

ACTIVE LISTENING

Forgiveness requires clear communication. When healing from trauma, expressing ourselves is essential. However, this is not a one-way street. It is vital that we not only listen, but that we also *deeply* listen. Listening is vital to growth and understanding other's perspectives. Active listening builds strong relationships, and these types of relationships are necessary for personal growth and achieving a quality life.

Inactive listening happens when we are physically there and technically listening, but our minds are on something else, often formulating our response. When we have focused on a distant object or mutter "uh-huh" absentmindedly, people usually sense that we are not actively involved with what they are saying. Perhaps we are thinking about how we will answer them, but that negates the entire process of communication, for we could be missing an essential part of what they are saying.

Active listening is a skill that is easy to understand intellectually but harder to do. It often takes a conscious effort to empathetically listen rather than listen while formulating our responses or making judgments about what is being said. At times, while someone is talking, our internal conversation about how wrong they are or how superior our point of view is prevents us from really hearing what they are saying. We need to resist the temptation to jump in and interrupt others.

While challenging, active listening brings deep healing for the person with whom we are speaking. By listening and not jumping in, we create a safe place for them to vent and express themselves fully. We validate the worth of those we choose to listen to.

A simple tool to help us become better listeners is *reflective listening*. This is where we do not comment on our thoughts or opinions at all but rather repeat back what we understand they have said. For example, we might say, "So, if I understand you correctly, you are saying..." or "While you were speaking, I noticed an expression on your face..." These techniques can be powerful ways to truly understand and show that another person's thoughts, feelings, and emotions are valued.

Another technique is to ask opened-ended questions, such as, "Can you expand upon that?" or "Tell me how that made you feel." Indeed, focusing upon feelings may be more important than just getting the facts and figures right. By consistently avoiding jumping back into your own story or things you want to say, you allow this person to talk it out. They will not only feel understood, but they will also feel cared for.

Our Stories of Forgiveness

DEBBIE

Debbie has not let her husband's secret life and suicide define her life. She forgave him for the pain he caused her and her children.

Years later, Debbie can discuss the experience without being triggered and can even use the ordeal to help others through their challenges. She is open, honest, and matter-of-fact about what happened and her process of healing.

JOHN

John is calm when the topic of the US government comes up, even though the US military detonated nuclear bombs at the nearby Bikini Atoll. He often thinks of his daughter and lives in a way that he feels she would be proud of.

When visitors come from the United States, John does not carry a grudge or get angry. He is kind and welcoming.

SUSAN

The idea of bestowing forgiveness on a vast, faceless entity like the City of Los Angeles is a bit daunting. Yes, the landslide was their fault, but it had not been the result of evil intent. It was just people—employees—who followed the directions of another employee which was, in turn, following the direction of someone above him. And that person probably got their directive from the City Council, who was, of course, elected by the populace. Susan realized that in this case, forgiving the City for its role in the destruction of her home was really so she and Peter would feel better.

Looking back now, Susan recalls the landslide that destroyed her family's home with a pragmatic perspective. Yes, it was heartbreaking to lose her home, and dealing with the aftermath was a horrific ordeal. The lawsuit against the City of Los Angeles tapped into every reserve of emotional strength she had.

Yet she no longer gets angry or depressed over it. Indeed, the landslide, she says, woke her up. It jump-started the process of re-evaluating her life. She learned that she was stronger than she thought and that she had what it took to navigate an incredibly stressful situation. If she could do that, she could undoubtedly explore improving parts of her life that she had only been daydreaming about before.

Now that she and Peter had the settlement money from the City of Los Angeles, they had a choice to make—they could rebuild their house in the same spot, set up Peter's business in the same way it had been before, and pick up the reins of their old life, or they could make their dreams—those that had been on the shelf so long—actually come true.

Susan started to scout out large parcels of land to build the retreat center she had envisioned. This brought even more healing and forgiveness.

SHAD

Shad forgave the United States government for getting America involved in the Vietnam War a long time ago. He does not look in the rearview mirror; his focus is helping veterans today. Even at 75 years old, Shad's energy and commitment to these soldiers are stronger than ever.

Shad's experience in Vietnam and the trauma he endured shaped his life. In addition to creating groundbreaking programs to help veterans recover from their trauma, he set out to educate the general public on what the soldiers who fought in Vietnam experienced.

In addition to his book, *Captain for Dark Mornings,* he has contributed to many books and professional articles. He has advised filmmakers to help the public understand what the Vietnam experience was genuinely like. He has been interviewed on countless television shows and has been a keynote speaker at events all over the world.

He shows no signs of slowing down at 75. He still goes to the office every day. He strategizes, develops programs, and takes many crisis calls. Not only has Shad's work for vets been extraordinary, but his efforts to get post-traumatic stress disorder recognized by health care professionals have brought healing to veterans and civilians.

GERI

Forgiveness is a crucial cornerstone of being able to move forward from the many injustices and unbearable pain that others have bestowed upon us. Geri believes that it is a process, and not everyone will be able to forgive others in the same time span. There is no set deadline for forgiveness, only that we consciously keep trying to do so daily. Remember, forgiveness not only helps to heal those forgiven but also helps to heal our hearts as well.

TANYA

Forgiveness is a daily decision. Tanya's mother forgave OJ for the role he played many years ago. She had to, she explained to Tanya, for the sake of her grandchildren, Justin and Sydney. It took longer for Tanya to forgive OJ. And when she did, she knew that forgiveness benefits herself as much as it does OJ—perhaps even more so.

Losing her sister in such a terrible way compounded the trauma she was already experiencing due to the other losses in her life. She began drinking excessively and, eventually, even attempted suicide. When she forgave OJ, she was able to let go of much of her pain.

Now, when Tanya talks about OJ Simpson, she is matter-of-fact.

She no longer hates him; she hates what she believes he did. She has researched domestic violence extensively and built a career in helping others find their freedom from the bonds of abuse that bind them.

JC

JC has forgiven his mother for the pain she put him through as a boy. He has forgiven others who have hurt him over the years, always preferring to practice forgiveness as the Bible dictates. He is still working on forgiving the former girlfriend whose betrayal helped cement his fate.

Part of it, he explains, is that she has never owned up to the lies she told to lessen the consequences of her actions. She told the police that killing her stepmother had been JC's idea—even though he was nowhere near the scene when it happened. But it was worse than that. She told law enforcement that JC had abused and threatened to kill her if she did not go along with his plan. None of it, not a single word, was true.

Her lies were successful. She ended up with a sentence of 15 years; JC was sentenced to 25-to-life.

A few months after JC was released, he ran into the former girlfriend at a fundraising event that JC was emceeing. A mutual friend had brought the two together. JC hoped that she would say something to him about what had happened, and why she had done what she had done. But he hoped in vain. She merely wished him well as the two of them shared an awkward moment. JC stood there silent, hoping that she would say more—that she would offer an explanation, and even an apology. But to no avail, JC walked away feeling betrayed, yet again.

LEO

Leo was reminded daily that he had lost an eye as he went through the routine of putting in a glass eye after brushing his teeth. Yet his mind was focused on something else—inventing guitars.

This focus paid off. Leo was not upset at God, the universe, humanity, or anyone else for his disabilities. He just accepted them and focused on his life's mission of making guitars and instruments for the people who God had called angels.

People had initially laughed at Leo Fender's guitars. Then, in 1950, when they started to sell, these same people tried to take credit. But Leo didn't care. Leo simply was not one to hold onto a grudge. He was on a mission, and besides, he held the patent! He grew out of his little radio shop on Harbor Boulevard, and he set up a manufacturing facility on Pomona Avenue. He outgrew that and built a larger facility on Raymond Avenue. There, Leo Fender invented the Stratocaster. This is easily the most successful guitar in the history of the world.

When *Guitar* came out with a list of the top 100 guitarists, over 90 percent had played one of Leo's guitars on stage. Today, Fender is a billion-dollar business. Fender guitars have been played by Buddy Holly, Willie Nelson, Elvis Presley, Jimi Hendrix, the Rolling Stones, Eric Clapton, Led Zeppelin, the Beatles, Heart, and just about everyone else. More importantly, Leo's guitars filled the entire world with music, which was precisely what he wanted! If you have ever heard a song, then Leo's accomplishments have impacted you.

JOE

Joe strives to follow Jesus' example and forgive those who have wronged him—and, on the flip side of the coin, ask for forgiveness from those that he has wronged.

Has Joe forgiven John Gotti for murdering his father? To a certain extent, he has. It was Joe's dad's murder that set Joe on a life path where he now can help countless people as an interventionist. Ironically, John Gotti's murder of Joe's father has helped Joe save lives.

On the other hand, Gotti destroyed Joe's opportunity to have a father in his life. Had his dad been around, Joe would have led a very different life and possibly ended up helping people anyway.

Or he could have fully embraced a life of crime. It is impossible to know. Joe continues to work on forgiveness. It is getting easier as time goes by.

ERICA

Erica will probably not forgive the Nazis for murdering her entire family, and she certainly will not forget it. However, she does have compassion for the young Nazi soldiers who were ordered to do horrific things day in and day out. She saw that these soldiers were young and scared too. She knew they would endure a lifetime of guilt and nightmares for what they were a part of. This was not something that they had wished for or orchestrated. They were ordered to do evil, and they did it.

TOM

Tom had to change his perspective. The cancellation of US involvement in the 1980 Olympics was no one's "fault." Instead, it was the perfect storm of international politics colliding against grandstanding by both the United States and the Soviet Union. The athletes were merely collateral damage.

Tom forgave the international leaders who caused such a disruption in his life. He admits it was hard, but at the end of the day, the only person suffering from his lack of forgiveness was himself.

MY STORY

My parents meant well by concealing the fact that I needed heart surgery until I was about 10. This was a difficult topic for them, too, and they were somewhat awkward in how they handled it. They were trying to protect me from the harsh realities. Frankly, they should have told me much earlier, rather than letting it accidentally slip out right before it was going to happen. For me, it was easy to forgive them for this. I understand that they were scared too, and parents want to spare their children bad news.

CHAPTER 14

Resilience

As we reframe our mindset, set goals, and look for new meaning, we find new energy to develop a newfound spirit.

RESILIENCE

RESILIENCE IS THE ABILITY to bounce back. To thrive, we use our hurts, fears, grief, and suffering to stay in motion. It is a valuable resource, not something to bury, hide, or be ashamed of. Face it. Own it. Use it. We paid the price for it, and it is one of the most significant assets we have. Healing from trauma is about being authentic regarding the hurt, but we still need to foster optimism. Henry Ford said, "Whether you think you can or cannot, you are right."

Some people will tell you the world is getting worse, and they are mistaken. Their world may be getting worse, but our world is getting better. People are getting kinder, smarter, and doing more and more wonderful things every day. Knowledge of the principles of post-traumatic thriving is spreading. People are healing. There is more to do, but the trend is certainly upward.

As we genuinely "sit in the fire" with our shock, anger, and depression, a new emotion slowly grows and emerges. Yes, we will not only survive, but also thrive! Survivors can manage their feelings, but thrivers can go a step further to use them as fuel, propelling them to places that they otherwise never imagined. This newfound, resilient power gives us the capacity to recover quickly from difficulties. We can recognize new opportunities that have emerged from the struggle and open ourselves to new possibilities that we never noticed before.

HOW TO GET HIGH

We all need to get high. Thrills come in many ways. When we get high, the brain secretes dopamine, endorphins, serotonin, and oxytocin. Don't be fooled by counterfeit buzzes like illegal drugs and excessive alcohol. Find your passion, and get a real high!

PICK YOUR POISON

PARTYING

DRUGS

ALCOHOL

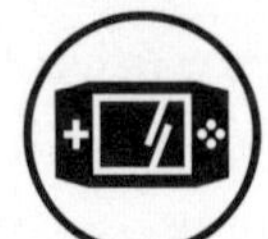
VIDEO GAMES

CHECKING OUT

JUNK FOOD

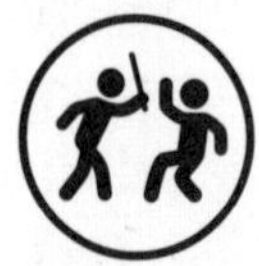
VIOLENCE

GOSSIP

PICK YOUR PASSION

MUSIC

READING

DANCE

DRAWING

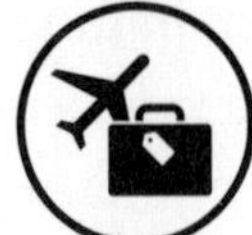
TRAVEL

SKIING

ROCK CLIMBING

COOKING

Understanding the underlying, full spectrum of effects from trauma is essential for healing. Trauma is not just an "it's in your head" thing, and it is certainly not a sign of mental weakness. Trauma is a physical issue involving chemical reactions in the brain. In other words, it is our biology and natural response to the fight-flight-freeze instinct. Not only do these reactions protect us, but they also unlock new dimensions of thinking.

Life's shocking and extraordinary events create measurable biological reactions. Scientists have identified the brain's pathways and chemical reactions to stress and trauma. There should never be shame or guilt associated with our natural responses to life's disasters and tragedies. Indeed, they open up new possibilities for us.

RESETTING THE NERVOUS SYSTEM

The concepts of sympathetic and parasympathetic nervous systems have been around for many decades. Since the Vietnam War, there have been considerable new insights into the fight-flight-freeze reactions. Some purport that there is actually a three-part nervous system. The Polyvagal Theory, developed by Dr. Stephen Porges, suggests that there is also a social component where safety and connection are important. Here, our mind-body connection includes social engagement, play, and intimacy. In essence, we "whistle while we work" and have a more nuanced and even playful approach to life and healing.

Indeed, the goal of healing trauma is to feel safe, connected, and be socially connected. We want to recalibrate our nervous system, and it can be reset through a variety of actions and approaches. The opposite of trauma is social connection. Talk therapy is a cognitive-based solution that is helpful for many reasons, including sharing our thoughts, fears, and experiences in a safe environment. By putting the experience into a narrative in a safe setting where we receive affirming social feedback, we can rewrite those memories and understand them in a new light. But, there is more. Since trauma is a sensory-based event, we also need sensory-based activities, such as meditation, cardio exercise, prayer, nature walks, and yoga.

If we are unable to address experiences and memories that are coming up at the moment, we can use containment exercises to put negative emotions in a mental "container" to be dealt with later, perhaps with a licensed therapist. In the meantime, we feel safe and separated from painful, intense emotions until they can be processed safely. This helps maintain distance from overwhelming trigger responses by offering ourselves the option for these negative emotions to be unpacked and processed at a better time. To temporarily contain overpowering emotions, think of an actual container that is large and strong enough to hold painful feelings and memories, then place your flashbacks or sensations in the box, and temporarily store it away. We remember that the box can be opened later when it is safe to do so. This can be an excellent means to deal with negative emotions productively, which is a trait of all thrivers.

Art, music, and community also bring healing. We can find rejuvenation from many sources. Look for what seems to work best for you. You can learn more from therapy, online or in-person support groups, literature, spiritual sources, a variety of meditation techniques, and even advice columns. Thriving does not result from the use of just one tool; it comes with an all-inclusive attitude involving a variety of cognitive and sensory-based activities.

THE NEW SCIENCE

Over just the last few decades, there has been a tremendous shift in understanding the human brain. As a result of trauma research, we can help people in all spectrums within society who are hurting. We can identify at-risk children and teenagers and get them the intervention they need. Victims of abuse can do this as well. Advancements in science can even help the perpetrators and offenders themselves deal with their traumas, such that they no longer want to do others harm. The savings and benefits to society can be enormous.

Not long ago, many scientists thought that the human brain remained fixed in adulthood. It was believed that the brain produced no new cells, nor could we alter our thinking or behavior in significant ways. For this reason, a lot of people assumed we could not rewire our thinking after adolescence. However, scientists have recently learned that the human brain is extremely flexible, capable of reshaping our thinking, and able to create new, neural structures throughout our lifetimes.

Every person is redeemable. While trauma does indeed have physiological effects on our brains that create specific negative and habitual responses, we can forge through new thinking pathways regardless of our age. Every person has value and is worthy of calm, peace, happiness, and love.

The notion has caught on, and the science has caught up. "When neurons fire together, they wire together." That is, mental activity creates new neural structures that match that activity. No matter our age, we can create new neurological pathways that enhance the quality of life and those around us. Numerous tools will improve our lives by helping to develop these pathways.

Thrivers aggressively employ any number of proven methods. Voluminous studies show that exercise has remarkable effects, both physically and neurologically. The field of interpersonal neurobiology is actively researching how one can develop better interpersonal relationships by being vulnerable and increasing trust. Social science has discovered that spirituality has measurable and positive impacts, which bring comfort, solace, and deeper meaning in life. This can happen through both religious and non-religious activities. Ultimately, it involves exploring religious traditions, spiritual paths, or philosophical practices that connect and move you.

There are times when it is right to sit in the fire and heal and when we do not need the distractions of uncomfortable emotions. These, and similar practices, can help us navigate these choices.

- Within appropriate boundaries, we can hug more people. Humans are built on personal touch and contact. Hugging and personal contact are comforting.
- Music has been proven, in numerous studies, to entirely

change one's mood or emotional state in a matter of only two to seven minutes.

- Joining community groups for playing sports, volunteering, playing games, singing, sharing interests or hobbies, creating music, or worshiping God are all known to help heal people from trauma.
- Expressive arts, such as music, writing, drama, and dance, or visual arts, such as painting and sculpture contribute to healing. Indeed, it has been said that the closest moments with our Creator are when we are creating.
- Group therapy can be remarkably validating for each participant as we listen to each other's experiences. Others have navigated the same challenges as we have, and we can share our stories and have them validated as well. Tiny habits and practices rewire the brain and create new neurological pathways over time, that add up to significant changes.
- One of the habits from my *MeWeDoBe* book, the one most talked about by the media, is to make our bed. This one habit statistically doubles our chances of becoming a millionaire! The real point is that the simple act of making our bed kicks in neurotransmitters from our brain that make us more productive throughout the day.
- There are mental exercises that are proven to be effective. For example, if we breathe in while thinking of a tense experience and exhale while thinking of a moment when we felt loved, we activate our calming parasympathetic nervous system.
- When a memory of a negative experience arises, consciously thinking of a positive experience or of a loving relationship that we enjoy is helpful. As we do this, the brain will emphasize fulfilling feelings and soften the unpleasant.

- Breathing exercises are simple and remarkably effective. The human brain can think of just one thing at a time, so if our attention is turned to our breathing, our mind is shifted away from a traumatic memory. When the physiological signs of sweaty palms or an elevated heart rate from a stress response arise, merely closing our eyes and taking slow, deep breaths can help tremendously.
- To steady the mind in down moments, we can deliberately think of moments or people who brought us prolonged feelings of happiness. This makes our brains secrete the neurotransmitters dopamine, which brings pleasure; oxytocin, which feels like a hug; or acetylcholine, which is calming and improves our mental focus.
- Personal affirmations are statements we can craft to remind ourselves of our core values and own worth. Remember, "We must be on our own side."
- Vision boards are posters we can create that reflect our dreams of the future. We can use personal photos or clip magazine photos. By looking at these pictures, our brains are rewired to think and act in ways that can make that dream a reality. If we use vision boards, it is essential to envision the process, not just "holding the trophy."
- When overseen by a qualified psychiatrist or doctor, medications can help balance brain chemistry and assist with the hard work we are doing. Some medicines are taken daily to achieve a steady baseline, and some are meant to be taken in the moment of an emotional crisis.

It only takes a relatively small number of conscious repetitions for a new behavior to become natural or nearly automatic because the neural pathways are now built-in. We don't have to do everything on the list.

"The problem is not the problem." The trauma is in the past, and the current problem is how we are going to manage it. In other words, when there is an event, there is also a response. It is that response that determines the outcome. We must practice self-care and other healing responses, rather than let gravity take us down a destructive path. In other words, we can react to trauma in harmful ways, or we can respond to injury in ways that are ultimately healing.

BROODING VS. PONDERING

Ruminative brooding is repetitively reviewing the trauma without finding resolution, developing any meaning, or taking any action. We are stuck, replaying the trauma over and over again in our minds, which prolongs the traumatic suffering. There we long for a world that no longer exists. Viktor Frankl said, "When we are no longer able to change the situation, we are challenged to change ourselves." There are a wide variety of traumas, yet all thrivers have one thing in common: they are adaptive and create new ways to survive and thrive.

We can change our situation by contemplating the trauma, seeking understanding, taking steps for self-care, and developing some understanding and meaning. When we actively take steps to cope and improve our situation, we avoid retraumatizing ourselves. When we seek resolution, even while we hurt, we channel our energy into productive and meaningful activities that heal. We can adjust our worldview as a result.

We all need independent points of view from outside ourselves to help us gain perspective on the situation. Through my visits to countless sites of tragedy and studies of the academic literature, I have needed independent, intelligent, and trustworthy coaches with whom to process my traumas. We all do. If you make life an entirely solo act, you will be stuck in your injury.

I HAVE A DREAM

In 1999, Dr. Lien B. Pham and Dr. Shelley E. Taylor of UCLA published a landmark study regarding vision boards, but it had a significant twist on prevailing assumptions. In their traditional form, vision boards may stunt our growth. Rather than motivating us to get to work, they can be a distraction because we over-fantasize about what we want.

It is far more effective to use them to visualize the *process* required to get the desired result. In other words, daydreaming does not just magically drop sunshine and happiness into our laps. We envision our goals, but we must also see the process of getting there.

In the UCLA Pham and Taylor study, one group of students was asked to visualize themselves getting a high grade on an exam. The other group imagined themselves studying for the exam. The students who envisioned themselves studying got higher scores on the test compared to those who visualized themselves getting a high grade. We perform better when we see ourselves taking steps to thrive. When we only daydream about the results, our brain reacts as if we already have it. We then experience a relaxation response, which lowers our energy and dampens our motivation.

A journey of a thousand miles begins with a single step. We need a map to see ourselves taking those steps, not just the practical tasks, but steps that heal our trauma and feed our soul, such as meditating, praying, taking nature walks, exercising, expressing ourselves, eating right, and getting enough sleep. To thrive, we identify and envision the small, short-term actions we need to take.

Envy, the last of the Ten Commandments, is a sin. All of commercialism is based on trying to look or behave like someone else. God created you to be you. Not somebody else. When we envy others, we leave ourselves and turn our backs on our individual purpose. They say there is nothing new under the sun and that it has all been said. But you have unique characteristics that nobody else has, so use them. You have a perspective based on your experiences that is special, which shapes a voice that only you can use. When used to craft a message, your unique perspective can reach people or create goodness in a way that no one else can.

A great secret of life is that the human brain does not distinguish significantly between an actual event and the picture of that same event. Good or bad, a picture elicits nearly the same neurological response as the actual event.

Goals are something that we write down. Intentions are good, but a vision is something that runs deeper. To envision something, shut your eyes, and imagine where you want to be in one, three, or five years. Think about it. Linger on the images. See, smell, touch, hear, and feel them. Dwell daily on your vision. Imagine it with crystal clarity!

This is a fun exercise, as the research clarifies that we are far more likely to achieve something we envision than something we do not. A great time to focus on our vision is as we go to sleep. See yourself in that place in life and on your way there. Envision the process, smell the smells, listen to the sounds, taste the foods, and feel the air. Envision it as clearly as you possibly can, and set a precise date for its arrival. This process sets both the conscious and unconscious mind into motion toward realizing that vision.

DON'T FORGET THE MUSIC

I am fortunate to know the family of Leo Fender, the inventor of the electric guitar. I grew up in Fullerton, California, in a home two blocks from Leo's. My dad worked for Fender as a mechanical engineer. As wannabe rockers, we looked to Leo as our local hero. Before him, every version of the electric guitar had some kind of hollow, acoustic chamber, but Leo was the first to make a guitar out of a solid piece of wood. The musical harmonics of this invention changed the world forever. At first, everyone laughed and called his guitars "boat paddles," but those who mocked him wanted to take the credit when sales took off. Leo got the last laugh, and today, Fender is a billion-dollar company.

Leo was a rare kind of person. He lived in our neighborhood, worked with my dad, and interacted with the entire community. In the decades he lived and worked, I never heard a single negative thing about him. He had impeccable honesty and integrity. The music world is wildly diverse, and Leo got along with everyone.

ADAPTING TO CHANGE JOURNEY

Learning new ideas and worthwhile concepts can be difficult. At first, external influences can result in denial and then personal resistance. Depending upon the character of the person, "open mindedness" and exploration will prevail and lead to eventual acceptance.

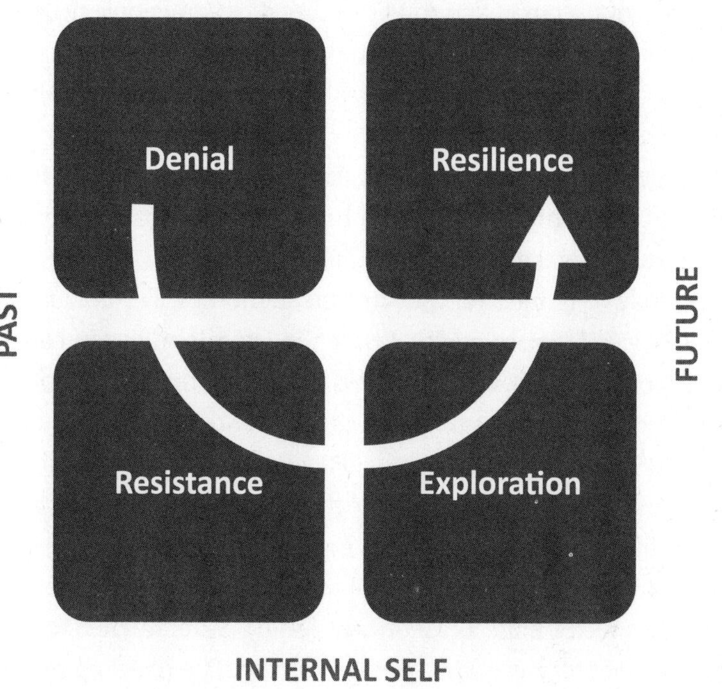

Leo was an exceptionally quiet person, but we are fortunate that his wife, Phyllis, has shared insights from the mind of this quiet giant. I will never forget the day when Mrs. Fender and I sat at a table at Polly's Pies in Fullerton, California, and she talked about what made Leo tick.

Leo was famously obsessed with designing electric guitars. While sitting at the captain's table on cruise ships, Leo was drawing guitars on the cloth napkins. His fixation just never stopped! Mrs. Fender said that one day, she stopped Leo in the kitchen, stared him down, and asked, "Leo, why? Leo, why are you so obsessed and always thinking about guitars?"

While a devout Christian herself, Leo was not religious. Quite reluctantly, Leo told Phyllis that when he was a young boy, he had a vivid dream. In that vision, Jesus said to him that his gift was not to be the magician he wanted to be. Instead, Jesus told Leo that this world is a tough place, and music makes it better. People need music, and musicians are angels who make life better. Jesus told Leo that his gift is to create instruments for these angels. Jesus told Leo that this is why he was on earth.

From that day forward, Leo focused on making guitars. He always felt that God was quietly behind his work, and near the end of his life, Leo also became a Christian.

A couple of years after that conversation, Mrs. Fender and I were invited to a rock concert. Mrs. Fender, my wife, and I went backstage, where we met Chas West, the lead singer for the classic rock band Foreigner. Chas is an interesting person, and we ended up chatting for some time. Then, Chas said, "Hey Randall, do you want to meet Nancy Wilson?" Of course, I did. After all, Nancy and her sister, Ann, formed Heart, one of the world's biggest rock bands.

Like zillions of others of her fans, I had a crush on Nancy when I worked at a record store as a teenager. I said, "Sure!" turned to my wife, and asked her to bring Mrs. Fender on over. The dressing room door swung open, and there in front of me was Nancy Wilson, easily one of the most significant female rock stars of all time. Nancy glanced up at Chas and me and said, "Hey guys, come on in!"

Frankly, I was tongue-tied, and I blurted out something stupid about shaking her hand at a concert when I was in college. I quickly turned to introduce Nancy to Mrs. Fender, but she and my wife were chasing a cart with roast beef sandwiches. I thought to myself, "Seriously? We are meeting with one of the greatest music legends of all time, and you are running after a sandwich!?!"

Once they got their roast beef fix, I had the privilege of introducing Mrs. Leo Fender to Nancy Wilson. It was epic seeing two iconic women in the world of music meet. Despite her wild fame, Nancy is a quiet, kind, and gentle soul, and the two of them had a long, beautiful visit. Mrs. Fender shared stories about Leo and his guitars. Later, Nancy went out on stage, and Mrs. Fender indulged in her very first rock concert. Nancy was one of the angels Leo talked about, and her love and musical gifts filled the hall. The whole night made us all smile.

Science shows us that music can immediately elevate our mood, while Leo's dream tells us that there is a deeper meaning behind it all. As we go through life, let us remember that the world can be a tough place, but music makes it so much better.

DOES ANYONE REMEMBER LAUGHTER?

It is no joke—laughter helps us heal from trauma! Comedy does a world of good. It not only helps emotionally, but humor also activates positive, physical changes in the body. Trauma is serious and can destroy our happiness, but laughter is a great way to reclaim it. Of course, we need to know what is appropriate. There may be nothing funny about our trauma itself, and we should never get a laugh at the expense of others. Yet, trauma aside, there are plenty of things to laugh about.

Humor is not only fun, but also beneficial. Neuropeptides are released by exercise or by being touched, but they are also released by laughter. Comedy triggers brain chemistry to counteract anxiety and tension. When we laugh, our brains release endorphins that bring good, relaxed feelings, make us feel better, and soothe our pain. Humor relieves our stress response, reduces our heart rate, stimulates circulation, relaxes our muscles, and reduces our blood pressure. A good laugh brings in oxygen-rich air and stimulates our heart, lungs, and muscles. Over the long term, humor can improve our immune systems. Just as negative thoughts trigger the release of cortisol, positive thoughts release endorphins that relieve that tension.

Laughter can bring our power back. It sends a message that this will not destroy us and that we are still alive and resilient. Laughter allows us to take a momentary break from it all. As we heal, we can smile and laugh again.

Improving our sense of humor is both fun and easy. It can be as simple as turning on a comedy channel or reading the comic strips that make us chuckle. We can hang up a funny saying on our bathroom mirror or refrigerator. We can choose funny movies over dramas or thrillers. The internet is full of funny websites. A wide array of scientific data shows that comedy clubs and sitcoms are good for us. So here we go:

Knock, knock
Who's there?
A little old lady
A little old lady who?
Wow, I didn't know you could yodel!

Laugh and the world laughs with you!

Our Stories of Resilience

DEBBIE

The pain of Debbie's husband's suicide—and his incredible betrayal—would never go away. Even as she moved forward with her life, the pain was always with her. At times she would cry alone, and at other times, she would cry with her children.

Even as she felt deep pain, she saw that the world kept spinning.

One of the things that helped her successfully work through her pain was imagining where she would be in a few years. It wasn't just a quick, mental snapshot. Debbie created a detailed image in her head, along with 3D color images and all the sounds, smells, and tastes. She saw herself living near the ocean and working as a therapist. After all, having been through this experience, she would have the humility and empathy to be an epic therapist.

JOHN

John still lives quietly on his island, which has been restored. Some of his children have immigrated to Hawaii and attended college, while others have stayed nearby. Though nothing will make up for the loss of his daughter, he has the quiet confidence that he took on the most powerful government on Earth—and won.

SUSAN

Susan took on the City of Los Angeles which was responsible for the landslide that destroyed her house. With the nightmare of the lawsuit behind her, she could now move on and do what she had been dreaming about. The realization that she had handled such a tough ordeal gave her newfound confidence.

And that confidence came shining through in every area of her life. Her whole demeanor was different. She was calm, sure of herself, and self-reliant. She was still as kind as ever. She had become a better version of herself. And everyone around her noticed—even her bosses at the network.

In her office on the Universal City lot, there is a vast vision board covering the entirety of two walls. I asked her about it, and she told me about a mix of personal and professional visions. They were all laid out, in detail, with precise facts, numbers, and dates. Susan was already remarkably successful, but it was clear that she was not going to rest there. The objective was to continue growing, evolving, and expanding.

Susan also knew that she had learned many lessons throughout the ordeal, experiences that helped her overcome what had happened to her and her husband. Lessons about keeping hope alive, looking at all the options, connecting with other people when she became depressed or sad, and always moving forward. She felt that she could help others through traumatic experiences now that she had had one of her own.

Susan decided to become a life coach—helping people cope with the things in life that overwhelmed them, made them feel "stuck," and prevented them from moving forward.

And soon, Susan was promoted. She was now an executive producer of a major television network.

SHAD

Shad's experience in Vietnam and the trauma he endured shaped his life. In addition to creating groundbreaking programs to help veterans recover from their trauma, he set out to educate the general public on what the soldiers who fought in Vietnam experienced.

In addition to his book, *Captain for Dark Mornings,* Shad has participated as a technical advisor to several films on the war and participated in several documentaries dealing with veterans coming home, notably *Until We Get Home* and *The Voices of Vietnam.* Currently, a documentary on his life work, *Mad Man* from Working Pictures, is slated for release.

GERI

Throughout her life, Geri met each challenge brought on by her disability with grace and grit. Her family did not shield her from the real world. Instead, they encouraged her to confront and embrace it, take all she could, and give back.

Barely out of her teens, Geri decided to leverage her considerable comedic skills to go onto the comedy stage. Getting into comedy is notoriously difficult. Agents scoff at newcomers. Auditions are often an exercise in humiliation. The performer is completely exposed and vulnerable. Even if you make it through the agent and onto the stage, the audiences can be ruthless.

Undaunted, Geri auditioned for the toughest gig possible on the comedy club circuit. She knew, deep in her heart, that she had what it took.

She was right. Geri got the gig and quickly became a sensation. In the days before the internet, Geri went "viral." Her unique routine and willingness to go places with her humor that others did not dare set her apart. She soon found herself traveling all over the country to play gigs in comedy clubs, hotels, and even on daytime talk shows.

Her comedy act caught the attention of major television producers. She was offered a recurring role in the immensely popular show *The Facts of Life.* For four years, Geri played, well, Geri. In one of her first appearances, she appeared on the show wearing a t-shirt that proclaimed, "I'm not drunk, I have cerebral palsy." The character of

"Geri" on the show was a huge hit. She was the first person in history with a visible disability to be cast in a network television show.

In an industry that can be brutal and where "fake friends" migrate, looking for that star to glom onto, Geri holds dear to the real friends who stuck with her through thick and thin. She has those real friends in the industry that Geri never takes for granted, like Fern Field, Norman Lear, David Milch, Laureen Arbus, and Robby Benson, to name a few. The friends Geri keeps close come from all walks in life, but all value honesty, love, and life.

Geri has guested on many shows over the years, and she also became a high-profile activist for the rights of people with disabilities, speaking at the White House on three different occasions—once in 1985 for the Reagan Administration, and then, years later, speaking twice for the Obama Administration.

Geri has not only pushed through her trauma, but she has also inspired millions of people.

TANYA

Tanya Brown looks back on her life and is, at times, astonished she survived. But survive she did. It is fair to say that Tanya is thriving. She is emotionally stronger than ever, thanks to her family's love, support from her friends, and guidance from caring therapists. They provided the tools she needed to overcome her trauma.

Today, Tanya speaks openly about her life experiences, from the loss of her sister to her substance abuse issues to her fight for her mental health. She appears on television and has been a keynote speaker at events around the world. She has inspired millions facing mental health issues, like depression or spousal abuse, to get the help they need, and has helped save countless lives.

JC

Looking over his life experiences and all he lived through—mental and physical abuse, poverty, his mother's drug addiction, foster care, sexual assault, homelessness, betrayal, and prison—JC chooses not to dwell on the past. His resilience is hard-earned. He's been through so much but has come out stronger.

That's not to say that JC did not have moments of deep pain and doubt. He recalls, while he was in prison, that there were times he felt deeply depressed and did not want to go on. At those times, he reached out to the people he had formed connections with and asked for their help getting through it. Sometimes, he says, you need to rely on others to remind you of who you are.

"Sometimes, a friend might say, 'You have come too far to quit now,'" JC recalls. "Other times, they would just sit with me silently. Some would bring me food or pray with me."

Just as others helped him, JC reaches out to those around him whenever they need help. He takes great comfort in knowing that being in prison put him on a path where he positively changed the lives of hundreds of men. It is quite humbling when he thinks about it. In his view, the credit goes to God and the many people along the way—like Claude—who helped him come through his darkest times, stronger than ever.

There is something else about JC as well—he has a strong desire to prove people wrong. Though he served his time and has worked hard to establish himself on the "outside," he knows that many people who learn his history will have certain feelings about him—not always positive feelings.

Some may be scared that he is a hardened criminal. Others may think that he will just end up in prison again and not want to invest their time or friendship in him. JC lets his actions show these people that their worries are unfounded. From volunteering at church, to mentoring young people, to working steadily towards his master's degree, every choice JC makes is one that will help him be the best person he can be.

LEO

Leo Fender never let a glass eye or hearing aids slow him down. He invented the electric guitar and became a household name. Yet, it never went to his head. He was living in a mobile home when $300 million, measured in current dollars, was put into his bank account. Leo just stayed in the mobile home. He liked its simplicity.

JOE

Joe has been to rehab twice over the years—opioid addiction is a harsh master, and for many, it takes multiple attempts to shake it.

After he got out of treatment for the second time, his sponsor, Steve, asked him what he wanted to do with his life.

Joe was an interventionist, helping thousands of people over the years. Yet there was something else he had always wanted to do but never really pursued—acting. As far back as third grade, he was writing plays. In high school, he was the lead in the school play and, according to all his friends, who admittedly may have been a bit biased, did a fantastic job. When he moved to California many years ago, Joe played with the idea of becoming an actor before finding out the truth about his father's murder.

The hit HBO series *The Sopranos* was filming in New York when he got out of rehab. He decided to audition. After all, they needed lots of extras. Besides, he knew he had a certain look. Tall, good-looking, thickly-built, and a perfectly shaved head—he was the embodiment of a New York gangster.

He went to an audition and got a small part in an episode. Encouraged, he went on more auditions. He got the lead part in the off-Broadway play, *The Sopranos' Last Spaghetti Dinner*, playing—who else? —Tony Soprano.

Since then, he has parlayed his acting success into a role on the Court television docudrama *Parco P.I.* playing a private investigator. He has also been featured on such reality television shows as *America's Psychic Challenge* and *Don't Forget the Lyrics*, where he won, incidentally, $200,000.

All the while, Joe has maintained his career as an interventionist because it feeds his soul. The acting roles feed his spirit.

ERICA

As of this writing, Erica is 99 years old and lives in a Jewish senior home, where she paints beautiful pictures of her childhood home in Europe. She inspires all that come in contact with her.

TOM

Tom moved on from his Olympic dreams. He earned his bachelor's and master's degrees and started a distribution company. Today, he has a beautiful wife and two successful sons, and his business has grown to 10 extensive distribution facilities around the world.

Not only is his business successful, but he also goes out of his way to know each employee and bless their lives in quiet but genuine ways. He believes that the situation with the Olympics, so long ago, helped him to learn humility, and accept that he isn't in control of everything. Looking back, he is almost, but not quite, grateful that it happened.

MY STORY

"The problem" is not the problem. For me, my heart surgery was not the problem. My problem was how I reacted to it. While I blew it by not playing high school basketball, I learned from that and pushed forward in areas where I had an aptitude.

Like a lot of kids, I loved sports and dreamed of making the major leagues. My heart surgery destroyed that dream. Other traumas have taken their hits as well, but we take the lessons and move on. Growing up, I, at times, struggled academically, and I have always been jealous of the kids who instantly understood everything. I just kept going, and one day I realized two things. First, if you stuck with a topic long enough, you would eventually not only understand it, but you could even master it.

Second, at times, I could relate to the lowest quarter of the class. I like things that are explained simply. I like teachers who can explain things in simple terms that people from various backgrounds can appreciate. That turns out to be an ideal attribute for being an expert witness—my chosen profession. I know that the jury is smarter than me, so I work to make sense and connect. This career has taken me all over the world and provided access to fascinating people and places.

CHAPTER 15

Gratitude

We cannot go back and change the beginning,
but we can start now and change the ending.

POST-TRAUMATIC THRIVING

MY EXPERIENCES HAVE RESULTED in the media calling me the *Master of Disaster.* I have never been interested in seeing bullet holes or blood. I am interested in solutions and getting people back on their feet. While I am not a big fan of the nickname, I figured that if this could help bring awareness to recovery and healing, then I would go with it.

Throughout my career, I have worked with people who have experienced nuclear fallout, terrorism, murder, war zones, mass suicides, hurricanes, fires, and landslides. These people have taught me that when trauma happens, we choose to dive, survive, or thrive. Thrivers stand out as the ones who use the energy from their ordeal to propel themselves into something that they would never have otherwise done.

Authentic thriving does not look or feel like many might expect. It is not flashy, sugar-coated, or particularly dazzling. We do not thrive by slapping on a Band-Aid, jumping on a unicorn, and galloping off with a bag of cotton candy. People often see the results in the lives of thrivers, but they have no idea about the price that was paid to get there.

ACHIEVEMENT VS SUCCESS
Success is actually a trend rather than a specific event. As this graph illustrates, everyone will have achievements and setbacks, but the real measure of success is the trend over time.
This is better termed an "achievement" than a "success"
Success
The "trend" is the real measure of value and success
This is better termed a "setback" than a "failure"
Time

Genuine, authentic thriving is stable, grounded, and resolute. It is hard-earned by spending long and painful hours in the pits of hell. We do not dodge or cheat the pain, but face shock, anger, regret, and depression head-on. The principles of thriving are simple, but it takes hard, clumsy work. It is ugly. It takes blood, sweat, and tears with a paced, day-to-day effort. We screw up, but we keep pushing

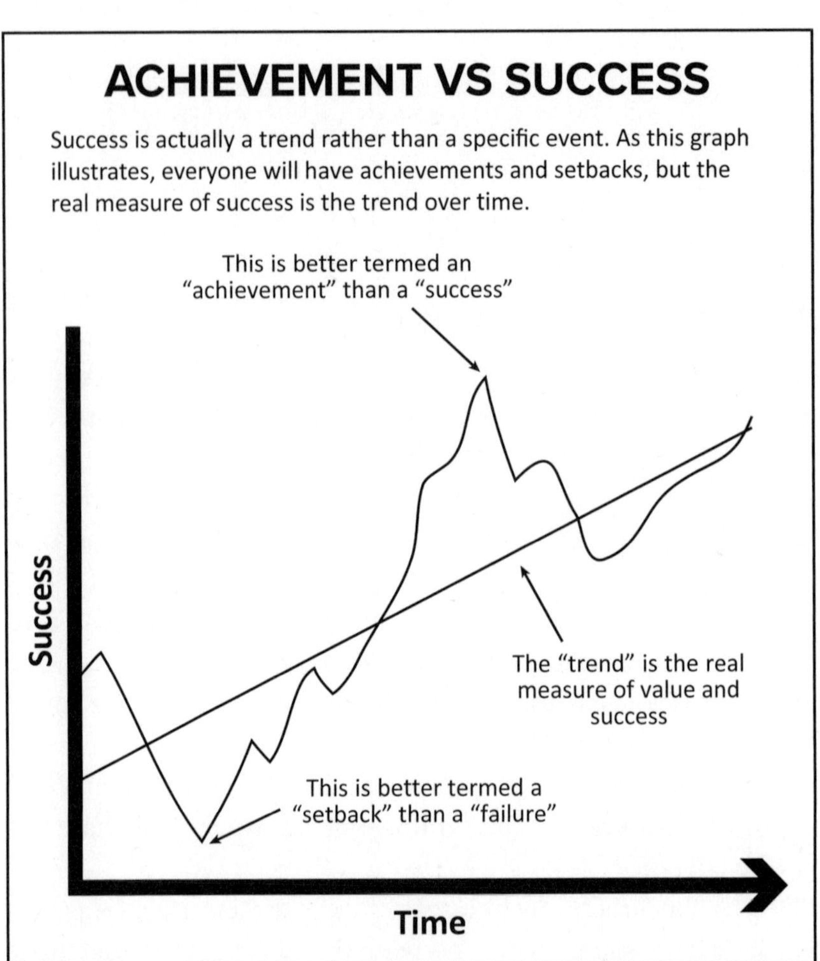

on. Thriving is sort of like making sausage. The process is not pretty, but in the end, it tastes pretty good.

There is also a certain maturity and wisdom in trauma recovery. We do not know all the answers. Gary Hamm is a thoughtful man who sat down with me and shared his experience of losing his 16-year-old son in an automobile accident on the way to a fishing trip. Gary told me about the grief, but he also said, "Once I understood that I would never understand, I began to heal."

We will never have all the answers. There will always be ups and downs along with achievements and setbacks, but we develop the wisdom to keep our eye on the overall trends. That is what matters.

We thrive by facing the harsh reality. We gain a new appreciation of our inner strength and personal awareness. Thriving is a quiet calm in knowing that we will meet our refiner's fire, and then convert that fire to fuel for something better than anything we could have done on our own power.

Those who dodge their trials may be scared, timid, frightened, or paralyzed with uncertainty. Of course, that is understandable, but to the great surprise of many, those who stare down their trials and overcome them are humble. Thrivers are empathetic and kind, but they are not suckers. Thrivers do not suck it up, bury their feelings, or forget about it. Thrivers dare to take it head-on. Thrivers draw in, harness their energy, and channel it in remarkable ways.

A THANKFUL HEART

Those who reach the pinnacle of healing always have a sense of gratitude. They do not appreciate the trauma but are forever grateful for the lessons. They have an appreciation for life and look for opportunities to contribute and be of service to others. Helen Keller said, "Many people have the wrong idea of what constitutes true happiness. It is not attained through self-gratification but through fidelity to a worthy purpose."

We all have much for which to be grateful. If you have a cell phone, food in your refrigerator, clothes on your back, a roof over your head, and a place to sleep, you are wealthier than 80 percent of the world. If you have a steady job, money in the bank, and some spare cash in your wallet, you are among the top 8 percent of the world's wealthy.

If you woke up this morning healthy, you are more blessed than the 1 million people who will not survive this week. If you have never experienced the dangers of battle, the agony of imprisonment or torture, or the horrible pains of starvation, you are luckier than 700 million people alive and suffering today. If you can read this message, you are more fortunate than 780 million people in the world who cannot read at all. None of this is intended to minimize our trauma, but as we navigate our path to healing, we must maintain a mindful perspective.

Thrivers are those of us who write letters of gratitude to our firefighters, police officers, and rescue workers. We give blood or volunteer in the community. We collect supplies to help alleviate another's tragedy, or we volunteer with society's marginalized. We use the fuel of our experience to make the world around us a tiny bit better. Thrivers step up to the opportunities for service all around us, and in the process, thrivers experience joy.

Our greatest defeats can be our greatest assets. The question is not, "Why did this happen *to* me?" but rather, "Why did this happen *for* me?" When we navigate through our trauma, we eventually realize that our injury can be seen as a gift.

Life is messy. Trauma rarely has a tidy resolution. One of the blessings of injury is that it opens the door to having more empathy for others. We do not need to imagine their pain; we have been there. The world can be a tough place, and it desperately needs kind and compassionate people who have been there. If life shuts a door, open it again, or open another door.

Compassion fatigue, however, is a condition where we have been exposed to too much of other people's trauma and pain, so we become exhausted, burned out, or numbed. This term was initially coined for first responders and mental or healthcare professionals, such as physicians or psychologists, who regularly see a parade of suffering.

Yet, it is also applicable to volunteers or anyone who spends time helping those who are in a dismal place.

Today, we live in a world where millions suffer. In one newscast, we can witness graphic images of unimaginable carnage with disasters, tragedies, and crimes all over the world. While we might be able to understand the suffering of a few people once in a while, we can easily be overwhelmed if we see too much at once. As we heal, we may want to moderate watching the news or going online.

The signs of compassion fatigue, or vicarious trauma, can mimic first-hand trauma and include anxiety, excessive complaining or alcohol consumption, feelings of hopelessness, sleeping disorders, problems concentrating, or depression. These realities are valid for the general population as well as healthcare professionals. We are all human, and we are all susceptible to fatigue. We all can burn out, so self-care is necessary for everyone.

I have a reasonably high threshold for trauma, yet I am aware of my limits. I have carefully considered the landscape of this work and have taken deliberate steps to practice self-care. I stop to look at the ocean and take frequent breaks to de-stress. I exercise and do grounding exercises daily. I have fun and goof off a lot. I connect with my family and friends frequently.

A SIMPLE CARD

Multitudes of scientific studies have identified gratitude as the single most important attitude. People who have an appreciation, even for their challenges, live longer, feel happier, make more friends, and enjoy life more. Another benefit is that gratitude chases out fear. It is impossible to be afraid and grateful at the same time. To thrive, it is essential that we, as a society, transition from *self-medication* to *self-care*. We have to be kind to ourselves and be grateful to others.

John Kralik was born in Cleveland, Ohio, and went to grade school there and in Pennsylvania. After graduating from high school, he attended the University of Michigan and earned both bachelor's and law degrees. He practiced law in Los Angeles, got married, and had a family.

At age 53, John found his life at a terrible, frightening low. He was 40 pounds overweight, his small law firm was failing, and he was struggling through a painful second divorce. He had grown apart from his two older children and was afraid he might lose contact with his young daughter.

In his tiny apartment, he froze in the winter and baked in the summer, and his girlfriend had just broken up with him. He was accused of being selfish and self-centered. John could not get along with his own family, let alone realize his dreams of becoming a judge.

Then, John did something small, but truly remarkable. He started saying, "Thank you." He decided to send one thank-you card every day for a year. He sent long overdue thanks to family, friends, clients, and colleagues for things they had done for him over the years. Every single day, he simply sent a card to someone to say, "Thanks."

Slowly, life started turning around. He began reconnecting with his family, old friends, and humanity. He started exercising, and that released even more neurotransmitters into his bloodstream.

In September 2009, the Governor of California appointed John as a Superior Court Judge. This is the power of gratitude.

HAVE A "WHY"

Alcoholics Anonymous provides another point of view that supports a belief in a higher power. Depending on who is asked, alcoholism affects about 5 to 10 percent of the population. It is a dishabituating disease, and the detoxification process is so ugly and severe that it should be done in a hospital.

Getting clear statistics is difficult, but I would estimate the success rate of a typical rehabilitation center at about 10 to 50 percent, in terms of a graduate being sober a year later. There are two primary reasons why scores of outdated drug and alcohol rehabilitation centers around the world have such a dismal, and frankly embarrassingly low, success rate.

First, out of political correctness, ignorance, or cowardice, many of today's recovery centers have eliminated any direct discussion of God, faith, or a higher power. In contrast, the success rate at Alcoholics Anonymous meetings, where there are hard-hitting discussions on our reliance on a higher power, is closer to 90 percent. One of the primary reasons is that God or a higher power, is a part of the discussion.

I am all for the benefits of secular science, yet when we strip God or a higher power out of the dialogue, our recovery success rates statistically plummet. The academic literature surrounding post-traumatic growth identifies spirituality as one of the essential components of healing. The numbers and science show the importance of faith and a higher power.

Second, the typical recovery program eliminates the step of providing service to others. In routine recovery, it is all about the patient. It is about massages, good food, and resort living. This is great up to a point, yet for complete healing, we must move beyond ourselves and contribute to society and humanity.

Our service to others raise our self-esteem and, in turn, generates additional healing and positive growth. When recovery centers and patients figure this out, they will be able to break out of the revolving door of perpetual treatment.

People who thrive never lose their drive for healthy self-esteem. They take responsibility for their thoughts and actions and own the stage of life they are in. They do not get stuck in non-action. They embrace critical thinking and are not threatened by opposing viewpoints. They ask themselves, "What root issues am I avoiding?" They hold themselves and others responsible for mistakes and use them as learning opportunities going forward. They do not ignore bad behaviors and pretend it did not happen, but respectfully assert themselves when needed. They embrace their gifts rather than focus on their flaws.

Thrivers speak with purpose, rather than from impulse. They take responsibility for their results rather than blame others. They use positive talk to build up others and themself. They keep a perspective and avoid becoming defensive. They recognize that they have the right to express their preferences, wants, needs, and desires, while allowing others to do the same. They respect themself and others and expect to be respected. They recognize that words matter. Words are powerful, and they choose them carefully. They keep their commitments and expect others to keep theirs as well.

When we have great pain, we need a great purpose. Today, better recovery treatment centers have incorporated both the need to render service and connecting to a higher power into the curriculum. Psychologist Rick Snyder, a pioneer in the field of positive psychology, sums up thriving as a feeling of motivation and a pathway for action. He dubbed these "willpower" and "why power." If we will identify the "why," we will always determine the "how." Thrivers have a calm but unbreakable passion for finding and fulfilling their "why."

HELPING A CHILD THROUGH TRAUMA

As we heal, thrive, and foster gratitude for our progress, we take on the responsibility to break the cycle and pass our knowledge down to future generations. In our roles as parents, teachers, therapists, and community leaders, we must understand the healing process for ourselves and the children under our care.

A child can sense who is on their side. A child cannot do the research, so it is up to us, as parents and caregivers, to study the facts, contact the right experts, find the right therapists, doctors, or government officials, call the police, ask the tough questions; and advocate for the child.

Faith is essential, but it should be kept in balance. Whatever your faith is, this is the time to use it. However, those who have a deep faith should not make the mistake that faith will cure everything. There is vast, considerable wisdom that is found in the secular world. Pray as if everything depends on God, but work as if everything depends on you.

Grounding exercises work at any age, including in childhood. Slow, deep breathing exercises help calm a child, just as they do for an adult. With the science-based evidence available today, it is clear that anyone facing a trauma should be doing daily grounding exercises, including children.

The conversation around trauma with children, as with anyone else, is remarkably meaningful. My parents were from the generation that was not particularly expressive, but society has progressed. Tell the truth in an age-appropriate way. As a child, I was smart enough to know that people kept unpleasant facts from me, and I did not like being kept in the dark. I always appreciated it when the doctors and nurses took a moment and explain things to me.

All people are sensitive, but children are particularly so. Kids love to play, and they should play a lot, but as a parent or caregiver, you should avoid making jokes or being sarcastic about their trauma. Many adults are uncomfortable about difficult situations, so they avoid any discussion or mask their feelings with sarcasm or excessive clowning around. Both are harmful. Children deserve a transparent, responsible, honest, and kind discussion about their situation. If parents are unsure of what to say or how to say it, they should engage a therapist specializing in childhood traumas.

Responsible parents are cautious in choosing whom to leave their children with, especially with one-on-one situations. Insist that therapists, clergy members, police officers, doctors, nurses, and hospital staff who interact with the child explain to the child who they are, what they are there for, and what they will be doing. The child should always be appropriately informed about the status of their condition.

With children, do not pretend that you do not see the problem. Quietly and appropriately acknowledge it. We do not have to fix it, but we do have to face it. Like adults, children sometimes just break down and cry from the shock and hurt of it all. I sure did. Just hug them. Just be there for them. It is what it is, and it hurts. Feeling understood and accepted, despite the hurt, is profoundly healing. For instance, we might say, "I understand that this is confusing and upsetting for you, Susie. I am here for you." Or, "Let's talk about it..."

Today, kids facing trauma may withdraw and get addicted to the "digital drugs" of video games and social media. They may retract from healthy activities such as outdoor sports and hiking. To the extent possible, we should encourage children to exercise, go outdoors, and engage with nature. This is good for all of us, and the academic studies show that it boosts our emotions.

At appropriate times, talk to the child about what their future looks like. Have them envision their options and process what is in front of them. Remember Geri, who was born with cerebral palsy following her mother's accident? When faced with her lifelong disability, Geri's parents told Geri that the world was alive with dazzling possibilities. Geri believed them and followed every dream. In doing so, she has inspired millions.

Through this, we teach healthy emotional habits to the children under our care. We give them the tools to thrive for a lifetime.

After my surgery, my parents proclaimed, "The doctors all said that went well, so you are good to go!" They were right, but I had been programmed for 11 years, my entire life until that point, to believe that I was physically impeded. This meant that I needed some emotional reprogramming that I, unfortunately, never received. Recovery is not just about the trauma, but also about conditioning the beliefs we build up around the trauma or that were instilled in us by an abuser. There is still a deconditioning aspect of our trauma. There are the beliefs that we have to consciously examine and change. Even when the physical trauma is over, it is vital to ensure that the child is getting the emotional support they need.

When I laid in my hospital bed day after day, I just adored the young student volunteers who came in. They quickly learned that I loved french fries, so they went out of their way to bring in a huge plate every night. I am sure that these people, who were just kids themselves, had no idea how much it meant to have someone come and chat. I loved it. They did that magical thing—they showed up.

My parents were always service-oriented, and they instilled that quality in me. When appropriate, teach a child the same concepts discussed here. Let them know that they now have a unique opportunity to "show up" to other people's traumas and help them. Allow your child to be there for others. Being of service is not just for adults.

Service can take many forms, and we should look inward to our innate talents and things we enjoy doing to find the best ways we can be of service. If we are aware of our inner world, it becomes easy to listen to our calling. Sometimes, service is described in narrow ways that make it difficult for some to relate. We may see service presented as a "people person" thing, such as taking cookies to the neighbor, baking casseroles, gardening, or cooking at a soup kitchen. Even if we cannot do these things, there are many ways to be of service, and our niche may be in social media activism or writing. There are many little ways that come easily to us, so do not try to fit a square peg into a round hole. There are many ways we can find our calling outside of the popular descriptions that are often pushed onto us. Permit yourself to write your own story.

We may consider art, in all forms, to be a great way to serve people. A fictional story, comic book, or painting, which expresses aspects of the human condition, can make a person feel seen, feel less alone, and feel inspired. There are many brilliant contributions to humanity. Just because something is "fun" to you does not mean it cannot be of service to others. In fact, the best service we can do will "feel right," even fun.

THE ARCHITECTURE OF THRIVING

It is Monday morning, and you open your calendar to see that at 9 a.m., you have an appointment to "Thrive." You know that the time has come to start thriving, but precisely what do you do?

As we look at this question, I am reminded of Blaise Pascal, who once said, "I would have written a shorter letter, but I did not have the time." This is a relatively long book, but it needs to be because this is a critically important topic.

All thrivers have one thing in common. They believe that they can. Let us bring it down to the essence of healing and thriving. One of the quotes posted in my firm's conference room is from Albert Einstein: "If you can't explain it simply, you don't understand it well enough." So, now I am going to make all of this as straight forward as possible.

If you want something you have never had, you need to do something you have never done.

Let me say that again.

If you want something you have never had, you need to do something you have never done.

Please, really let that sink in. Do you just want to read another book, or do you want real change and a new life? Gratitude includes appreciating and benefiting from acts of both self-care and caring for others. Gratitude puts us in the moment. It reframes whatever past and future we think about. Gratitude is presence. We get dopamine from anticipation, and dopamine is the neurotransmitter that propels and motivates us to act. A combination of gratitude and intention toward improving our lives is powerful.

To thrive, we must put in small acts of self-care, even when they are seemingly insignificant. In other words, if you finally want to heal from trauma, you need to do some new things. These activities I have listed are not strenuous, but they do take some focus. Each one has been previously discussed, but I will put them all together and summarize them. Never sacrifice what you want most for what you want now. If you consistently implement these core practices, *you will heal and thrive.*

THE ARCHITECTURE OF THRIVING

This is a blueprint for constructing a fulfilling life and is based on published social-science research.

Grounding: Deep breathing exercises (mindfulness, mediation, yoga, focused breathing) resets the brain's fight-flight-freeze mode, connects with our inner voice, and brings focus. Do this 10 minutes a day.

80 • 10 • 10: Thriving requires stable finances. Live on 80% of all income. Save 10% to create security. Give 10% to those in need. If in debt, live on 70% and use 10% to pay it off

Faith: It takes faith to cross a street. Those with faith in a higher power (God, nature, humanity, intelligent design, meaning, and so forth) fare better. Maintain a daily practice that builds faith and hope.

Movement: A sedentary lifestyle breeds depression. Studies reveal a connection between mental fitness and exercise. With a doctor's approval, do cardio exercise 10 minutes a day.

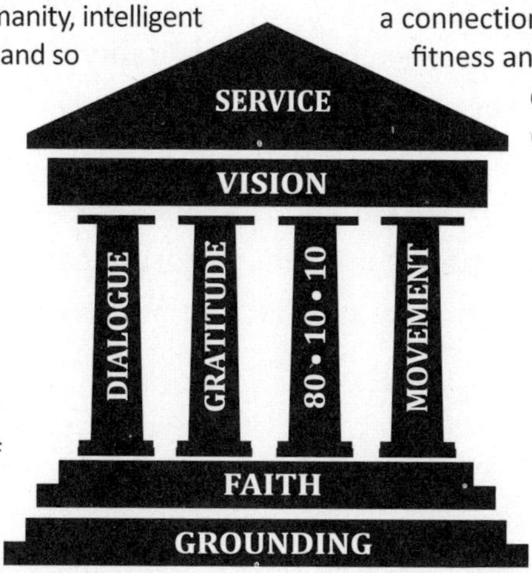

SERVICE

VISION

DIALOGUE

GRATITUDE

80 • 10 • 10

MOVEMENT

FAITH

GROUNDING

Dialogue: We cannot "bottle up" feelings and thrive. Be part of a community. "Sit in the fire" and confide in a trusted person, licensed therapist, or write in a journal. Do this once a week.

Vision: This is more than a goal; it is our soul's voice. See, touch, hear, smell, taste, and feel the dream. Convert a trauma's energy to fuel. Envision a timeline and the steps to get there.

Gratitude: A thankful heart is kind and charitable. Gratitude is the highest form of humanity. Visit, call, or send a note to say "thank you" once a week.

Service: We have a purpose that is greater than ourselves. It could be creating art, charity work, literature, music, or other talents. Meaningful service, aligned with our inner voice, is the pinnacle of thriving.

FAITH:

Those with faith in a higher power—God, nature, humanity, or intelligent design—fare better. Faith is not to deny reality; it is to move forward despite the reality.

If you do not know your core values, you cannot live them. Connect with your higher power. For some, this is God, and for others, this is nature, the universe, or humanity. Albert Einstein said, "There are only two ways to live your life. One is as though nothing is a miracle. The other is as though everything is a miracle." If you are not in awe, you are not paying attention. We should be in awe of all of it. We feel spiritual in the wonder of it all, the questions that have no answers. It is all just so vast and marvelous. Simple acts, like looking at a flower, playing with a child, or laying on our back and watching the sky, can all bring overwhelming feelings of spirituality.

Faith gives us a beautiful hope. Mrs. Phyllis Fender has a sublime faith in God. We were having lunch one day, and she told me, "I am almost excited to go to Heaven!" She radiates faith. However you define your higher power, make an effort to connect in a real and meaningful way daily. This can be a deeply personal topic, so let us leave it there.

GROUNDING:

Deep breathing exercises—mindfulness, meditation, focused-breathing, and yoga—have profound benefits and reset the brain's fight-flight-freeze mode. Dr. Sara Lazar of Harvard Medical School has published numerous articles that show brain scans and the measurable benefits of grounding, meditation, and mindfulness. The science coming out on this is irrefutable.

Grounding is linked to a host of benefits. It measurably reduces our blood pressure and anxiety. But it does more than that. The word "integrity" is derived from the word "integrate." Grounding integrates our mind and body and connects us to our inner voice. Grounding turns on our internal GPS.

Do a grounding exercise 10 minutes a day. This could be breathing exercises, meditation, or mindfulness practices. This will help clear our monkey-mind of anxieties and distractions. The scientifically-proven benefits also include reduction of pain, heart disease, anxiety, anger, and depression. It increases our immune system function, clears our thinking, and brings better blood flow and moods.

The secret of success is found in our daily routines. The single most powerful habit is to get spiritually grounded each morning, and then decide on one thing we will do to help someone that day. Grounding can also be used to ease emotions as issues arise. Eventually, you may find yourself grounding automatically throughout the day.

GRATITUDE:

The antidote for depression is gratitude. There are many wonderful virtues, yet the one that stands out above them all is gratitude. Simply writing one thank-you card or thinking about the good things in life can have profound, positive consequences.

DIALOGUE:

We cannot "bottle up" our feelings and thrive. We must find an avenue to tell our story fully. We must lay out our complete narrative and be heard. Express the full details of your wound to a trusted therapist, family member or friend, or at least journal until such a person is found. Bottling up trauma amplifies the damage. It increases the internal pressure like a volcano.

It is dangerous to confide in the wrong person, as confidentiality and gentleness are essential. It is also important to confide in someone who does not want to "fix" you but can listen as you spill it all out. Avoid confiding in anyone who gossips, an untrained minister, or someone you do not know well. This can be retraumatizing. The person should be someone who does not mind hearing some of the same things repeatedly, as processing the trauma can be long and repetitive.

While I have openly discussed my childhood trauma, a congenital heart defect at birth that required open-heart surgery, I do not share all of my traumas publicly. Nor should you. I do not suggest that you should openly discuss all your traumas. That is your decision. But, at a minimum, your traumas should be between you and a trusted person. We open up to the full measure of our hurts and wrongs. Where we were wronged, we confront it. Where we were wrong, we make amends.

80-10-10:

Many people obsess over what they are living *on,* rather than what they are living *for.* Money is only weakly connected to happiness, but it is connected. We must be disciplined. Our salaries do not make us rich, our spending habits do. Thriving requires basic, stable finances so that our essential needs are met. If we have enough money to pay for our necessities, we are statistically as likely to be as happy as a billionaire. To thrive, we must have reasonable financial stability. When I was on NBC's *Today Show* in New York, I surprised everyone when I said, "Money does buy happiness, but it is not expensive!"

The rules of money are simple. Live on 80 percent of your income. Save and invest 10 percent of your income, no matter how small. This builds security. Give 10 percent to others in need. If you are in debt, cut costs and live on 70 percent, and use 10 percent to pay the debt off.

Keep money in perspective. We are not on earth to just buy more things for ourselves. Your life is a gift to the world. I have never met someone who gave 10 percent of their income to the needy and did not receive it back tenfold. I prefer to give my charitable dollars directly to the needy. No middle man for me. I want to see the benefits first hand.

MOVEMENT:

Studies reveal a clear connection between mental fitness and exercise. A sedentary lifestyle breeds depression, and you cannot hire someone to do your pushups for you.

With the approval of your healthcare provider, get 10 minutes of cardiovascular exercise a day, every day. You have 10 minutes.

VISION:

This is more than a goal; it is your soul's voice. Dr. Martin Luther King, Jr. did not inspire the world by delivering the speech, "I have a complaint!" He encouraged the world with his dream and sense of vision! Maintain a timeline and steps to get there. The brain uses trauma's fuel to ignite passion.

It is just as easy to dream a big dream as a small one. Envision your future life that is healthy and healed. Envision where you want to be and the process needed to get there. Commit your agenda and lists to writing. Create a breakthrough vision. This generates hope and appreciation for the future.

Regularly dream about a point in the future when memories of your trauma can pass through your mind without causing damage. It means actively envisioning the life you want, and as you envision it, you can not only see it, but also touch it, smell it, taste it, and hear it. You go in with all your senses. A vision loves specifics, so give it as many details as you can. This being said, we don't have to go overboard. Our vision should be specific enough to land us in the right general zip code. It does not need to land us at the right street or house. Think of your vision as you go to sleep or create a vision board using images and place it where you will see it often. Don't just see yourself with the trophy, but also the process of getting there. As we envision our actions for a complete, healed, and healthy state, it naturally grows and develops into a reality.

The human brain reacts to pictures, images, and other imagined senses the same way it responds to reality. As we continually put positive images in our minds, both our conscious and unconscious minds will react and set actions in motion to make that vision a reality. It does not happen overnight, but it happens.

SERVICE:

You are not here just to get more stuff. You have a purpose that is greater than yourself. Service comes in many forms, based on your talents, including art, literature, music, or another gift. Service that is aligned with your inner voice is the pinnacle of thriving. Humanity needs your talent in the form of the volunteering you do, the poem that you write, or the child that you teach. Everyone wants to matter and be significant. That is a prime reason why people join gangs and high-demand religions. These are just counterfeits, and we want the real thing.

Our importance is never determined by our status, salary, or success. Our level of service determines how rich and fulfilling our life is. Desmond Tutu said, "Do your little bit of good where you are; it's those little bits of good put together that overwhelm the world." The great secret of life is that it is impossible to be of service to others without helping ourselves even more. We should not give service out of guilt or obligation, as that is not genuine. Authentic service is what nobody asked us to do or what we do when nobody is watching. It is something we are inspired to do, not what someone asks us to do. Albert Pike stated, "What we have done for ourselves alone dies with us; what we have done for others and the world remains and is immortal." The great secret of life is that we cannot deplete abundance. It is difficult to give when we think there isn't enough for ourselves. Service best comes from a feeling of abundance, and it shifts us from a scarcity mentality to a belief that there is enough, not just for ourselves, but for those around us. Ultimately, we only get to keep what we give away.

There's a "grow where you're planted" vibe to service. Our unique experiences, talents, and interests are key to finding our best call to service. We want to not only help others, but also bring ourselves joy.

Not all service will turn into a huge thing, and it doesn't matter if it does or doesn't. Maybe we help one person feel safe and fulfilled, and that is huge. What matters most is that we can hear that inner voice and find a path that will bring us joy. It might require a lot of trial and error. Finding our calling is an iterative process. Rinse and repeat. We may still not be even exactly sure what our calling is, but we can feel like we are on the right track because we are listening and opening ourselves up so we can take action.

In the aftermath of life's train wrecks, our capacity for learning and growth increases exponentially. Opportunities exist for new attitudes and profound wisdom. Those who take each step in this path to healing and recovery will become stronger, wiser, more connected, and more determined to make a difference.

These principles work; however, they are like brushing our teeth. We don't do it on January 1 and expect results for the rest of the year. If you are only *interested* in thriving, then this is the end of the line. If you are *committed* to thriving, then this is the ticket down the whole track. So, ask yourself, are you *interested* in thriving, or are you *committed?*

Have a big vision, but act small. Break down your game plan into small steps. These eight principles are so high-octane that it is unnecessary to do all of them at once. Leo Fender invented the electric guitar with only a vision. John Kralik became a superior court judge with a single focus on gratitude. The men in San Quentin focus on grounding and dialogue. Just these two items generate a profound change of heart. Don't overwhelm yourself. However, you now have the formula to put "thrive" on your calendar and get going.

As Forrest Gump said, "Helping helps the helper." I have seen a woman and man who have lost a daughter to a violent murder use that grief and energy to bless the lives of millions. I have seen homeless women and men get back on their feet, become employed, and reconnect with their children. I have seen the addict climb out from under the freeway overpass, get sober, stay sober, get married, and create a beautiful family. I have seen the alcoholic stay sober, become a lovely person, and earn advanced college degrees. I have seen inmates emerge from prison, committed to a decent and honorable life, and they have kept those commitments. I have seen all of these people thrive, along with thousands of others. This is the recipe to thrive.

* * *

There is no question that trauma will hit us all; it is an inevitable element of human experience. It is a part of our story. It is a part of our legacy. The only question is, "What will we do with it?" Do we make the classic mistake of stuffing it down deep? Or do we take the healthier approach of facing each stage of healing as it unfolds? Do we use it to fuel our resentment and blame? Or do we harness its high-octane fuel to do something meaningful? A great secret is that trauma provides the opportunity to do something remarkably meaningful that we otherwise never would have done.

At times, we grieve and dive. Other times, we get back on our feet and survive. Still other times, we feel the intense energy, blast off, and thrive. The process is to wash, rinse, and repeat. Our resolve is to face each layer as it unfolds. We may not be grateful for trauma, but we can be thankful for its many dimensions of learning.

Disasters result in many insurance claims and lawsuits and studying them has taught me how to collect and analyze data. It has taught me how to go into a courtroom and slug it out with the world's great legal minds. I have learned how to expose the tricks and logical fallacies that my opponents try to use to fool judges and juries. Disasters have taught me how to organize compelling arguments, defend my position, fight, and, ultimately, prevail. I have learned how to organize a case and do the research that results in million and billion-dollar verdicts.

These are good lessons, but they are not life's great lessons. Far more important, this experience has taught me to appreciate the people behind the statistics. For decades, I have been sitting at coffee shops, park benches, kitchen tables, boardrooms, and coconut tree logs listening to their stories.

Traumas reveal life's supreme meaning. Traumas teach us to cut ourselves some slack, be kind, and even love ourselves. Traumas teach us to be compassionate and love others. Traumas teach us that everyone is in the same struggle, which is an opportunity to understand

and love humanity. Traumas teach us to show our love by being more gentle, caring, and considerate. Traumas teach us to follow our bliss, appreciate our joy, laugh, and love more. Traumas remind us to show our love for society's marginalized. Traumas teach us to love the victim and never let them walk their journey alone. Traumas teach us to hold perpetrators accountable and still love them enough to help them in their rehabilitation. Traumas remind us to love and protect every child. Traumas tell us to take our eyes off the ground, look up at the sky, and thank the God who created and loves us. Traumas hurt, but they teach us life's most profound lessons, and those lessons always include love.

Our Stories of Gratitude

DEBBIE

Debbie, whose husband died by his own hand, lost the life she believed she had. She suffered a betrayal so deep that it nearly made her completely give up. But she not only survived her trauma—she thrived. Now working as a family therapist, Debbie has a reputation as a genuinely caring person who has an exceptional connection with her clients. She is extraordinarily empathetic and authentically caring as she provides the support, insight, and perspective people need to overcome their trauma and live the life they were meant to have.

Debbie has found her life's mission. And, just as she envisioned, she lives by the beach. Her children and grandchildren are doing well.

JOHN

John prefers to live quietly and nearly anonymously on his ancestral islands. He frequently meditates by the ocean. John quietly channeled his grief from losing his daughter into a cause he champions—to have his islands cleaned from the environmental contamination and restored so that they can be reinhabited. While a simple island man, his relentless work and quiet leadership were instrumental in taking on the United States federal government and obtaining a $2 billion settlement. This was the largest verdict for an environmental case in the world.

Was the loss of John's daughter worth $2 billion? No. She was worth far more, but John's effort honored her short, sweet life and has made life a bit better for his family, friends, and community. John fulfilled his vision and provided service to all around him.

SUSAN

"Looking back," Susan says, "the landslide was an 'aha' moment, what some people would call my 'bottom.'"

It was the most catastrophic event of her life, yet she learned that she could not only survive but also attain something even better. In her case, she gained a new awareness of the creative process. She permitted herself not only to explore it for her benefit but also to see how she could share this knowledge with others.

Interestingly, Susan and her husband, Peter, were trapped in a comfortable luxury that kept them from their real purpose. Peter said, "That landslide was the best thing that ever happened to us. It broke us out of our comfort zone and got us going on the dreams we always had." Susan said, "So many people do not realize that they have the power to create their dreams. They say they want to make a change but fail to follow through in their actions—and that makes all the difference."

Susan Sherayko is the executive in charge of production of Hallmark Channel's *Home & Family*, one of television's most popular shows. Peter now has his ranch with 20 buildings. It outfits 40 to 50 Western movies a year with authentic saddles, boots, clothes, guns, and more. Susan and Peter realized their dream of establishing a 140-acre ranch and retreat. Susan's inspirational book, *Rainbows Over Ruins,* is found online and at bookstores.

SHAD

On a horrible night more than 50 years ago, Captain Floyd "Shad" Meshad was the officer on duty in a MASH unit where 35 brave, young men died of their injuries after a battle with the Viet Cong. It was a nightmarish experience that horrified him and changed who he was forever. The experience galvanized him to help Vietnam veterans and all vets.

In the last 50 years, Shad has made an indelible mark on the world. He fought to have post-traumatic stress disorder recognized by the *Diagnostic and Statistical Manual for Mental Disorders* as a genuine mental health issue. This is a profound accomplishment for two reasons: First, this is the authoritative reference for all mental health professionals, and second, the research stemming from this is the foundation for voluminous research that has helped millions of vets and non-vets alike.

Shad created Veterans Administration programs that are still used today to treat people with PTSD. Through the National Veterans Foundation, he has made it possible for more than 450,000 veterans and their family members to get the help they need to overcome the trauma they experienced and to thrive.

No one told Shad that this was his path. He figured it out based on where he landed and the things that came to him naturally. He went with the flow, which took him in a direction where he met the right people. He followed his inner voice. He did what came naturally to him, and his work was instrumental in developing a huge field which is so important.

When he started, Shad never knew how important his work would be, but many of us owe him a personal debt of gratitude.

GERI

Geri Jewell has built upon her career as a comedy club star and actor in her role on NBC's hit *Facts of Life*. More recently, she starred in the HBO series *Deadwood*. She is the first person in history with a visible disability to star in a network television series.

For all she has accomplished, one of her triumphs is something of a wish come true. When she was just a girl, she spent hours visualizing the day when she would someday meet her childhood "star" crush—singer David Cassidy. Sure enough, a little more than a decade later, she heard that he was going to appear on a particular daytime talk show. By now, Geri was well-known in the entertainment industry and was able to finagle a backstage meeting with the former "boy of her dreams." She was nervous when she met him and couldn't help but blurt out that he had been her "fantasy boyfriend" when she was a preteen.

David was gracious and kind, and they both laughed over her schoolgirl crush. For Geri, the girl who spent all her time bouncing a tennis ball against a concrete wall and envisioning the day she would meet the boy of her dreams, getting to meet David Cassidy was just about the best thing that ever happened to her—to that point, at least.

Today, Geri lives a life of dignity and class, and her example continues to entertain and inspire millions around the world. Geri's excellent book, *I'm Walking as Straight as I Can,* is found at bookstores and online.

TANYA

In the years that followed Nicole's death, Tanya's struggle with her unprocessed, multi-layered trauma led to addiction, a series of abusive relationships, eventually a suicide attempt, followed by a behavioral health diagnosis and a stay in a mental health facility. Through it all, though, Tanya still fought to help others by writing books; speaking at events to help abused women and those struggling with mental illness or mental health challenges, and supporting all the people in her full social circle.

Tanya earned her master's degree in psychology and now works with an organization that helps people with addiction and behavioral health issues to overcome their problems and find a path to a better life. She is stronger than she has ever been, but she acknowledges that the trauma—all the traumas—she has been through have taken her life in directions she would have never imagined. She shares her story openly and honestly with anyone who asks.

She also practices mediation and exercises regularly to maintain

THE T.A.N.Y.A. FORMULA

T

TALK ABOUT IT
Walk through the Tornado of Chaos to prevent becoming overwhelmed, exhausted, or even depressed.
TECHNOLOGICAL DETOX
We are too connected to things instead of to those who matter.

A

ATTENTION ON THE POSITIVE
There is always a silver lining in chaos. Be still to see and hear it.

N

NURTURE YOURSELF
Do something every day, even for just 10 minutes, that nurtures your soul.

Y

"YOU" TIME
Schedule self-care time daily! You are no good to others if you are not putting your well-being first. Remember, you must put the oxygen mask on yourself first.

A

ATTITUDE OF GRATITUDE
There is always something to be grateful for, even in the darkest of times.

Concept developed by Tanya Brown.

balance in her life. "You can," she says, "learn to love life again after the trauma."

Tanya has learned a great many truths over the years and has used them to help others overcome their trauma. She applied her own advice when she tested positive for COVID-19, which she survived. She has distilled these truths down to a concept called the T.A.N.Y.A. Formula.

JC

With dignity, JC served his time for murder. He led a clean life in prison, bettered himself through classes, earned two degrees, was ordained as a minister, and founded or co-founded several organizations within the prison system designed to help inmates.

One of the most important of the prison programs he helped found is The Last Mile. This unique program was designed for those close to their release date. When it first started, The Last Mile helped men learn how to write business plans so that when they were released from prison, they could start their businesses or go to work for a company. Over time, the program curriculum shifted to coding so that upon release, they had an instantly marketable, high-demand skill that would help them get good-paying jobs.

JC and other Last Mile leaders reached out to area businesses to pitch the idea of hiring these new graduates. Local companies learned of the program and clamored to hire the people who were recently released.

The Last Mile has been in existence for 10 years and is now in prisons in six states. In the last decade, thousands of inmates have been impacted by the program. Some of the program graduates have been hired by companies within a few months of their release.

JC is proud of what The Last Mile has accomplished, but he is even more proud of the men who have successfully completed the program, found good jobs, and made a positive contribution to society. "These men are all examples of what transformation and redemption look like," stated JC.

JC also has the distinction of being the first person in history to give a TED talk from inside a prison. In addition to everything else, JC is also a gifted writer and poet. Singer John Legend, who is passionate about transforming the criminal justice system, learned about JC's poetry. Legend invited JC to join him, from prison, in a TED talk. JC recalls this as an incredible experience. You can watch this on YouTube by entering John Legend with JC Cavitt.

JC looks forward to the changes ahead. At just under 40 years old, JC graduated with a bachelor's degree with honors and is now working towards his master's degree and PhD. He's married and is an active volunteer with his church, works as a corporate trainer, and has a son. He is involved with a number of organizations that offer support and guidance to those who have been impacted by the criminal justice system.

LEO

Leo Fender pushed through a strict upbringing on a small farm in Fullerton, California. He struggled through the loss of his eye as a young boy and the damage to his hearing, blown out by an amplifier as a young adult. He kept going to school, learning, working, and persisting. With his one good eye, he carefully observed others and their struggles and one night at a war bond dance, he noticed the guitar players were struggling to be heard.

Up until that time, "electric guitars" were acoustic guitars with microphones or pickups in the chamber. Leo was the first to eliminate these acoustic chambers and build a guitar out of a solid piece of wood.

Driven by his passion and a vision from God, Leo kept going. Finally, in 1950, his guitars took off. They have sold like hotcakes ever since. One of the impacts of the Fender guitar is it allowed bands to play to huge audiences instead of what once were artists limited to small venues or audiences of a few hundred. It allowed musicians to play to large concert halls filled with thousands. It facilitated the rise of the rock star, something which previously was impossible.

He changed the face of music forever. His original inventions sit in museums. In Leo's dream, God told him that the world was a tough place, and we needed more music to make it better. Leo fulfilled his mission and today, Fender is a billion-dollar company and a household name around the world. More importantly, the world is full of beautiful music from his guitars and the angels who play them.

JOE

Joe was not destroyed by anger and depression, opioid and alcohol addiction, prison time, or even his father's death. Instead, Joe's life experiences have simultaneously strengthened him, while at the same time humbled him, and made him a more caring, loving, empathetic person. He spends his time now helping other people conquer their trauma so that each one can be the person they were meant to be.

Joe recently launched a YouTube channel that focuses on helping people change their lives for the better. We can connect with Joe at joebrat.tv.

ERICA

After surviving World War II and the Holocaust, Erica Leon immigrated to the United States and got married. After her husband passed away, she was shocked to learn that the fiancé of her youth was still alive. They met and got married, and they lived many beautiful years together. Living in Los Angeles, Erica recently celebrated her 99th birthday. She paints gorgeous oil and watercolor paintings of her homeland, all from memory.

TOM

Tom (which is not his real name as he wishes to remain anonymous) moved past his crushed Olympic dreams and used his athletic abilities to obtain college scholarships and earn two degrees. He is the CEO of a global distribution company with 10 facilities around the world. He knows each employee by name and enjoys the fact that his business operation allows many to work and support their families.

MY STORY

I will never be happy that I was born with a congenital heart defect and that I had to have heart surgery as a kid. However, I am grateful for the lessons I learned and how it built some character. Today, when I see a child in a hospital, in a wheelchair, or on a bench during the game because of a disease or illness, I am grateful for that tear that comes to my eye. I am thankful that I do not have to imagine what that kid feels like. I paid a high price for that tear, and it has great value to me. I am that kid. I know exactly how he or she feels. I do not have to imagine. I know the feeling of shame, hurt, and embarrassment that they feel.

In a way, I am grateful that I was born with my trauma, as so many have to wait years before they experience their trauma and wake up. There is much more to be grateful for. I am thankful for parents who worked so hard and found the very best doctors and hospital in the country for my condition. I am grateful to those doctors and nurses who dedicated their studies and careers to helping kids like me. I am grateful for all the volunteers who came to my hospital bedside to cheer me up. I am grateful to my teacher, Mrs. Thatcher, who gave me a pack of magic cards to play with in the hospital. I am thankful for friends who took a look at my colossal scar down at the beach, shrugged, and said that it was no big deal.

If there is a pinnacle moment when one knows they are a post-traumatic thriver, it is when they realize all that they are grateful for. Yes, I had open-heart surgery at age 11, and much later in life, I learned that I suffered from PTSD from it, and had it treated.

At age 60, I was told that I needed heart surgery again. I found the right doctor and followed her wise advice. I began doing grounding exercises every morning, and I have been regularly running five to ten miles since. At the age of 60, when a lot of people are letting themselves go, I got going.

Then a small miracle happened. A buddy of mine invited me to hike Mt. Kilimanjaro in Africa, which is the tallest, non-technical mountain in the world. I was not too bright, and without doing any homework or knowing what I was getting into, I said, "Yes." I trained hard by running for months. I followed all of my doctor's orders. I thought I was ready to go.

The hike started, and I quickly saw that I was in over my head. It was brutally hard, and day after day, we saw young people in their 20's and 30's going down the mountain defeated, and some even went down on stretchers. Hiking up and up and up for thousands of feet took its toll. It was cold and wet, and honestly, the food was not gourmet. Many times, I was out of breath, straining to get some oxygen into my system. It was grungy work. Excuses flooded my mind. Our little group, after all, were the oldest guys out there. I wanted just to surrender and join the parade of people being carried down in stretchers. But I would think about that little boy who endured open-heart surgery, and that gave me the fuel to keep pushing up and up and up.

We kept hiking day after day. Finally, at 8:27 a.m. on June 4, 2019, my three colleagues and I summited at 19,341 feet. We were all surprised by the most brilliant sunrise we had ever seen. At that moment, I realized that all this stuff we are talking about really works. At that moment, in my small way, I knew I had faced my childhood trauma and joined the ranks of other post-traumatic thrivers.

Do not fake your joy. Do not fake happy. Do not go down the rabbit hole of a perfectionist, materialistic lifestyle. Go for the real thing. Many people are walking around and pretending to be perfect. Why are we pretending to be perfect? It is okay to have negative feelings. It is okay to hold onto suffering, as long as we do not use it to hurt ourselves or others. We can use our pain to our advantage. Do not try to toss it out or suppress it. After all, sugarcoating our suffering never works in the long run. It is best to face it, tap into its energy, and even embrace our hurt as the pure fuel that it is. The great secret is that the greater our suffering, the greater our capacity to excel in something that matters. Suffering amplifies our joy.

We suffered trauma and paid an enormous price. Rather than flushing that precious fuel down the drain, let us harness that high-octane energy and do something remarkable. Instead of following society's norms of "shaking it off" and "stuffing" our emotions, let us do something smarter. Let us stop pretending and patching things over with our favorite brand of self-medication, and, instead, practice self-care. A wise and anonymous person once said, "We cannot go back and change the beginning, but we can start now and change the ending." With this new perspective and these tools, we will change the world. And if that does not happen, at least we will change our world.

APPENDIX A

The 15 Stages of Post-Traumatic Thriving

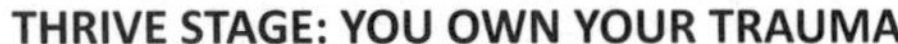

15 STAGES OF THRIVING

THRIVE STAGE: YOU OWN YOUR TRAUMA

15. **Gratitude:** Wisdom and appreciation for life; contribute, love, and give back
14. **Resilience:** Reframe, set goals, new meaning, and a new-found spirit
13. **Forgiveness:** Let go of past; work and grow to realize new possibilities
12. **Connection:** Accept support; form new ways to love and relate to others
11. **Faith:** Passion in God or higher power; spiritual or existential awareness

SURVIVE STAGE: YOU STABILIZE

10. **Awareness:** Mindfulness of personal strength and transformation
9. **Acceptance:** Character to hold ourselves and others accountable
8. **Experiment:** Test new life skills to cope; show self-care and love
7. **Sort Out:** Untangle guilt (wrongdoing) vs shame (circumstances)
6. **Confront:** "Sit in the fire," and identify the pain head on

DIVE STAGE: THE TRAUMA OWNS YOU

5. **Depression**: Feelings of utter hopelessness and despair
4. **Bargain**: Negotiating or seeking ways around trauma
3. **Anger**: Filled with rage, hate, resentment, or blame
2. **Denial**: Dodging, hiding, and avoiding the inevitable
1. **Shock:** Feeling stunning disbelief and paralyzed to the core

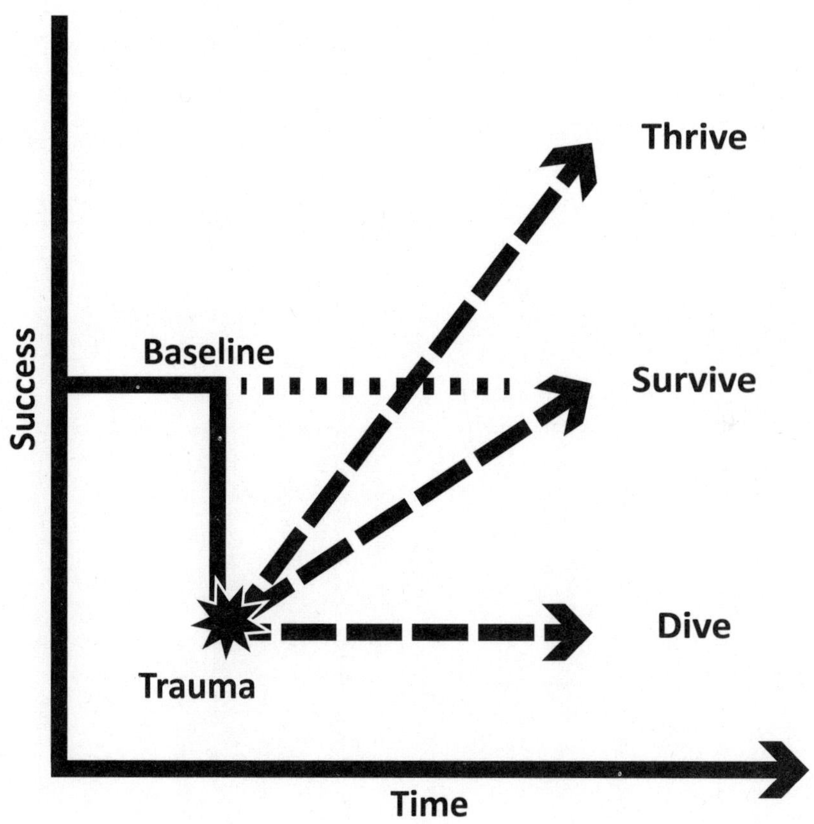
POST-TRAUMATIC THRIVING
Thrive
Baseline
Survive
Success
Dive
Trauma
Time

APPENDIX B

Exercises for Further Exploration

There is a life-force within your soul; seek that life.
There is a gem in the mountain of your body; seek that mine.
O traveler, if you are in search of that, don't look outside.
Look inside yourself, and seek that.
-Mewlana Jalaluddin Rumi

EACH OF THE PRECEDING CHAPTERS introduces us to powerful concepts that compel us to look deep inside. The exercises on the following pages help guide us through the process. As we complete them, we will come to understand our reaction to the trauma we have experienced. More importantly, we will identify the best way to approach our journey and heal.

To achieve the full benefit of these soul-searching exercises, it's essential to carefully read the directions for each one, and then thoughtfully answer each question or scenario in full.

We may want to write out our answers in a journal. Perhaps we will use these exercises as a way to explore our memories in a more focused way. If we are reading *Post-Traumatic Thriving* as a part of a class, seminar, or therapy program, these questions can serve as a launchpad for a therapeutic discussion with our colleagues or therapists.

Remember, there is no need to complete each exercise in one

sitting. Allow time to process the emotions, whether it takes a few minutes, weeks, or longer. Once we give ourselves the time to access our feelings, we can come back and complete the next exercise.

As a word of caution, please do not push yourself or anyone else too hard through these exercises. On the one hand, we want to grow. Yet, on the other hand, we do not want to retraumatize ourselves. There is an optimal level of moving beyond our comfort zone. If we are pushing ourselves to the point of panic or mental anguish, that's going too far.

Be patient. Healing takes time. Be confident knowing that when we follow the principles we have discussed, we will heal. We will change our world. We will *thrive*.

CHAPTER 1: SHOCK EXERCISE

Think of a trauma you have experienced. Make a note of your shock and emotional and physical responses you experienced at the time of the trauma. Through this exercise, I hope you will become more aware of your reactions to shock and note how these reactions are nature's way of protecting you and your loved ones.

1. What was your trauma?
2. What did you notice about your heart rate?
3. What was your breathing like? Did you hyperventilate?
4. What was your emotional state? Were you angry, scared, or anxious?
5. Did you take fight, flight, freeze, or appease?
6. Did you request help? Who responded?
7. Hold long did your shock last?
8. What would you have done differently?
9. What would you do the same?
10. Do you feel the same physical reactions today, or has the shock subsided?

CHAPTER 2: DENIAL EXERCISE

This exercise is designed to identify the issues of denial and your trauma.

1. What am I avoiding, and what is the root cause?
2. Have I fully admitted the impact of the trauma to myself today?
3. Have I admitted the trauma to others?
4. How long did my denial or minimizations last?
5. How was I protecting myself or others with my denials?
6. Are my denials still protecting me from something?
7. If not, is it time to let them go and face what I need to face?

CHAPTER 3: ANGER EXERCISE

1. How mad and upset were you as a result of your trauma?
2. Did you bottle your feelings up, or did you let it out?
3. Did your anger unnecessarily hurt anyone?
4. Did your anger result in you doing something that you now regret?
5. What is your level of anger today?
6. What are some ways you could direct the anger to use it as fuel to resolve the issue or help others with similar issues?

CHAPTER 4: BARGAIN EXERCISE

1. How did you bargain with your trauma?
2. Did it work?
3. Are you still bargaining?
4. Are you bargaining with any toxic groups?
5. Is your inner voice aligned with your outer world?
6. Is your inner voice aligned with any group that you belong to?

CHAPTER 5: DEPRESSION EXERCISE

1. Do you feel sad, blue, hopeless, or down? If so, how long have you felt this way?
2. Has your behavior changed? Are you sleeping more or less, avoiding activities you once found fun, or struggling to accomplish desired tasks?
3. Is any depression subsiding, remaining the same, or getting worse?
4. Have you been diagnosed as having depression?
5. Do sad feelings interfere with leading a healthy life?
6. If you are feeling depressed for a prolonged period, are you seeking professional help?

CHAPTER 6: CONFRONTING EXERCISE

Have you "sat in the fire" and faced your trauma? What is your level of awareness? Let us confront both our bright and dark sides. Circle all of the words, good or bad, which describe where you are now in your life:

Absent
Abusive
Academic
Affectionate
Aggressive
Alcoholic
Angry
Animated
Anxious
Arrogant
Authoritarian
Available
Bitter
Blaming
Boring
Brutal
Bullying
Busy
Calculating
Calm
Caregiver
Center of Attention
Centered
Childish
Cold
Compassionate
Competitive
Confused
Controlling
Critically harsh
Cruel
Curious
Degrading
Democratic
Dependent
Depressed
Disapproving
Disrespectful
Distrustful

Dominating
Egotistical
Empathetic
Envious
Excited
Exhausted
Extroverted
Fake
Flashy
Forgetful
Forgiving
Fragile
Friendly
Frightened
Frustrated
Fulfilled
Fun-loving
Grandiose
Greedy
Harmonious
Helpful
Honest
Hopeful
Hostile
Humorous
Hurtful
Impatient
Inattentive
Inconsistent
Indecisive
Intelligent
Interested
Intolerant
Invalidating
Involved
Jealous
Joyful
Judgmental
Kindhearted
Lazy
Lively
Loud
Loving
Martyr-like
Materialistic
Mean
Mellow
Moody
Naïve
Narcissistic
Negative
Non-judgmental
Obstinate
Open-hearted
Optimistic
Overly protective
Paranoid
Passionate
Passive
Peaceful
People pleaser
Perfectionist
Promiscuous
Racist
Rageful
Regretful
Relentless
Resentful
Righteous
Rude
Sad
Satisfied
Self-centered
Sensitive
Serene
Stable
Stingy
Submissive
Suspicious
Sympathetic
Tender
Thoughtful
Timid
Tired
Tranquil
Trusting
Truthful
Unavailable
Unforgiving
Uninterested
Unkind
Unreliable
Vain
Vengeful
Violent
Warm
Weak
Workaholic
Worrier

CHAPTER 7: SORT OUT EXERCISE

1. What shame do you feel in your life?
2. What guilt do you feel in your life?
3. Do you have a trusted person you can confide in?

CHAPTER 8: EXPERIMENT EXERCISE

1. What have you tried, since the trauma, that you now see as unhealthy?
2. What have you tried, since your trauma, that you now see as healthy?
3. What would you like to try that could help you heal from your trauma?

CHAPTER 9: ACCEPTANCE EXERCISE

1. What have you had a difficult time accepting?
2. What do you now accept?
3. What do you do now to prove to yourself that you have accepted your reality?

CHAPTER 10: MINDFULNESS EXERCISE

Grounding, also known as meditation, contemplation, focused breathing, or yoga, is a natural, simple, and effective technique. It can have dramatic effects on lowering our blood pressure, stabilizing brainwaves, and calming anxiety in as little as five to ten minutes. The essence of meditation is to not think about the past or the future but to focus on the here and now. Here is one approach to meditation that you can try:

- Sit down in a comfortable, quiet place, either on a chair or on the floor.
- Close your eyes or focus on an object in the center of the

room. Take a few deep breaths. If concentrating on your breathing causes anxiety, focus on a person or place that brings peace.

- Start taking normal breaths while focusing on your breathing.
- Some prefer to repeat the word "So" silently. Exhale through your nose while silently repeating the word "Hum."
- It is okay if you're distracted by outside sounds or your attention drifts. When it happens, passively observe the thought until it dissipates, and then gently return to your breathing.
- Do this for 10 minutes a day, and lengthen the time if you want. The objective for many people is to meditate half an hour a day. You can do this in complete silence, or you can add soft music. There are also apps and guided meditations you can use.
- When you finish, open your eyes, and sit for a few moments in the stillness and silence. You will notice that your mind and body are calmed, which will naturally extend throughout the day.

Similar to grounding is a "safe place" exercise. This is calming for many people who mentally visit a comforting or "safe place." Create an image in your mind that you can visit when you want to relax. It can be a beach, cabin, meadow, or any place, real or imagined, that you love and makes you feel calm. Spend time developing this place in your imagination in as full a sensory way as you can.

- How does it look?
- What does the sky look like?
- How does the air feel?
- What are the smells?

- When you are sitting, how does the grass, dirt, or sand feel?
- What sounds do you hear?

When emotions threaten to overwhelm, you can visit this place, remember as many of the sensations as possible, and relax into them.

CHAPTER 11: FAITH EXERCISE

1. What are your beliefs about a higher power or sense of that which is greater than yourself?
2. What inspires the greatest sense of awe and wonder for you?
3. What thoughts make you feel most centered and at peace with yourself?
4. What do you do to cultivate your beliefs in the divine and your admiration of nature?
5. What daily act or ritual do you use to connect to God, nature, or your inner sense of spirituality?
6. Where do you feel the greatest sense of excitement and purpose?
7. Are there sources of information, literature, music, art, poetry, or other works that inspire you? What are you doing to foster that sense of inspiration?
8. Have you ever felt "drawn"? What events or thoughts have given you a feeling of being pulled towards greater things? What does your inner voice sound like?

CHAPTER 12: CONNECTION EXERCISES

Quietly consider each of the following questions, and assess where your predominant communication style lies:

1. Do you have to yell to be heard?
2. Do you have a hard time saying no?
3. Are your feelings about your trauma bottled up?
4. Do you clam up when you are being criticized?

5. Do you feel upset and angry with others?
6. Is it essential that you "win" a conversation with others?
7. Do you try to blend in with the conversation?
8. Do you feel shamed or shunned by people you should be close to?
9. Do you feel uncomfortable when people disagree with you?
10. Do you try too hard to avoid conflict?
11. Do you regret not speaking up and saying something after conversations?
12. Do you feel overly anxious about telling others how you feel?
13. Is peace at any cost vital to you?

If you answered yes to any of these questions, you might be communicating passively, aggressively, or passive-aggressively. Consider how you can turn from these old behaviors to a healthy, assertive style of communication if it is safe to do so.

1. Do you keep a journal and keep it in a safe and secure place?
2. Have you identified a trustworthy friend or family member in whom you can confide?
3. Do you have a licensed and competent therapist in whom you can confide?

The more you can answer "yes" to these questions, the better.

CHAPTER 13: FORGIVENESS EXERCISE

1. What memories cause you to become emotionally charged?
2. What does forgiveness mean to you?
3. Who in your life do you need to forgive?
4. Who do you owe an apology to?
5. Who in your life do you need forgiveness from?
6. Do you harbor bad feelings toward yourself or others over the trauma?

7. What do you do to burn off steam?
8. Will you commit to seeing a healthcare provider about getting the okay to do 10 minutes of cardio a day—six days a week?

CHAPTER 14: RESILIENCE EXERCISE

1. Do you bounce back easily from difficult emotions, or does it take a while?
2. What activities or thoughts help you get emotionally evened out?
3. What do you envision yourself doing in six months?
4. What stands in your way?
5. Build a vision board with a timeline and all the steps to get there.

CHAPTER 15: GRATITUDE EXERCISE

Trauma, while unpleasant, can yield gratitude to those who allow it. We are usually not grateful for an injury itself, but write a "gratitude letter" expressing your thankfulness for the lessons you have learned from your trauma and detailing how your trauma has allowed you to gain wisdom and help others.

Answer these questions honestly:

1. What was your trauma?
2. Summarize the key points you have learned so far.
3. List three specific things you learned about yourself.
4. List three specific things you learned about your trauma.
5. What healing thoughts have you used in the past?
6. What healing thoughts will you use in the future?
7. What situations are triggers or high-risk for you now?
8. What tools have you found to be most helpful?
9. What areas of work do you still need or would like to do regarding your ongoing healing?

10. Who are the people who can help you achieve your current goals?
11. If you could do anything, what would be the one thing you would do to heal yourself?
12. What can you do to serve others or your community?

If you are comfortable and so inclined, email a copy of your letter to me at Bell@CoreIQ.com. Please let me know if I may share your thoughts or if you wish for me to keep them confidential.

APPENDIX C

How Was School Today?

SOME OF US STUDY TRAUMA for the purpose of helping a child. The following questions are designed to help stimulate an in-depth conversation with a child, rather than just asking, "How was school today?" Go through the list and pick a couple of questions that best suit the child:

1. What was the best thing that happened at school today?
2. What was the strangest thing you heard at school today?
3. What was the worst part of school today?
4. How did somebody help you today?
5. How did you help somebody today?
6. If I called your teacher tonight, what would she tell me about you?
7. If you could choose, who would you like to sit by in class? Why?
8. If you could switch seats with anyone in the class, who would you trade with? Why?
9. If you got to be the teacher tomorrow, what would you do?
10. If you were principal for a day, what would you do?
11. Is there anyone in your class that needs a time out?

12. Tell me one thing that you learned today.
13. Tell me something good that happened today.
14. Tell me something that made you laugh today.
15. What do you think you should do less of at school?
16. What do you think you should do more of at school?
17. What was your favorite part of lunch?
18. What word did your teacher say most today?
19. When were you bored today?
20. When were you the happiest today?
21. Where do you play the most at recess?
22. Where is the most relaxing place at the school?
23. Who in your class do you think you could be more helpful to?
24. Who is the funniest person in your class? What makes them so funny?
25. Who is the most helpful student at your school?
26. Who is the nicest teacher at your school?
27. Who would you like to play with at recess that you have never played with before?
28. Who would you not want to sit by in class? Why?

APPENDIX D

24 Things I Learned in San Quentin

GOING INSIDE OF PRISONS and jails has been a life-altering experience. There is no time for sugar-coated remedies. If we want to help someone turn their lives around, we need to get to the core of what is effective and what is not.

1. **Meditate.** I learned how to meditate for the first time in prison.Meditation (or "grounding") lays the cornerstone for transforming the cold heart of a criminal. It is the first step for an offender to take full responsibility for the harm and damage they have caused and transition into becoming a person of integrity. As I learned about meditation, I discovered that it focuses the mind on "now," rather than the regrets of the past or the worry of the future. This alleviates what Eastern society calls "monkey mind" and Western society calls "anxiety." Later, my cardiologist explained how brain waves work and prescribed ten minutes of meditation a day—every day. In its simplest form, we sit comfortably, close our eyes, and focus on breathing. It was easy, and my

blood pressure dropped. That is when it hit me: Meditation heals broken hearts.

2. **Deal with Unprocessed Trauma.** Life is tough. According to one university study, 66 to 85 percent of all people have faced at least one trauma by college age. Unprocessed trauma is at the core of crime, alcohol abuse, drug abuse, fringe politics, fringe religion, overeating, and other forms of self-medication. Any of these gives a counterfeit high but is not a solution. Self-medication numbs reality, and we cannot heal from something we avoid. A better choice is to face the issues, seek help, and get authentic highs through exercise, meditation, prayer, music, charitable service, sports, hobbies, healthy relationships, and pursuit of our passions.
3. **Don't Rank Crime.** Crime is crime. Sin is sin. Abuse is abuse. My crimes, sins, and abuses are no better than yours. Your crimes, sins, and abuses are no better than mine. They all hurt people, and it is all wrong. When we rank our sins and crimes, we constantly compare ourselves to others to see where we measure up. This results in false feelings of superiority or inferiority. When we remove the ranking and judgment, we align with reality.
4. **Understand "Grounded Theory."** In prison, people have hit rock bottom. In academics, we recognize that sometimes, we learn better when we throw out everything and just start over. In business school, we called it "frame-breaking." In essence, we just scrap everything and start from the ground up. When we hit bottom, it shakes us to the core. Yet rock bottom is a wonderful place from which to build.
5. **Know Everyone Is Redeemable.** My volunteer work is through a program called "Insight Prison Project." One of its leaders said, "Human life is a miracle, but human transformation may be even more miraculous." In the right environment, I have seen the most hardened criminals, who flash gang signs and put on the whole macho act, melt like

butter. Everyone can turn their life around, even with a life sentence. I have seen it happen many times. Ultimately, true character is measured by the ability to navigate through a crisis successfully.

6. **You Can't "Teach" Deep Transformation.** The power for transformation comes from inside. Profound transformation takes a Socratic approach (questioning dialogue), not a conventional, didactic, teacher-student model. External solutions do not solve internal problems. Books, lectures, seminars, and sermons can help, but ultimately the answers are not out there. They are buried in the last place people often look—deep inside the heart.
7. **Meet People Where They Are.** You cannot find people more broken than those in prison. While I am trained and qualified to facilitate group meetings, I cannot fix anyone else. Frankly, you cannot either. What we can do is to simply meet people where they are. If they are angry, ask why they are angry. If they hurt, ask if you can help. If they lie, don't call them out, but realize that it is a protection against something they are not yet ready to share. Just being there at their level helps them process their trauma and heal in their own time and way. Trying to fix, diagnose, convert, or repair a person is a waste of time and can even be damaging. Simply show up and meet people where they are.
8. **Don't Judge Others.** Sometimes I have judged an inmate and realized I was completely wrong once I got to know them. When I learned their backstories, I thought that they were doing better than I ever could. Eventually, I just admitted that I am terrible at judging, so I no longer bother. We never know what battles people are fighting. Judgmental and self-righteous behaviors are enemies of healing and healthy lifestyles.
9. **Diversify.** You will never see a more racially-charged place than prison. Even today, Blacks, Whites, Hispanics, Asians,

and others are strictly segregated. Yet real progress is only achieved when everyone is included. We must directly challenge the ignorant precedents of racism and instill a spirit of absolute teamwork and mutual respect. Smart investors diversify their portfolio, and intelligent people and businesses diversify their teams. In prison, we face this issue head-on and address the depravity of racism. Every person has inherent value. We intentionally form diversified groups so we can draw on everybody's strengths.

10. **Be Trustworthy.** In our prison program, we form a circle and discuss topics that could get the speaker killed in the prison yard or jeopardize their possibility of being paroled. Gossip and idle talk are a life and death matter. It is critical we keep these conversations confidential and never talk about them outside the group. Ever. The inmates and victims are asked to trust the process and stick to the established curriculum, as it has been proven to work. Once a safe place is established, the offenders are asked to be brave, vulnerable, and willing to take a risk. This same principle applies to everyone. We can be vulnerable and find a trustworthy person to confide in. If we have been trusted, we must maintain that integrity. It is critical to build a safe place where healing can happen. Trust and vulnerability are key elements when coming clean and freeing ourselves from unresolved trauma and pain.
11. **Cut Some Slack.** Life is messy. Anyone who "knows" all the answers to life's biggest questions is kidding themselves. The world is a broken place and people mess up. In this kind of work, there is no checklist, and there is no script. Inmates will make mistakes, and so will I as a group facilitator. We just agree to pick ourselves up and move forward.
12. **Don't Be a Sucker.** There are con artists in prison. Frankly, they are so good that they fool me; however, they can't con the other inmates in the circle. Of course, con artists are not

just in prison; they are everywhere. Harvard sociologist Dr. Martha Stout estimates that one out of 24 people is an everyday sociopath. The simple rule of thumb is that if you catch someone in three lies, they have a problem. Some con artists set up phony charities, do fake work at their jobs, and enjoy abusing others. We want to be kind, but we do not ever want to be a sucker.

13. **Don't Motivate by Fear.** Fear is the cheapest and sleaziest way to influence people. It may work at first, but at a cost, and there is a risk of negative fallout. A far more effective way is to engage people and accept them. Show respect, whether it is earned or not. Love the unloved. Care for those who do not care. This is a higher way.
14. **Understand Guilt vs. Shame.** Guilt and shame are very different, and understanding this is a game-changer. Guilt comes from doing something bad. Shame is feeling ashamed for something for which we had no responsibility or control over. In other words, guilt is what I did, while shame is who I am. For example, some of us feel shame for growing up poor, being abused or bullied, not understanding school subjects, the color of our skin, having a disability, being attracted to the same gender, and so on. In my life, I felt shame about having open heart surgery when I was a kid. Unprocessed shame can build up like a volcano and explode when triggered. The solution is to talk about feelings of shame with a trusted person. A remedy may or may not be possible, but these discussions help relieve the pressure. That way, when we are triggered, we don't explode.
15. **Listen.** This is the single most important principle. In prison, people tell horrible stories of their crimes, and their backstories are heartbreaking. We simply listen as the inmates talk about these terrible events and the guilt, rage, and anger. We cannot scream and run out of the room. We learn to "sit in the fire," and quietly listen. We listen to

things that are repulsive to the core. Yet, just being there, while people speak from the soul and pour out their guilt and shame in a safe environment, allows them to heal. Listening will enable others to feel heard, seen, and validated. Not only is the violence and ugliness discussed, but we also see joy, excitement, and happiness. The process is not all "doom and gloom." Time and time again, there are beautiful transformations that take place in those sacred circles.

16. **Have Open Conversations.** We will never find more fallout from trauma than in prison. The only way inmates heal is from real conversations about the rough stuff. It does not happen overnight. It takes many months or years. But the objective, inside and outside prison, is to have open and honest conversations on any topic with people we trust. Toxic people say, "Forgive and forget," or "Let us not talk about it." On the other hand, healthy people say, "Let us have that conversation," "I will listen to whatever you say," or "That is wrong; let's call the police." The objective of any healthy relationship, family, or organization is to maintain a place where there are open conversations on any relevant topic. Healthy people do not hide, duck, or bury their feelings, avoid opposing views, or dodge inconvenient truths.
17. **Embrace Your Joys and Hurts.** Buddha said, "Life is suffering," and I think he was half right. Life is an adventure that brings both suffering and joy. The lows in prison are apparent, but many inmates engage in activities that bring them joy, such as music, art, work, and writing. Sometimes, I get so busy that I forget to stop and enjoy those things that make me happy. For example, I love to play the guitar. I am not that good, and I have no interest in performing, but I just love it. Sometimes I realize that I am working too hard and have not picked up my guitar for months. I suppress my joys. On the other hand, my past traumas hurt, so I want to

suppress them. We all have joys and traumas.

Yet when we face and embrace both, we heal, grow, and live.

18. **Own It.** In prison, you cannot heal from trauma until you own it. It is the same outside. Only a fool would say, "I am never wrong." Only a toxic leader would say, "We do not make apologies." If we are wrong, we need to own it. If we feel shame, we need to own it. That is the only way to respect others and ourselves. That is how we go from arrogance, insecurity, and being desperate to becoming authentic, genuine, and real.
19. **Understand Religion Has Its Limits.** I am religious, but religion can get in the way of healing unresolved trauma. Healing takes real work, and the process is difficult. Some people dodge and say, "I already dealt with this with my pastor (priest, rabbi, cleric, bishop, minister, etc.)." It is great to have those conversations, but it does not provide a free pass from doing the work any more than it would allow you to dodge having a doctor reset a broken bone. Research and social science show the process for healing, so follow the proven path.
20. **Show Up.** My first visits to prison were tainted by my curiosity and ego. After the shock and novelty wore off, I took an in-depth look inside and realized I was still authentically drawn to the work. Somehow I knew my journey was tied to it. So I just kept showing up. One day, an inmate came up to me and said, "Thank you for coming in here. You being here makes me feel like a human. What I did was horrible, but I have committed to living a good and honorable life from now on—even if the rest of my life is inside a prison." That man inspired me to keep showing up. Just showing up is a big part of any solution.
21. **Practice Unconditional Empathy.** When new inmates come in, some are hard to appreciate because of their rough, defensive, even aggressive exterior. Many people say, "I will respect you

when..." or "I love you, if..." but these are conditions. If we only love others based on how we see them or how we wish they would be and not how they see themselves, it is conditional love. When we listen quietly and with no judgment, it allows others to unlock that intuitive ability to process the damage, heal, and grow. We are there to "sit in the fire" of uncomfortable feelings and stories. From that, we often develop a sense of "unconditional empathy." Ultimately, I came to appreciate and respect every inmate that showed up and stuck with the program.

22. **Know How Sinners and Saints Operate.** On the extremes, sinners can suffer from a "guilt complex," while saints carry a "martyr complex." Neither is fully equipped to respond to logic, facts, or figures—yet they do respond to kindness. Guilt and self-righteousness are obstacles to growth; we must be teachable. Some "saints" have put on a beautiful show that turns out to be a fraud. Remarkably, the "sinners" in prison taught me about integrity. Face the truth. I would rather live an uncomfortable truth than a comfortable lie.
23. **Give Credit.** Give credit to those who inspire you. Insight Prison Project is a secular restorative justice program, but it presents the most profound spiritual principles I have ever seen. As the inmates and victims share their stories, it brings tears to my eyes every time. I give them all the credit for doing the work and inspiring me. Looking back on my journey, my visits to prison were not inspired by groups or authorities, Republicans, Democrats, organized religions, nor university professors. While this program is secular, my volunteer efforts are credited to the unfiltered words of Jesus who taught people to visit those in prison. Now I know why.
24. **Appreciate That This Stuff Works.** Prisons present the most complex challenges known to humanity. At least 90 percent of all prison inmates will be released or paroled at some time. The questions is, "How do we want them released?

Do we want men and women paroled who are cold, angry, and bitter or who have taken the responsibility to be healed, kind, and productive?" Prisons are the ideal setting to sort out what is fake and what is real. When the prevailing systems fail, these principles work. This program is in dozens of prisons, and of the hundreds of inmates who have completed it and have been released, the recidivism rate is near zero. I am not sure who else can say that. Not only do these principles work in prisons, they help anyone who wishes to evolve.

APPENDIX E

What You Should Never Say vs. What You Should Say

When we communicate, we want to express how we feel, as well as validate how others are feeling. These simple phases help us adapt a new language that does that:

Avoid saying ...

- Do not be silly.
- Do not be so negative.
- Do not be ungrateful.
- Everything happens for a reason.
- Get over it.
- Grow up, and stop living in the past.
- Have you prayed about it?
- I know how you feel.

- I have been through worse.
- It was not that bad.
- It is all part of God's plan.
- It is not like he hit you.
- Just let it go.
- Suck it up.
- That was so long ago.
- Think of all the people who have it worse.
- Time heals all wounds.
- Well, did you provoke it?
- You need to just forgive them.
- You were not worthy.
- You are an adult. You cannot blame your parents for your problems anymore.
- Your parents did the best they could.

Show understanding and say ...

- It is safe to show your feelings to me.
- I have no solutions, only sympathy.
- I hear you.
- I am sorry.
- I wish it was not this way.
- I wish I could make you feel better.
- If you did not recognize that you were being abused, you are not alone.
- It was not your fault.

- It was not your job to be “the adult” as a kid.
- It is not your job to protect all the grownups. It is their job to protect you.
- I believe you.
- It is okay to be angry.
- It is okay to cry.
- It is okay to talk about it.
- Of course, you would feel that way.
- Tell me more.
- Tell me what happened.
- It was not okay what they did to you.
- What you heard is not true.
- You are a warrior.
- You are beautiful.
- You are not the worthless mistake you were told you are.
- You are strong, and recovery is possible.
- You are stronger than you think.
- You are worthy of love.
- You are not a sexual object.
- You can do this.
- You can stop the cycle of abuse.
- You deserve to talk about it.
- You did not deserve that.
- Your feelings are real and valid.

APPENDIX F

Psychological War Zones

When we hear about PTSD, we may think of combat war veterans. While this can be true, PTSD actually affects millions of people from a wide spectrum of traumatic backgrounds. PTSD can be behind any of the following conditions, and if it is, professional assistance is advisable:

- Aggression
- Avoidance of situations that bring back memories
- Depression
- Difficulty concentrating
- Drawn to unhealthy relationships
- Easily startled
- Emotional outbursts
- Excessive "inner critic"
- Excessive feelings of shame or guilt
- Excessive ruminations
- Feeling defective

- Flashbacks where we relive the traumatic experience
- Hyperarousal
- Hypervigilance
- Irritability
- Isolation
- Lack of interest in activities we once enjoyed
- Low self-esteem
- Memory loss
- Negative self-talk
- Panic attacks
- Risky behavior
- Self-blame
- Self-doubt
- Self-harm
- Sleeping disorders
- Substance abuse and addictions
- Suicidal thoughts

APPENDIX G

Daily Affirmations

HAVING A QUOTE OR DAILY affirmation in our purse or wallet or on our bathroom mirror can be an effective way to building a good attitude. Affirmations help release beneficial neurotransmitters and inspire our minds to actively work at making the phrase be true. Here are some ideas:

- I am loving.
- I am kind.
- I am grateful.
- I have value.
- I am humble.
- I have integrity.
- I am generous.
- I have a sense of humor.
- I am healing day by day.
- The world is evolving from greed and fear to peace and love, and I am part of this.

- I am the captain of my soul. –"Invictus" by William Ernest Henley
- The sun will come up in the morning. Simply showing up is a big part of the solution. I will show up for breakfast, my family, my friends, my self-care, my interests and hobbies, my therapist, and my tribe.
- I am persistent. A river cuts through solid rock not because of its power, but by its persistence.
- You can watch me, mock me, or join me. But you cannot stop me!
- I may not solve the world's problems, but I can make a difference one kind act at a time.
- When things get real, it exposes who is real and who is phony.
  I am real!
- It is okay not to be okay.
- The best things in life are not things.
- Hurt people hurt people, but healed people heal people.
  As I heal, I will help those around me.
- I look good. I feel good. I have the goods!
- God has a plan for my life, but so does everybody else. I will pick the plan that is right for me.
- I have character. I will not take my career, car, or cash to heaven.
  The only thing I can take is my character.
- A negative mind will never give me a positive life.
- I am grateful for the rude and obnoxious people in my life—as they serve as examples of what I do not want to do.
- It is okay to be angry, but it is never okay to be cruel.
- I remember those who love me, even when I felt unlovable.

- I am nice to rude people, not because they are not nice, but because I am.
- I will not stay silent so that you can stay comfortable.
- Rock bottom teaches me lessons that mountain tops never will.
  Rock bottom is a beautiful place from which to build.
- The person on top of the mountain did not fall there.
- A person who never made a mistake never tried anything new.
- Integrity is everything.
- Yesterday was fine, but the future is all that I have time for.
- If I have the power to make someone happy, I will do it.
- Peace is the result of integrity. The very word "integrity" comes from the word "integrated," where my inner voice aligns with my choices.
- I am a person of integrity. I follow my moral compass, no matter what any authority tells me.
- Just because I am kind to people does not mean that I must spend extra time with them.
- The short-term pain of the truth is better than the long-term pain of illusion.
- The best use of my life is to love.

APPENDIX G

Trauma Tree

TRAUMA TREE

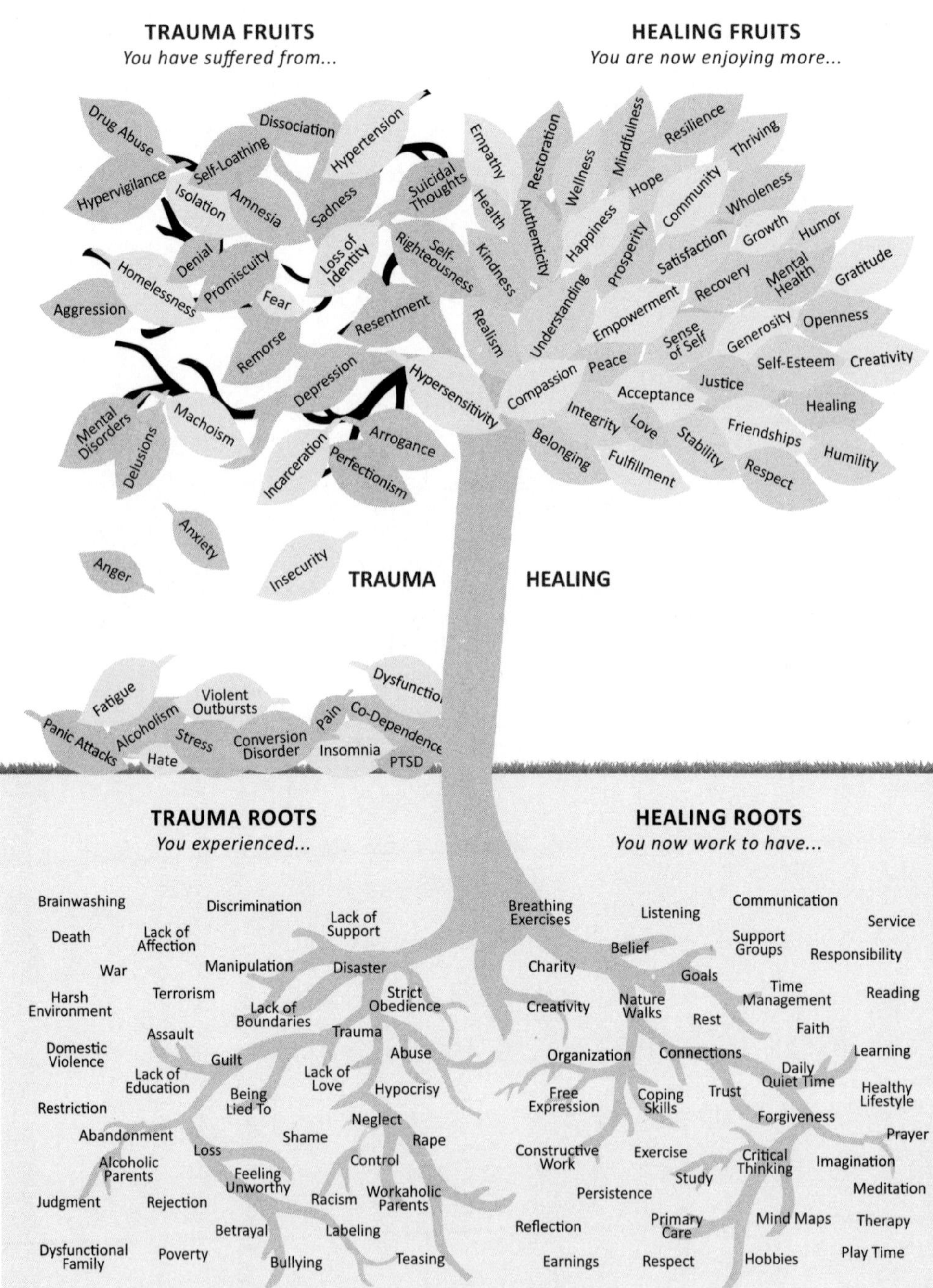

TRAUMA FRUITS
You have suffered from...
HEALING FRUITS
You are now enjoying more...
Drug Abuse
Dissociation
Hypertension
Self-Loathing
Hypervigilance
Isolation
Amnesia
Sadness
Suicidal Thoughts
Denial
Promiscuity
Loss of Identity
Self-Righteousness
Homelessness
Fear
Aggression
Resentment
Remorse
Depression
Hypersensitivity
Mental Disorders
Delusions
Machoism
Arrogance
Incarceration
Perfectionism
Anxiety
Anger
Insecurity
Empathy
Restoration
Wellness
Mindfulness
Resilience
Thriving
Health
Authenticity
Hope
Community
Wholeness
Kindness
Happiness
Prosperity
Satisfaction
Growth
Humor
Realism
Understanding
Empowerment
Recovery
Mental Health
Gratitude
Sense of Self
Generosity
Openness
Compassion
Peace
Justice
Self-Esteem
Creativity
Acceptance
Healing
Integrity
Love
Stability
Friendships
Belonging
Fulfillment
Respect
Humility
TRAUMA
HEALING
Fatigue
Violent Outbursts
Dysfunctio
Panic Attacks
Alcoholism
Stress
Conversion Disorder
Pain
Co-Dependence
Hate
Insomnia
PTSD
TRAUMA ROOTS
You experienced...
HEALING ROOTS
You now work to have...
Brainwashing
Discrimination
Lack of Support
Death
Lack of Affection
War
Manipulation
Disaster
Harsh Environment
Terrorism
Strict Obedience
Lack of Boundaries
Assault
Trauma
Domestic Violence
Abuse
Guilt
Lack of Education
Lack of Love
Being Lied To
Hypocrisy
Restriction
Neglect
Abandonment
Shame
Rape
Loss
Alcoholic Parents
Control
Feeling Unworthy
Judgment
Rejection
Racism
Workaholic Parents
Betrayal
Labeling
Dysfunctional Family
Poverty
Bullying
Teasing
Breathing Exercises
Listening
Communication
Service
Support Groups
Belief
Responsibility
Charity
Goals
Time Management
Reading
Creativity
Nature Walks
Rest
Faith
Organization
Connections
Learning
Daily Quiet Time
Free Expression
Coping Skills
Trust
Healthy Lifestyle
Forgiveness
Prayer
Constructive Work
Exercise
Critical Thinking
Imagination
Study
Persistence
Meditation
Reflection
Primary Care
Mind Maps
Therapy
Earnings
Respect
Hobbies
Play Time

References

1. Affleck, Glenn, Howard Tennen, and Jonelle Rowe. Infants in Crisis: How Parents Cope with Newborn Intensive Care and Its Aftermath. New York, NY, US: Springer-Verlag Publishing, 1991. https://doi.org/10.1007/978-1-4612-3050-2.

2. Afonso, Rui F., Joana B. Balardin, Sara Lazar, João R. Sato, Nadja Igarashi, Danilo F. Santaella, Shirley S. Lacerda, Edson Amaro Jr., and Elisa H. Kozasa. Greater Cortical Thickness in Elderly Female Yoga Practitioners—A Cross-Sectional Study. Vol. 9. Frontiers in Aging Neuroscience, 2017. http://journal.frontiersin.org/article/10.3389/fnagi.2017.00201/full.

3. Alexander, Michelle. The New Jim Crow: Mass Incarceration in the Age of Colorblindness. New York: The New Press, 2010.

4. Allen, Jon G. Coping with Trauma: Hope through Understanding. 2nd Edition. Arlington, VA, US: American Psychiatric Publishing, Inc., 2004.

5. Bains, Tina (@tina_bains). "And then it happens...One day you wake up and you're in this place. You're in this place where everything feels right. Your heart is calm. Your soul is lit. Your thoughts are positive. Your vision is clear. You're at peace...." 2/17/18, 5:36 AM. Tweet.

6. Bajpai, Shweta, Monika Semwal, Ram Bajpai, Josip Car, and Andy Hau Yan Ho. "Health Professions' Digital Education: Review of Learning Theories in Randomized Controlled Trials by the Digital Health Education Collaboration." Journal of Medical Internet Research 21, no. 3 2019 https://doi.org/10.2196/12912.

7. Bar-On, Reuven. Bar-On Emotional Quotient Inventory, Technical Manual (A Measure of Emotional Intelligence). Toronto: UK/Edgepress US/ Multi-Health Systems Center for Research in Critical Thinking, 1997.

8. Beckett, Lois. "The PTSD Crisis That's Being Ignored: Americans Wounded in Their Own Neighborhoods." ProPublica, February 3, 2014. https://www.propublica.org/article/the-ptsd-crisis-thats-being-ignored-americans-wounded-in-their-own-neighbor?token=dobN47zSt-vHcmbER7GvkvKAYTIy9JN7t.

9. Bell, Randall. MeWeDoBe: The Four Cornerstones of Success. Berkeley: Leadership Institute Press, 2017.

10. Benson, Herbert. The Relaxation Response. New York: William Morrow, 1976.

11. Bower, Matt. "Technology-Mediated Learning Theory." British Journal of Educational Technology 50, no. 3 (May 1, 2019): 1035–48. https://doi.org/10.1111/bjet.12771.

12. Bowlby, John. A Secure Base: Parent-Child Attachment and Healthy Human Development. 2nd Edition. New York: Basic Books, 1988.

13. Bradshaw, John. Healing the Shame That Binds You. Deerfield Beach, FL: Health Communications, Inc., 1988.

14. Briere, John N., and Catherine Scott. Principles of Trauma Therapy: A Guide to Symptoms, Evaluation, and Treatment (DSM-5 Update). Second Edition. Thousand Oaks, California: SAGE Publications, Inc., 2015.

15. Brown, Austin McNeill, and Robert Ashford. "Recovery-Informed Theory: Situating the Subjective in the Science of Substance Use Disorder Recovery." ResearchGate, January 2019. https://doi.org/10.31886/jors.13.2019.38.

16. Brown, Tanya, and William Croyle. Finding Peace Amid the Chaos: My Escape from Depression and Suicide. Austin, TX: LangMarc Publishing, 2013.

17. Buchheit, Carl, and Ellie Schamber. Transformational NLP: A New Psychology. Ashland, OR: White Cloud Press, 2017.

18. ChildTrauma Academy. "The Childtrauma Academy A Learning Community," n.d. https://www.childtrauma.org.

19. Cieslak, Roman, Charles Benight, Norine Schmidt, Aleksandra Luszczynska, Erin Curtin, Rebecca A. Clark, and Patricia Kissinger. "Predicting Posttraumatic Growth among Hurricane Katrina Survivors Living with HIV: The Role of Self-Efficacy, Social Support, and PTSD Symptoms." Anxiety, Stress, and Coping 22, no. 4 (July 2009): 449–63. https://doi.org/10.1080/10615800802403815.

20. Comte-Sponville, Andre. A Small Treatise on the Great Virtues: The Uses of Philosophy in Everyday Life. Translated by Catherine Temerson. New York: Metropolitan Books/Henry Holt and Company, 2002.

21. Constantinescu, Azizeh Elias, and Newton B. Moore. "Applying Adult Learning Principles, Technology, and Agile Methodology to a Course Redesign Project." The Journal for Quality & Participation, January 2019, 26–29.

22. Cranshaw, Cheryl, Barbara A. Staten, and Tami Jo Halverson. "Conscious Voices Curriculum: A Provider's Tool for Prevention, Early Intervention and Healing Trauma in the African American Community." June 21, 2015. https://issuu.com/innovationsta/docs/rconscious_voices_-_covo_-_innovati..

23. Csikszentmihalyi, Mihaly. Flow: The Psychology of Optimal Experience. New York: HarperCollins Publishers, 1990.

24. Curran, Vernon, Diana L Gustafson, Karla Simmons, Heather Lannon, Chenfang Wang, Mahyar Garmsiri, Lisa Fleet, and Lyle Wetsch. "Adult Learners' Perceptions of Self-Directed Learning and Digital Technology Usage in Continuing Professional Education: An Update for the Digital Age." Journal of Adult and Continuing Education 25, no. 1 (May 1, 2019): 74–93. https://doi.org/10.1177/1477971419827318.21.

25. Curtin, Melanie. "Neuroscience Shows That 50-Year-Olds Can Have the Brains of 25-Year-Olds If They Do This 1 Thing." Inc.com. Accessed October 15, 2019. https://www.inc.com/melanie-curtin/neuroscience-shows-that-50-year-olds-can-have-brains-of-25-year-olds-if-they-do-this.html.

26. Dauer, Francis Watanabe. Critical Thinking: An Introduction to Reasoning. Oxford: Oxford University Press, 1989.

27. Debbie Hecht. "The ART OF RESILIENCE and the LESSON of the JAPANESE BOWL." Debbie Hecht: Thoughts & Theories (blog), November 23, 2018. https://debbiehecht.com/2018/11/23/the-art-of-resilience-re-birth-and-the-lesson-of-the-japanese-bowl-2/.

28. Dement, William C. The Promise of Sleep. New York: Random House, 2000.

29. Desbordes, Gaelle, Tim Gard, Elizabeth A Hoge, Catherine Kerr, Sara W Lazar, Andrew Olendzki, and David R Vago. Moving Beyond Mindfulness: Defining Equanimity as an Outcome Measure in Meditation and Contemplative Research. Mindfulness, 2015.

30. Diagnostic and Statistical Manual of Mental Disorders. 5th Edition. Arlington, VA, US: American Psychiatric Publishing, 2013.

31. Doerfler, David. "Concentric Journeys." Concentric Journeys, n.d. http://www.concentricjourneys.com/.

32. Doyle, John Sean. "Resilience, Growth & Kintsukuroi." Psychology Today, October 3, 2015. https://www.psychologytoday.com/blog/luminous-things/201510/resilience-growth-kintsukuroi.

33. Eastern Mennonite University. "STAR: Strategies for Trauma Awareness & Resilience," n.d. https://emu.edu/cjp/star/.

34. Ekman, Paul. Emotions Revealed: Recognizing Faces and Feelings to Improve Communication and Emotional Life. New York: Henry Holt and Company, LLC, 2003.

35. "ERASE Racism," n.d. http://eraseracismny.org/index.php.

36. Facione, Peter. "Critical Thinking: What It Is and Why It Counts." Insight Assessment, 2007.

37. Fisher, Alec, and Michael Scriven. Critical Thinking: Its Definition and Assessment. Norwich, England: University of East Anglia, Centre for Research in Critical Thinking, 2017.

38. Gard, Tim, Britta K. Hölzel, and Sara W Lazar. The Potential Effects of Meditation on Age□related Cognitive Decline: A Systematic Review. Annals of the New York Academy of Sciences, 2014.

39. Gard, Tim, Maxime Taquet, Rohan Dixit, Britta K. Hölzel, Bradford C. Dickerson, and Sara W. Lazar. Greater Widespread Functional Connectivity of the Caudate in Older Adults Who Practice Kripalu Yoga and Vipassana Meditation than in Controls. Frontiers in Human Neuroscience, 2015. http://www.frontiersin.org/Human_Neuroscience/10.3389/fnhum.2015.00137/abstract.

40. Gard, Tim, Maxime Taquet, Rohan Dixit, Britta K. Hölzel, Yves-Alexandre de Montjoye, Narayan Brach, David H. Salat, Bradford C. Dickerson, Jeremy R. Gray, and Sara W. Lazar. Fluid Intelligence and Brain Functional Organization in Aging Yoga and Meditation Practitioners. Frontiers in Aging Neuroscience, 2014. http://journal.frontiersin.org/article/10.3389/fnagi.2014.00076/abstract.

41. Goldstein, Avram. Addiction: From Biology to Drug Policy. New York: Oxford University Press, 2001.

42. Goleman, Daniel. Emotional Intelligence: Why It Can Matter More Than IQ. New York: Bantam Books, 1995.

43. Good, Darren J, Christopher J Lyddy, Theresa M. Glomb, Joyce E Bono, Kirk Warren Brown, Michelle K Duffy, Ruth A Baer, Judson A Brewer, and Sara W Lazar. Contemplating Mindfulness at Work: An Integrative Review. Journal of Management, 2015.

44. Greenberg, J, TD Braun, ML Schneider, L Finkelstein-Fox, LA Conboy, ED Schifano, C Park, and SW Lazar. Is Less More? A Randomized Comparison of Home Practice in a Mind-Body Program. Behaviour Research and Therapy, 2018.

45. Greenberg, Jonathan, Tanya Datta, Benjamin G. Shapero, Gunes Sevinc, David Mischoulon, and Sara W. Lazar. Compassionate Hearts Protect against Wandering Minds: Self-Compassion Moderates the Effect of Mind-Wandering on Depression. Spirituality in Clinical Practice, 2018. http://doi.apa.org/getdoi.cfm?doi=10.1037/scp0000168.

46. Greenberg, Jonathan, Victoria L. Romero, Seth Elkin-Frankston, Matthew A. Bezdek, Eric H. Schumacher, and Sara W. Lazar. Reduced Interference in Working Memory Following Mindfulness Training Is Associated with Increases in Hippocampal Volume. Vol. 13. Brain Imaging and Behavior, 2019. http://link.springer.com/10.1007/s11682-018-9858-4.

47. Greenberg, Jonathan, Benjamin G. Shapero, David Mischoulon, and Sara W. Lazar. Mindfulness-Based Cognitive Therapy for Depressed Individuals Improves Suppression of Irrelevant Mental-Sets. Vol. 267. European Archives of Psychiatry and Clinical Neuroscience, 2016. http://link.springer.com/10.1007/s00406-016-0746-x.

48. Groopman, Jerome. The Anatomy of Hope: How People Prevail in the Face of Illness. New York: Random House, 2004.

49. Hamish, Sinclair. "VIP-ManAlive." VIP-ManAlive, n.d. https://www.vip-manalive.com/.

50. Hanh, Thich Nhat. Peace Is Every Step: The Path of Mindfulness in Everyday Life. New York: Bantam Books, 1991.

51. Hanson, Rick. Buddha's Brain: The Practical Neuroscience of Happiness, Love, and Wisdom. Oakland, CA: New Harbinger Publications, Inc., 2009.

52. Hassen, Steven. Combating Cult Mind Control: The #1 Best-Selling Guide to Protection, Rescue and Recovery from Destructive Cults. Fourth Edition. Newton, MA: Freedom of Mind Press, 2018.

53. Hauri, Peter. No More Sleepless Nights. New York: John Wiley & Sons, Inc., 1996.

54. Hedlund, Thomas. "Thomas Hedlund: 'Integrating Science into the Healing of Heart and Mind.'" Thomas Hedlund, n.d. http://www.thomashedlund.com/.

55. Herman, Judith. Trauma and Recovery: The Aftermath of Violence—from Domestic Abuse to Political Terror. New York: Basic Books, 1997.

56. Holland, Alison S. "Effective Principles of Informal Online Learning Design: A Theory-Building Metasynthesis of Qualitative Research." Computers & Education, 2019.

57. Hölzel, Britta K., Vincent Brunsch, Tim Gard, Douglas N. Greve, Kathrin Koch, Christian Sorg, Sara W. Lazar, and Mohammed R. Milad. Mindfulness-Based Stress Reduction, Fear Conditioning, and The Uncinate Fasciculus: A Pilot Study. Vol. 10. Frontiers in Behavioral Neuroscience, 2016. http://journal.frontiersin.org/Article/10.3389/fnbeh.2016.00124/abstract.

58. INSIGHT PRISON PROJECT. "Trainings," n.d. http://www.insightprisonproject.org/trainings.html.

59. Jong, Marasha de, Sara W. Lazar, Kiran Hug, Wolf E. Mehling, Britta K. Hölzel, Alexander T. Sack, Frenk Peeters, Heidi Ashih, David Mischoulon, and Tim Gard. Effects of Mindfulness-Based Cognitive Therapy on Body Awareness in Patients with Chronic Pain and Comorbid Depression. Vol. 7. Frontiers in Psychology, 2016. http://journal.frontiersin.org/Article/10.3389/fpsyg.2016.00967/abstract.

60. Jong, Marasha de, Frenk Peeters, Tim Gard, Heidi Ashih, Jim Doorley, Rosemary Walker, Laurie Rhoades, et al. A Randomized Controlled Pilot Study on Mindfulness-Based Cognitive Therapy for Unipolar Depression in Patients With Chronic Pain. Vol. 79. The Journal of Clinical Psychiatry, 2018. http://www.psychiatrist.com/JCP/article/Pages/2018/v79n01/15m10160.aspx.

61. Kabat-Zinn, Jon. Full Catastrophe Living: Using the Wisdom of Your Body and Mind to Face Stress, Pain, and Illness. New York: Bantam Books, 1990.

62. Kaufman, Scott Barry. "Are You Mentally Tough?" Scientific America, March 19, 2014. https://blogs.scientificamerican.com/beautiful-minds/are-you-mentally-tough/.

63. Kim, Soonja. "Mothering Women." Mothering Women, n.d. http://motheringwomen.com/.

64. "Kintsugi." In Wikipedia, September 28, 2015. https://en.wikipedia.org/w/index.php?title=Kintsugi&oldid=683186968.

65. Kolk, Bessel van der. The Body Keeps the Score: Brain, Mind, and Body in the Healing of Trauma. New York: Penguin Books, 2014.

66. Kornfield, Jack. A Path with Heart: A Guide Through the Perils and Promises of Spiritual Life. New York: Bantam Books, 1993.

67. Korzybski, Alfred. Selections From Science and Sanity: An Introduction to Non-Aristotelian Systems and General Semantics. Second Edition. Fort Worth, Texas: Institute of General Semantics, 2010.

68. Krouska, Akrivi, Christos Troussas, and Maria Virvou. "Advancing Adult Online Education through a SN-Learning Environment," 2019. https://doi.org/10.1109/IISA.2019.8900705.

69. Kübler-Ross, Elisabeth. On Death and Dying: What the Dying Have to Teach Doctors, Nurses, Clergy and Their Own Families. New York: Scribner, 1969.

70. Kushner, Harold S. When Bad Things Happen to Good People. New York: Schocken Books, Inc., 1981.

71. Levine, Peter A. Healing Trauma: A Pioneering Program for Restoring the Wisdom of Your Body. Boulder, CO: Sounds True, Inc., 2008.

72. Lewis, Lisa, Kay Kelly, and Jon G. Allen. Restoring Hope and Trust: An Illustrated Guide to Mastering Trauma. Baltimore: Sidran Institute Press, 2004.

73. Lombardo, Elizabeth. A Happy You: Your Ultimate Prescription for Happiness. Garden City, NY: Morgan James Publishing, LLC, 2010.

74. Lombardo, Elizabeth. Better than Perfect: 7 Strategies to Crush Your Inner Critic and Create a Life You Love. Berkeley, CA: Seal Press, 2014.

75. Lowe, Sarah R., Emily E. Manove, and Jean E. Rhodes. "Posttraumatic Stress and Posttraumatic Growth among Low-Income Mothers Who Survived Hurricane Katrina." Journal of Consulting and Clinical Psychology 81, no. 5 (2013): 877–89. https://doi.org/10.1037/a0033252.

76. MacNair, Rachel M. Perpetration-Induced Traumatic Stress: The Psychological Consequences of Killing. Westport, CT: Praeger/Greenwood Publishing Group, 2002.

77. Mayo Clinic Staff. "Denial: When It Helps, When It Hurts." Mayo Clinic, April 9, 2020. https://www.mayoclinic.org/healthy-lifestyle/adult-health/in-depth/denial/art-20047926.

78. McEwen, Bruce S., and Elizabeth N. Lasley. The End of Stress As We Know It. Washington, DC: Joseph Henry Press, 2002.

79. McGraw, Phil. "Dr. Phil." Dr. Phil, n.d. https://www.drphil.com/.

80. McMillen, J. C., E. M. Smith, and R. H. Fisher. "Perceived Benefit and Mental Health after Three Types of Disaster." Journal of Consulting and Clinical Psychology 65, no. 5 (October 1997): 733–39. https://doi.org/10.1037//0022-006x.65.5.733.

81. Merriam, Sharan B., and Lisa M. Baumgartner. Learning in Adulthood: A Comprehensive Guide. Hoboken, New Jersey: John Wiley & Sons, Inc., 2020.

82. Mikal-Flynn, Joyce. Turning Tragedy Into Triumph. JMF Company, 2012.

83. Moore, Christian. The Resilience Breakthrough: 27 Tools for Turning Adversity into Action. Austin, TX: Greenleaf Book Group Press, 2014.

84. Morgan, Oliver J. Addiction, Attachment, Trauma and Recovery: The Power of Connection. Norton Series on Interpersonal Neurobiology. New York: W. W. Norton & Company, Inc., 2019.

85. National Institute of Mental Health. "Post-Traumatic Stress Disorder," May 2019. https://www.nimh.nih.gov/health/topics/post-traumatic-stress-disorder-ptsd/index.shtml.

86. Norris, Fran H., Susan P. Stevens, Betty Pfefferbaum, Karen F. Wyche, and Rose L. Pfefferbaum. "Community Resilience as a Metaphor, Theory, Set of Capacities, and Strategy for Disaster Readiness." American Journal of Community Psychology 41, no. 1–2 (March 2008): 127–50. https://doi.org/10.1007/s10464-007-9156-6.

87. Nygaard, Egil, and Trond Heir. "World Assumptions, Posttraumatic Stress and Quality of Life after a Natural Disaster: A Longitudinal Study." Health and Quality of Life Outcomes 10, no. 1 (June 28, 2012): 76. https://doi.org/10.1186/1477-7525-10-76.

88. Porges, Stephen W. The Polyvagal Theory: Neurophysiological Foundations of Emotions, Attachment, Communication, and Self-Regulation. Norton Series on Interpersonal Neurobiology. New York: W. W. Norton & Company, Inc., 2011.

89. PsychAlive. "Psychalive - Psychology for Everyday Life," n.d. https://www.psychalive.org/.

90. Psychology Today. "Empathy," n.d. https://www.psychologytoday.com/us/basics/empathy.

91. PTSD: National Center for PTSD. "PTSD Basics," n.d. https://www.ptsd.va.gov/understand/what/ptsd_basics.asp.

92. PuddleDancer Press. "Nonviolent Communication and Restorative Justice," n.d. https://www.nonviolentcommunication.com/learn-nonviolent-communication/nvc-restorative-justice/.

93. Read, Jennifer P., Paige Ouimette, Jacquelyn White, Craig Colder, and Sherry Farrow. "Rates of DSM-IV-TR Trauma Exposure and Posttraumatic Stress Disorder Among Newly Matriculated College Students." Psychological Trauma: Theory, Research, Practice and Policy 3, no. 2 (2011): 148–56. https://doi.org/10.1037/a0021260.

94. RJOY. "RJOY – Restorative Justice For Oakland," n.d. http://rjoyoakland.org/.

95. Roth, Susan, Elana Newman, David Pelcovitz, Bessel van der Kolk, and Francine S. Mandel. "Complex PTSD in Victims Exposed to Sexual and Physical Abuse: Results from the DSM-IV Field Trial for Posttraumatic Stress Disorder." Journal of Traumatic Stress 10, no. 4 (October 1997): 539–55. https://doi.org/10.1023/a:1024837617768.

96. Sandford, Paula. Healing Victims of Sexual Abuse: How to Counsel and Minister to Hearts Wounded by Abuse. Lake Mary, FL: Charisma House, 2009.

97. Saraiya, Tanya C., Margaret Swarbrick, Liza Franklin, Sara Kass, Aimee N. C. Campbell, and Denise A. Hien. "Perspectives on Trauma and the Design of a Technology-Based Trauma-Informed Intervention for Women Receiving Medications for Addiction Treatment in Community-Based Settings." Journal of Substance Abuse Treatment 112 (May 1, 2020): 92–101. https://doi.org/10.1016/j.jsat.2020.01.011.

98. Schacter, Daniel L. Searching for Memory: The Brain, the Mind, and the Past. New York: Basic Books, 1996.

99. Schiraldi, Glenn R. The Post-Traumatic Stress Disorder Sourcebook: A Guide to Healing, Recovery, and Growth. Second Edition. McGraw-Hill Companies, 2009.

100. Schwartz, Sunny. Dreams from the Monster Factory: A Tale of Prison, Redemption and One Woman's Fight to Restore Justice to All. New York: Scribner, 2009.

101. Sevinc, Gunes, Britta K. Hölzel, Jonathan Greenberg, Tim Gard, Vincent Brunsch, Javeria A. Hashmi, Mark Vangel, Scott P. Orr, Mohammed R. Milad, and Sara W. Lazar. Strengthened Hippocampal Circuits Underlie Enhanced Retrieval of Extinguished Fear Memories Following Mindfulness Training. Vol. 86. Society of Biological Psychiatry, 2019. https://linkinghub.elsevier.com/retrieve/pii/S0006322319314076.

102. Sevinc, Gunes, Britta K. Hölzel, Javeria Hashmi, Jonathan Greenberg, Adrienne McCallister, Michael Treadway, Marissa L. Schneider, Jeffery A. Dusek, James Carmody, and Sara W. Lazar. Common and Dissociable Neural Activity After Mindfulness-Based Stress Reduction and Relaxation Response Programs: Vol. 80. Psychosomatic Medicine, 2018. http://journals.lww.com/00006842-201806000-00006.

103. Sevinc, Gunes, and Sara W. Lazar. How Does Mindfulness Training Improve Moral Cognition: A Theoretical and Experimental Framework for the Study of Embodied Ethics. Vol. 28. Current opinion in psychology, 2019. https://www.ncbi.nlm.nih.gov/pmc/articles/PMC6706316/.

104. Shapero, Benjamin G., Jonathan Greenberg, David Mischoulon, Paola Pedrelli, Kathryn Meade, and Sara W. Lazar. Mindfulness-Based Cognitive Therapy Improves Cognitive Functioning and Flexibility Among Individuals with Elevated Depressive Symptoms. Vol. 9. Mindfulness, 2018. http://link.springer.com/10.1007/s12671-018-0889-0.

105. Sharpe, Susan. Restorative Justice: A Vision for Healing and Change. Edmonton, Alberta, CA: Edmonton Victim Offender Mediation Society, 1998.

106. Shirtzinger, Tony. "Help Yourself Therapy." Help Yourself Therapy, n.d. https://helpyourselftherapy.com/.

107. Smyth, Joshua M., Jill R. Hockemeyer, Kristin E. Heron, Stephen A. Wonderlich, and James W. Pennebaker. "Prevalence, Type, Disclosure, and Severity of Adverse Life Events in College Students." Journal of American College Health: J of ACH 57, no. 1 (August 2008): 69–76. https://doi.org/10.3200/JACH.57.1.69-76.

108. Snyder, C. R. The Psychology of Hope: You Can Get There from Here. New York: The Free Press, 1994.

109. Steinberg, Marlene, and Maxine Schnall. The Stranger in the Mirror: Dissociation—the Hidden Epidemic. New York: HarperCollins Publishers, 2001.

110. Tedeschi, Richard G., and Lawrence G. Calhoun. "Posttraumatic Growth: Conceptual Foundations and Empirical Evidence." Psychological Inquiry 15, no. 1 (2004): 1–18. https://doi.org/10.1207/s15327965pli1501_01.

111. Tedeschi, Richard G., and Lawrence G. Calhoun. "The Posttraumatic Growth Inventory: Measuring the Positive Legacy of Trauma." Journal of Traumatic Stress 9, no. 3 (1996): 455–72. https://doi.org/10.1002/jts.2490090305.

112. Tedeschi, Richard G., Elizabeth Addington, Arnie Cann, and Lawrence G. Calhoun. "Post-Traumatic Growth: Some Needed Corrections and Reminders." European Association of Personality Psychology, 2014, 350–51.

113. Thayer, Robert E. Calm Energy: How People Regulate Mood with Food and Exercise. New York: Oxford University Press, 2001.

114. Trauma Resource Institute. "Trauma Resiliency Model®," n.d. https://www.traumaresourceinstitute.com/new-page-1.

115. Turning Point. "Turning Point," n.d. https://www.turningpointservices.org.

116. Umbreit, Mark S. The Handbook of Victim Offender Mediation: An Essential Guide to Practice and Research. San Francisco: Jossey-Bass Inc., 2001.

117. Vago, David R, Resh S Gupta, and Sara W Lazar. Measuring Cognitive Outcomes in Mindfulness-Based Intervention Research: A Reflection on Confounding Factors and Methodological Limitations. Vol. 28. Current Opinion in Psychology, 2019. https://linkinghub.elsevier.com/retrieve/pii/S2352250X18302367.

118. Van Dam, Nicholas T., Marieke K. van Vugt, David R. Vago, Laura Schmalzl, Clifford D. Saron, Andrew Olendzki, Ted Meissner, et al. Mind the Hype: A Critical Evaluation and Prescriptive Agenda for Research on Mindfulness and Meditation. Vol. 13. Perspectives on Psychological Science, 2018. http://journals.sagepub.com/doi/10.1177/1745691617709589.

119. Van Dam, Nicholas T., Marieke K. van Vugt, David R. Vago, Laura Schmalzl, Clifford D. Saron, Andrew Olendzki, Ted Meissner, et al. Reiterated Concerns and Further Challenges for Mindfulness and Meditation Research: A Reply to Davidson and Dahl. Vol. 13. Perspectives on Psychological Science, 2018. http://journals.sagepub.com/doi/10.1177/1745691617727529.

120. Vermilyea, Elizabeth G. Growing Beyond Survival: A Self-Help Toolkit for Managing Traumatic Stress. Baltimore: Sidran Press, 2000.

121. Von Culin, Katherine R., Eli Tsukayama, and Angela L. Duckworth. "Unpacking Grit: Motivational Correlates of Perseverance and Passion for Long-Term Goals." The Journal of Positive Psychology 9, no. 4 (2014): 306–12. https://doi.org/10.1080/17439760.2014.898320.

122. Walker, Lenore E. The Battered Woman. New York: Harper & Row, Publishers, Inc., 1979.

123. Walker, Pete. Complex PTSD: From Surviving to Thriving: A Guide and Map for Recovering from Childhood Trauma. Lafayette, CA: Azure Coyote, 2013.

124. Walker, Pete. "Frequently Asked Questions About Complex PTSD." Pete Walker, M.A., MFT, n.d. http://pete-walker.com/fAQsComplexPTSD.html.

125. Wells, Dawn, and Steve Stinson. What Would Mary Ann Do?: A Guide to Life. Lanham, Maryland: Taylor Trade Publishing, 2014.

126. Westerlund, Elaine. Women's Sexuality after Childhood Incest. Women's Sexuality after Childhood Incest. New York, NY, US: W. W. Norton & Company, Inc., 1992.

127. Williams, Mark London. Cry of Pain: Understanding Suicide and Self-Harm. London: Penguin Books, 1997.

128. Winell, Marlene. Leaving the Fold: A Guide for Former Fundamentalists and Others Leaving Their Religion. Berkeley: Apocryphile Press, 2007.

129. Xu, Zhihong, Manjari Banerjee, Gilbert Ramirez, Gang Zhu, and Kausalai (Kay) Wijekumar. "The Effectiveness of Educational Technology Applications on Adult English Language Learners' Writing Quality: A Meta-Analysis." Computer Assisted Language Learning 32, no. 1–2 (January 2, 2019): 132–62. https://doi.org/10.1080/09588221.2018.1501069.

130. Zerbe, Kathryn J. The Body Betrayed: Women, Eating Disorders, and Treatment. Washington, DC: American Psychiatric Press, Inc., 1993.

About the Author

RANDALL BELL, PHD, is a sociologist and economist who specializes in disaster recovery projects. No stranger to how harsh the world is, Dr. Bell has consulted in more tragedies around the world than anyone. He was retained for the World Trade Center, Flight 93, Sandy Hook, BP Oil Spill, Hurricane Katrina, the Bikini Atoll Nuclear Test sites, the Northridge earthquake, OJ Simpson, Jon Benet Ramsey, Heaven's Gate, and hundreds of other cases. He has been retained by the Federal Governments of the United States, Canada, and Australia to help resolve numerous crises, and his work has generated billions of dollars to rebuild damaged communities.

Dr. Bell's investigations have taken him to 50 states, and seven continents. Having met with countless victims, he earned the nickname of *Master of Disaster.* In every case, Dr. Bell observed the emotional consequences and how some fared better than others. He was inspired to put his unique research skills to work and study the cycle of trauma.

A frequent guest of the media, Dr. Bell is the featured expert in Topic's "Distressed Real Estate" documentary series streamed on Apple TV and Amazon Prime. His career has been profiled by *NBC's Today Show, Rolling Stone Magazine, The Wall Street Journal, People Magazine, ABC's 20/20, Hallmark's Home & Family,* and many others.

Dr. Bell is the author of *MeWeDoBe* and the founder of *Core IQ,* a non-profit educational foundation that provides free online training on life skills. He is certified through the *Insight Prison Project* to facilitate group discussions with victims and offenders at San Quentin Prison. He has been active in jail ministries and a volunteer in homeless shelters.

In *Post-Traumatic Thriving,* Dr. Bell lays out the academic research and speaks freely about his trauma of being born with a congenital heart defect. Diagnosed with PTSD, he utilized these principles to heal from his childhood trauma and summit Africa's Mt. Kilimanjaro at 60.